D1480377

Rethinking the Ethics of Clinical Research

Rethinking the Ethics of Clinical Research

Widening the Lens

Alan Wertheimer

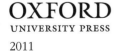

OXFORD
UNIVERSITY PRESS
2011

OXFORD
UNIVERSITY PRESS

Oxford University Press, Inc., publishes works that further
Oxford University's objective of excellence
in research, scholarship, and education.

Oxford   New York
Auckland   Cape Town   Dar es Salaam   Hong Kong   Karachi
Kuala Lumpur   Madrid   Melbourne   Mexico City   Nairobi
New Delhi   Shanghai   Taipei   Toronto

With offices in
Argentina   Austria   Brazil   Chile   Czech Republic   France   Greece
Guatemala   Hungary   Italy   Japan   Poland   Portugal   Singapore
South Korea   Switzerland   Thailand   Turkey   Ukraine   Vietnam

Published by Oxford University Press, Inc.
198 Madison Avenue, New York, New York 10016
www.oup.com

Oxford is a registered trademark of Oxford University Press

Library of Congress Cataloging-in-Publication Data
Wertheimer, Alan.
Rethinking the ethics of clinical research: widening the lens /
by Alan Wertheimer.
   p. cm.
Includes bibliographical references and index.
ISBN 978-0-19-974351-3
1. Medical ethics. 2. Human experimentation in medicine. I. Title.
R724.W37 2010
174.2'8—dc22   2010009527

*The views expressed here are those of the author. They do not necessarily represent any position
or policy of the National Institutes of Health or the Department of Health and Human Services.*

9 8 7 6 5 4 3 2 1

Printed in the United States of America
on acid-free paper

For Eliot Morton Wertheimer

Preface

This is the first extended work of my second career. At seminars in my current academic home, it is customary for the attendees to introduce themselves to the guest speaker. On one occasion, I uttered what has since become my mantra: "I'm Alan Wertheimer. I am a retired political philosopher from the University of Vermont, where my research focused on the concepts of coercion, exploitation, and consent. I'm now on the faculty at NIH where I'm working on the concepts of coercion, exploitation, and consent." Plus ça change, plus c'est la même chose.

My affiliation with the Department of Bioethics began in 2005-06, when I had the privilege of spending a post-retirement year as a visiting scholar. Fortunately (for *me*), knowledge of medicine or bioethics is not a requirement of that position. My only obligations were to engage in research, attend departmental events, and to make myself available to my colleagues and departmental fellows. Nice work if you can get it. For reasons I still do not fully understand, I was invited to become a member of the faculty where my responsibilities remain pretty much the same. Still nice work.

By happenstance (path-dependence?) more than design, my work has focused on the moral status of dyadic relations: when is one coerced in a way that compromises one's responsibility for one's actions? When does someone exploit another? What is the moral force of that exploitation? When does a person give valid consent to sexual relations? Having no major projects on my back burner when I arrived at NIH, I waded into the literature on the ethics of research with human subjects, only to find what I would have known had I thought about it, namely, that the concepts about which I had been obsessing for many years were central to that discourse. Can offers of financial payments to participate in research be coercive if they are too good to refuse? Are researchers exploiting subjects in less developed countries when participation in research is their only way of obtaining medical care? Do research subjects give valid consent when they do not fully understand or appreciate that they will not be receiving personalized medical care? Even though I found my name (yes, I looked) occasionally appearing in the literature, I found much of the analysis of these issues unsatisfying. And so I started working along lines with which I was familiar but in a context that was entirely new to me and which has led me to extend and revise my views.

The philosophical focus of this book is mostly limited to the dyadic relations between researchers and subjects or, on occasion, between IRBs (institutional review boards are committees that are charged to approve, monitor, and review research with human subjects) and researchers or IRBs and subjects. There is no context with which I am familiar that so clearly involves the use of some individuals for benevolent purposes and so vividly exhibits the tension "between the individual good and the common good, between private and public welfare" and which puts our views as to how to resolve or manage that tension to such an explicit test.[1] The moral status of those relations is put to a more severe test when—as is increasingly common—research is conducted by for-profit organizations with subjects who live under non-ideal and grossly unjust conditions.

Much of this book can be understood as a non-ideal exercise in non-ideal theory. Broadly speaking, non-ideal theory asks two different questions: (1) What principles should govern actions within a context of misfortune or injustice? (2) How should we chart a path towards a more just society, starting from a position of social injustice? This book is an exercise in non-ideal theory because much of it seeks to respond to (1) with respect to the recruitment and use of research subjects. This book is a decidedly non-ideal exercise in non-ideal theory because it has little to say about (2). I focus on (1) not because I regard it as more important than (2) but because I think the issues posed by (1) are large enough and because I fear that I have nothing original and sound to say about (2). In bioethics as elsewhere, there's room for a division of labor.

The Department of Bioethics at NIH has been an ideal place in which to undertake this type of non-ideal moral theory. The department represents the best of academia without the downside—fantastic pre-doctoral and post-doctoral fellows; smart, knowledgeable, and accessible colleagues with a variety of professional backgrounds; time for research; congenial space; a culture of discussion and collaboration; high intellectual standards yet little cynicism; ample and helpful administrative support. And, lest I forget, no grading.

Prior to my arrival at NIH, I had always written the old fashioned way—by myself with a lot of help from my friends. I have now entered the world of scholarly collaboration. Earlier versions of Chapters 2 and 3 were written with my colleague, Franklin Miller. Our collaboration has convinced me that synergy is not (always) a buzz word.

I have received numerous suggestions and comments on parts of this manuscript from my colleagues and fellows. I have also received extremely helpful comments from John Arras and an anonymous reviewer for Oxford University Press.

Although I have burdened the reader by sparing myself the advantages of Susan's sharp editorial assistance, my wife and best friend has made all this possible in more ways than I can count.

January 12, 2010

Contents

Rethinking the Ethics of
Clinical Research

1 Introduction

With apologies to Hans Jonas, this book provides decidedly non-systematic philosophical reflections on the ethics of the recruitment and use of research subjects. Apologies are necessary, because my philosophical reflections often lead me in a direction and to conclusions that Jonas would reject and might find distasteful. I say reflections. This book does not aim to provide the philosophical *foundations* of research ethics. Research ethics is a practical enterprise that has developed in response to specific historical events. It is not built on any general or overarching theory. The reigning principles—there are plural principles and they are reigning principles—respond to the desire to square the genuine need for biomedical research with the protection of human subjects in the context of a history that contains several episodes of serious abuse and exploitation of subjects. The question is which principles can be given sound philosophical support. I shall argue that some commonly accepted principles or worries are harder to defend than is often supposed and that some principles are best defended in ways that many bioethicists have been inclined to resist.

Jonas has said that experimentation (one says "experimentation" rather than "research" if one is hostile) with human subjects involves the "selective abrogation of personal inviolability and the ritualized exposure to gratuitous risk of health and life, justified by a presumed greater, social good."[1]

This sentence contains at least three problematic claims. First, Jonas is too quick to assume that his conception of personal inviolability is sound. Second, he is too quick to assume that exposing subjects to risk of health and life in research is necessarily (or even often) gratuitous. Third, and as I shall argue at several points, it is misleading (although not inaccurate) to think that exposing individual subjects to risk activity is justified by a greater "social" good, an adjective that obscures the obvious fact that there are discrete individuals on both sides of the equation.

But Jonas is right to think that the ethics of medical research with human subjects raises genuine moral worries not to be found in the ethics of medical care. At the most general level, the core problem of medical (therapeutic) ethics is to determine what we can ethically do to people *for their benefit*. By contrast, the core problem of research ethics with human subjects is to determine what we can ethically do to people for the *benefit of others*. So compared, medical ethics is relatively easy. I do not mean that the theoretical problems of medical ethics are easier to resolve. I mean that medical ethics does not exhibit a deep ethical tension at its core. To the contrary, there is a fundamental identity of interest between physician and patient at the core of medical practice. There are, of course, difficult theoretical issues about the permissibility of medical paternalism. Is it permissible to deceive patients for their own good? Is it permissible to prescribe placebos? There are important issues with respect to end-of-life care. Is voluntary euthanasia or physician-assisted suicide permissible? Should we respect an earlier competent self's advance directive about (non)treatment that a later demented self now rejects? There are important issues about rationing or the allocation of scarce resources such as organs. In addition, a physician's duty to her patients may, at times, conflict with the interests of public health. All that said, the fundamental principles of medical care are relatively unproblematic because appropriate medical care is an unalloyed good.

By contrast, the ethics of research exhibits a deep tension at its core between the interests of participants who are used as means by researchers and the interests of those who seek or are served by the pursuit of generalizable knowledge. And clinical research really uses people as means (I don't say "merely" as means). No Kantian abstractions necessary here. Researchers inject substances, draw blood, perform lumbar punctures, intubate trachea, perform sham arthroscopic surgery, and extract and store tissue. Researchers expose healthy volunteers to toxicity in order to determine possible dosage. In challenge studies of vaccines, researchers deliberately expose healthy volunteers to malaria-infected mosquitoes. Researchers have subjects with schizophrenia withdraw from their medication and then scan their brains with positron emission tomography in order to better understand the physiological basis of the disease. Although subjects may occasionally or even often receive medical or collateral benefits from participating in research, they emphatically do not benefit from many component procedures (for example, blood draws, lumbar punctures) that are designed to test study hypotheses. Some such procedures may not be particularly risky, but they can be burdensome or inconvenient, and are not done for the welfare of the subject. What justifies using people in these ways?

It is often said that medical research exhibits a tension between science or progress or a "greater social good" and the interests or rights of the individual. Although that way of putting things is not wrong, it is also misleading. After all, "society," and "science," and "progress" do not describe metaphysical entities that are not reducible to the interests of individuals. Rather, they are different ways of describing the interests of discrete, albeit statistical, individuals. There may sometimes be a tension between the interests of individuals who serve as research subjects and the interests of individuals who stand to gain from such research. But its individuals versus individuals all the way down. This is *not* to suggest that we should always be prepared to sacrifice some individuals for the sake of a greater number of other individuals. It is to suggest that we squarely face the implications of the choices we make in determining whether and when we are justified in using people as research subjects.

Some medical research does not "use" subjects as that term is ordinarily understood. Some research uses observational data, as when we study the relationship between obesity and type II diabetes or the relationship between male circumcision and HIV-transmission rates. Some research uses stored tissues previously extracted from subjects or patients, but does not use *them*. There are interesting questions as to whether people should be able to prevent researchers from using data about them or from using their tissues. For present purposes, however, I will focus on clinical research that involves the direct use of people.

To set the stage for the theoretical discussion, it will be useful to briefly distinguish between four stages of clinical research. (*Warning*: knowledgeable readers can skim this and the next paragraph). What is known as Phase I research is designed to test the toxicity or side effects of a novel intervention, often with a view to determine the maximal safe dosage. It is typically performed with a small number of subjects and often involves healthy volunteers, although Phase I oncology trials typically use patients for whom other treatments have not proved successful. Phase II research is designed to test the efficacy and safety of an intervention and typically uses a somewhat larger but still relatively small number of patient-subjects. If an intervention shows sufficient promise in Phase II research, investigators will embark on Phase III research, which is designed to test the safety and efficacy of an intervention with a large number of subjects. Randomized controlled trials are the "gold standard" of Phase III clinical research. In some cases, researchers will conduct a placebo controlled trial; they will compare an intervention with no treatment. In other cases, researchers will conduct an active controlled trial; an experimental intervention will be compared with an existing intervention. In one of the 20th century's most important Phase III active controlled trials, women with breast cancer were randomized into two treatment groups. One group received the (then) standard treatment of a modified radical mastectomy which involves the removal of the entire breast and some surrounding tissue. Another group received the less disfiguring lumpectomy (followed by radiation), which involves the removal of the cancerous tissue, but which leaves much of the breast intact. These studies demonstrated that the survival rate of the mastectomy group was no greater than the lumpectomy group and dramatically changed standard medical practice.[2]

Phase IV, or post-marketing surveillance trials, involves the study of efficacy and safety after a drug receives permission to be sold. A recent Phase IV study concerned the safety and efficacy of hormone replacement therapy (HRT).[3] When post-approval evidence revealed that HRTs increased the risk of heart disease and breast cancer, the use of HRTs dropped dramatically.

We should not exaggerate the contributions of clinical research to the reduction of mortality in the developed world. On that front, it is possible that the major mortality-reducing scientific discoveries have already been made. At the same time, we should also not underestimate the importance of clinical research. Marginal improvements in mortality are important—particularly to those on the margins. Improvements in the quality of life matter, even if they do not affect longevity. And medical treatments often generate the need for *new* medical treatments. For example, the widespread use of antibiotics has given rise to the evolution of an increasing number of "superbugs" or drug-resistant bacteria, so we now need to develop drugs that can treat the effects of other successful drugs.[4]

Apart from seeking reductions in mortality and morbidity, there are important economic reasons to do clinical research. We should not spend resources on interventions that are inefficacious or provide too little benefit relative to the cost. It was of both medical and economic importance to determine that autologous bone marrow transplant following high dose chemotherapy was not effective in treating breast cancer even though it showed promise in early cases (and there was great pressure on insurance companies to cover this very expensive procedure).[5] It was important to determine that arthroscopic surgery for osteoarthritis of the knee is often useless, not because it is particularly risky, but because it uses scarce health care resources.[6]

By contrast with the developed world, medical research (and the delivery of ordinary medical care) has a long way to go in the developing world. It is said that 90% of the global research budget aims at illnesses (or conditions) that cause 10% of the world's disease burden, whereas only 10% of worldwide expenditure on health research and development is devoted to the problems that primarily affect the poorest 90 per cent of the world's population.[7] In some cases, we need to develop vaccines or treatments that are simply not available. But even when effective prophylactics or treatments are available in affluent countries, they may be unaffordable or administratively infeasible in developing societies, and so we need research to develop interventions that are affordable and feasible for resource-poor countries.

Of arguably lesser moral importance, but of greater relevance to the present project, a large and increasing proportion of research on interventions that will be used primarily in affluent societies takes place in less developed countries. Just as developed societies have moved data processing, help-lines, medical record keeping, x-ray analysis, and the manufacture of athletic shoes and cell phones to less developed countries, the outsourcing or, more accurately, the off-shoring, of clinical research to developing societies is a widespread and growing industry.[8] Major pharmaceutical corporations frequently outsource their research to "contract research organizations" that conduct such research in developing nations where participation in research is a way for people to obtain some medical care and screening. As one company advertises, "A huge population with a diversity of diseases that are untreated—yes, that is the "India advantage."[9] And so we have a world in which malaria continues to cause millions of deaths per year in Asia and Africa, while people there "line up for experimental doses of arthritis, heart disease, and obesity drugs."[10]

I believe that the allocation of resources for research may be the big—macro—issue of research ethics. This book focuses on a smaller (not small)—micro—dimension of research ethics, namely, the recruitment and use of research participants. For whether the research in question serves the needs of developed nations or the citizens of underdeveloped nations, and whether the participants come from developed or developing nations, we must still ask: When is it ethically justifiable to recruit and use people as research subjects?

The standard view in bioethics is that research is ethically permissible *only if* (1) the risks of participation are reasonable in relation to the anticipated benefits *to the subjects or to others* (the "reasonable risk criterion") and (2) if the subjects have given their competent, voluntary, and appropriately informed consent (the "informed consent criterion").[11] I say "only if" because research may have to satisfy additional criteria (such as scientific validity) if it is truly to pass ethical muster.[12] But these are the most important criteria and, by themselves, would be sufficient to exclude most or all of the poster children of unethical medical research such as the Nazi experiments, the Tuskegee study, the Jewish Chronic Disease Hospital case, and the examples cited in Henry Beecher's famous article.[13]

Within the class of studies that meet both of these criteria, we can distinguish between what Jerry Menikoff calls "good choice studies" and "bad choice studies."[14] *The labels may mislead.* The distinction between "good choice" and "bad choice" studies refers to the subject's *self-interest*, and not to the moral quality of the choice. A good choice study is one in which a person could reasonably participate for self-interested reasons because the expected medical benefits *to the subject* are greater than the expected personal risks and burdens from participation. A bad choice study is one in which a person could not reasonably participate for self-interested reasons because the expected personal risks and burdens exceed the expected personal benefits even though those risks may be outweighed by the anticipated benefits to others. It may be *morally* praiseworthy or even obligatory to participate in a bad choice study. But, by definition, it is not, *ex ante*, in the medical interest of an individual to participate in a bad choice study.

There are some randomized trials in which the interventions (or the intervention and a placebo) are in strict equipoise, where there is no reason, *ex ante*, to think that one of the interventions is more efficacious (or safer) than the other. Setting aside the burdens of participation in research and a general desire not to have one's treatment determined, in effect, by the flip of a coin, it would not be unreasonable to participate in such a study for self-interested reasons. But even when there is genuine uncertainty about the comparative efficacy of a novel intervention, there may be good probabilistic reasons to think that it is superior to placebo or standard treatment intervention. Participation in such a trial may be a "good choice" if the novel intervention is not available outside the trial, but a "bad choice," *ex ante*, if the probabilistically preferred intervention is available outside the trial, even if it turns out, *ex post*, that one received the superior intervention. After all, if there were probabilistic reason to think (*ex ante*) that mastectomies would have greater survival rates than lumpectomies, then participation in a randomized trial was arguably a bad choice even if, *ex post*, it turned out that lumpectomies were no less effective and those who received mastectomies had the more disfiguring surgery without any compensating benefit.

Good choice studies present no serious problems of recruitment, as the interests of investigators are in line with the interests of participants. Indeed, participation in a Phase I oncology study of an experimental treatment may be a "good choice" for a terminal cancer patient who has exhausted standard treatments even though the study is designed only to test toxicity and even if there is little evidence that the intervention is effective. The drug is unlikely to help, but it may still be the patient's best hope.

But how can subjects be recruited when participation is a bad choice as will almost always be so in Phase I trials, often so in Phase II trials, and frequently so in Phase III trials? Here we face a form of the prisoners' dilemma. Suppose that the best available information suggests that it is 60% likely that intervention X is superior to intervention Y. Although it is in the *ex ante* interest of each individual not to participate in research and to simply receive X, it is in the interest of many others (including future persons) that a sufficient number participate in research to determine whether X is superior to Y with a greater level of certainty. Moreover, even if it were 50/50 as to whether X is superior to Y, it would be a bad choice to enter such a trial if one has to undergo procedures that were not clinically indicated or one were otherwise inconvenienced by participation. How can we deal with this dilemma in a manner that is ethically permissible?

First, we could decide that we should not try—at least not too hard—to solve the dilemma and that we should generally avoid using individuals in bad choice research. Hans Jonas argued that whereas it was permissible to quarantine contagious persons because they represent a *danger* to others, it was typically not permissible to subject individuals to medical risks in order to *benefit* others even with their consent. On Jonas's view, the mere issuing of the appeal, "the calling for volunteers, with the moral and social pressures it inevitably generates, amounts even under the most meticulous rules of consent to a sort of *conscripting*."[15] Jonas believes that the benefits of scientific progress are "optional," whereas avoiding harm to subjects is not. And if this means that research progresses more slowly, so be it. The price of slower research and the avoidable morbidity and mortality it entails "may have to be paid for the preservation of the most precious capital of higher communal life."[16]

Second, we could bite Jonas's bullet and go the other way entirely. We could abandon the requirement of informed consent and view participation in socially valuable research as an obligation to society for which it is permissible to conscript people on some fair basis. Just as we may conscript people for military service or require people to pay taxes or serve on juries or testify as witnesses, we could require people to participate in bad choice research if the interests of society so demanded. In effect, society might say, "We need to determine whether lumpectomies have lower survival rates than mastectomies, so your treatment for breast cancer will be determined by randomization." (See Chapter 3)

Third, we could retain our commitment to the principle that participation in research should be consensual and try to promote more altruistic participation. Whether we assume that participation in research is *prima facie* obligatory or supererogatory, we could adopt educational or persuasive strategies aimed at increasing the number of persons who voluntarily choose to participate in bad choice studies. Just as the prisoners' dilemma is a dilemma because people often do not act altruistically, it is unlikely that altruism alone is or will be in sufficient supply to keep the research enterprise going at a healthy speed. Although some persons will choose to put themselves at risk for the benefit of future patients, and although the desire to contribute to medical science is frequently cited as one motivation for participation in research even when participants are paid or participate for other reasons, the widespread use of incentives implies that altruism alone will not suffice.

Fourth, and as noted above, we can use incentives to recruit research subjects. Although participation in a bad choice study is contrary to a subject's *medical* interests (by definition), a subject may believe that receipt of payment renders participation compatible with his interests, all things considered. In effect, investigators use money to convert what would otherwise be a "bad choice" into a "good choice" from the subject's point of view.

How else to get a sufficient number of healthy people to participate voluntarily in a Phase I trial of toxicity or to expose themselves to infection in a challenge study of a malaria vaccine? Some regard the use of financial incentives as a "morally unacceptable" method for getting people to participate in clinical trials.[17] Many others would not go that far, but find it troubling or worrying. I consider this issue in Chapter 4.

Fifth, and related to the previous point, investigators can (and do) take advantage of the background fact that whereas participation in a study may be a bad choice for someone like myself who has access to high quality personal medical care, participation may be a good *medical* choice for others. Participation may provide free medical examinations or treatment for the uninsured. Participation may also provide access to higher quality treatment and closer monitoring than a patient would otherwise receive or access to novel interventions that would otherwise be unavailable.

The approach to recruitment just described lies behind the increasing offshoring of medical research from developed societies to less developed countries, where few people have access to what we regard as acceptable medical care. It is often argued that this mode of recruitment is deeply problematic, that researchers are engaged in wrongful exploitation when they take advantage of the fact that what would be a bad choice for most persons in affluent societies is a good choice for many persons in less developed countries. Sonia Shah notes that whereas Americans buy lots of drugs, they are "loathe to participate in clinical trials" without which such drugs would not be available.[18] Of course, Americans also buy lots of wine even though most wine drinkers are loathe to pick the grapes without which such wine would not be available. Picking grapes is a bad choice for me, but unfortunate though it may be, it may be a good choice for others. Is it unfair if researchers and sponsors take advantage of such conditions if participation is, in fact, a good choice for the participants? I consider this issue in Chapter 5 and extend the analysis in Chapter 6.

Finally, there are worries about the validity of consent. Subjects may consent to participate in bad choice trials because they mistakenly believe they are participating in good choice trials or they wrongly believe that the value of the financial incentives outweighs the burdens and risks of participation. In the first case, participants wrongly believe that participation is in their medical interest. They are not conscripted or coerced. They are not altruists. And the investigators may not have engaged in active deception. Indeed, investigators may have disclosed facts that would lead a rational subject to reject participation. Nonetheless, subjects may be in the grips of the "therapeutic misconception," where they mistakenly believe that they are receiving personalized medical care when the truth is that the intervention and its dosage is randomly chosen and will not be adjusted to the subject's condition. I consider this issue in Chapter 3.

There are other worries about consent. Subjects may consent to participate in research because they have no reasonable alternative. And, it may be said, their consent is not truly voluntary because they are coerced by their circumstances. And even if subjects are not coerced to participate, it may be thought that payment may constitute an "undue inducement" that compromises the validity of their consent. I touch on these issues in Chapter 3 and consider them at more length in Chapter 4.

On a broad level, these options establish the background for the analysis to follow. I shall not engage them all. I will say relatively little as to whether we should follow Hans Jonas and be prepared to accept less research as the price for a more robust respect for the interests of prospective subjects, save to note that one person's "optional progress" is another person's life or body. Interestingly, if doctors impose unnecessary risks on *all* patients, we call it treatment. But as Leon Eisenberg points out, tonsillectomies were regarded as routine procedures in many locales well into the twentieth century, but are now regarded as generally useless and not without risk. These procedures produced more deaths per 100,000 each year than the total deaths from all non-therapeutic research.[19] Thousands of women have undergone less mutilating lumpectomies rather than radical mastectomies because "optional" scientific progress showed that lumpectomies did not increase the risk of mortality. Of course, allowing avoidable suffering is the inevitable price for any non-maximizing consequentialist ethics that respects individual autonomy and requires informed consent. Nonetheless, we should not be insensitive to the considerable human and economic cost of *not* doing research.

Those are the concerns that motivate this project. This is the plan of the book. In Chapter 2, I explore the institutional structure of research ethics. Why not simply require informed consent by participants? Why is it necessary that IRBs first determine that the risks of participation are reasonable in relation to their anticipated benefits before prospective subjects are given the opportunity to consent? Chapter 2 argues that bioethics has failed to acknowledge that the entire institutional structure of the regulation of research is fundamentally paternalistic, perhaps because paternalism is viewed with opprobrium and is thought to be inconsistent with respect for persons and a commitment to the value of autonomy. I also argue that this paternalism is eminently defensible and that, properly understood, is actually quite consistent with respect for the values with which it may be thought to conflict.

Although the principle of informed consent is the most famous and most well examined principle in research ethics, Chapter 3 argues that our understanding of that principle should be recast. The dominant view is that it is permissible for investigators to proceed only if the subject's consent is "valid" and that the validity of the subject's consent is based on the subject's mental state. And thus it is often argued that if subjects are in the grips of the therapeutic misconception—the mistaken belief that therapy and research are governed by the same primary goal: to advance the individual patient's interest—their consent is not valid because they do not understand that to which they are consenting. It may also be argued that when researchers offer financial payment as inducements to participate, this puts pressure on people to enroll and that such pressure compromises voluntariness and may be incompatible with valid consent. Although "valid consent" is now the coin of the realm, Chapter 3 argues that the fundamental ethical question is not whether the subject has the appropriate mental state, but whether the consent *transaction* is fair to both the giver and recipient of consent. In most cases, the answers to these questions will converge. But when they diverge, it is the fairness of the consent transaction that is crucial. When we approach consent from a bilateral perspective, it turns out that it may be permissible for investigators to proceed even if the subject's consent is not valid. Somewhat paradoxically, it may not be permissible for investigators to proceed even if the subject's consent is valid.

I noted above that researchers frequently use financial incentives to recruit research subjects, but that this practice is viewed with considerable moral suspicion.[20] Moreover, even when it is thought ethically permissible to offer financial incentives if an IRB has established that the risks of the research are reasonable in relation to the anticipated benefits, the standard and virtually unquestioned view is that payments to the subject should not be regarded as a benefit of research for the purpose of making that determination. In Chapter 4, I argue that most of the ethical worries about financial payment are not well grounded. I consider and reject arguments based on the alleged coerciveness of financial payments, the commodification of research subjects, and the non-representativeness of the subject pool. I suggest that financial payments may constitute undue inducements and thereby compromise the status of consent if, but only if, they distort the subject's decision-making.

In addition, and more controversially, I argue that to the extent that we are concerned with the protection of subjects, we should *reject* the standard view that payments should not be regarded as a benefit in determining whether the risks of research are reasonable in relation to the anticipated benefits.

As I noted above, an increasing proportion of clinical research is being off-shored to developing countries. Chapter 5 considers the claim that much of this research is fundamentally exploitative. To pursue the theoretical issues, the discussion is framed around the question as to whether it is permissible to conduct placebo-controlled trials with participants who would otherwise receive no treatment if there is an established and effective intervention available in developed countries. Such research is barred by some (not all) codes of research ethics, such as the Declaration of Helsinki and is opposed by many prominent bioethicists. Building on some earlier work, I argue that it is important to distinguish between exploitative interactions that are harmful and nonconsensual and those that are mutually advantageous and consensual.[21] I also argue that it is difficult to specify when a mutually advantageous and consensual transaction is actually unfair and exploitative, but that even if such a transaction is exploitative, it is difficult to justify interfering with an interaction to which the exploited party consents and which is beneficial to her. Difficult, but not impossible. And so I also consider what would justify preventing persons from entering into what would be a mutually advantageous and consensual agreement.

In developing my analysis of exploitation in clinical research, I came to believe that worries about exploitation are but one manifestation of what I call *"The Interaction Principle"* (IP). The Interaction Principle maintains that people often acquire special obligations to those with whom they interact and particularly when they have benefitted from that interaction. Although not generally (or ever) articulated in quite these terms, I believe that IP (or something close to it) underlies much ordinary ethical thinking and, in particular, that it underlies much thinking about the obligations of researchers. In the research context, IP maintains that even though researchers may have no obligations to conduct research or use persons as research subjects, once researchers enter into a relationship with research subjects, they may thereby acquire an obligation to provide additional benefits to those subjects even though the subjects benefit from their participation in research and consent or would consent to such participation *without* those additional benefits. For example, it may be argued that researchers acquire an obligation to provide post-trial treatment to subjects or to provide "ancillary care" for illnesses that are discovered in the course of research but which are not the subject of the research.

Despite its intuitive appeal, IP has some important counter-intuitive implications. It implies that it may be worse to interact with another person in a way that benefits that person than not to interact with her at all. And it implies that one may have greater obligations to those who have already benefitted from an interaction than to those who have not benefitted at all and are worse off than those with whom one has interacted. I will argue that IP is more difficult to defend than might be supposed, and that several arguments in defense of IP simply do not work. Although there is at least one plausible argument in defense of IP, its implications for research are not entirely clear. Ultimately, I will argue that some principles of research ethics that receive support from IP may need to be abandoned or at least revised.

The previous paragraphs describe the organization of the book. Although I do not aim to provide a comprehensive and systematic treatment of the philosophical underpinnings of the principles of research ethics, the analysis is tied together by several strands of thought.

First, as a latecomer and still quasi-outsider to the world of bioethics, I have been struck by the extent to which the literature of research ethics tacitly (and sometimes explicitly) adopts a type of "medical exceptionalism," the view that participation in research is a distinctive activity that requires moral principles that we do not adopt or reject in other social contexts. Here are a few examples. Bioethics often proceeds as if the idea of consent were somehow unique to the medical context and that it is obvious that morally transformative consent be preceded by an elaborate disclosure of information. Yet we make no such assumption in many other areas of life, such as sexual relations and employment, where we speak of consent but not *informed* consent. It is generally assumed that if one agrees to participate in research, one retains a right to withdraw at virtually any point without penalty. Yet in many other areas of life, people may waive their rights in exchange for benefits and make binding commitments. Why not here? It is often said that it is morally problematic to provide financial inducements to prospective subjects to get them to accept risks to their life or health that they would not otherwise accept. On the other hand, we pay people to accept risks all the time, be it as soldiers, loggers, fishermen, fire fighters, structural steel workers, or pizza deliverers. It's called employment. Is there something morally distinct about the risks of research? If so, what is it?

Or consider the "off-shoring" of medical research. Although the benefits of "free trade" are somewhat controversial, it is generally thought that "off-shoring" of manufacturing and services is a net good for countries and workers abroad and for those who consume those products and services (at lower prices) here. It may be thought that it is relatively unproblematic to employ Indians to answer telephones, but morally troublesome to employ them as research subjects for testing drugs. But why is that so?

Although some versions or instantiations of medical exceptionalism may turn out to be correct, I suspect this will be in virtue of contingent features of clinical research and not the simple fact that it is "medical." If consent to participate must be more robust than a person's consent to gamble or have sex or buy a car or take a job, this will be in virtue of factors such as asymmetry or complexity of information, and not the fact that "medicine is different." If, for example, we should *not* treat participation in research as a form of employment, we must identify the features of participation in virtue of which it is different. And so my various analyses will often proceed by stepping back from the context of clinical research to examine the relevant principles in a wider context. Hence the need to widen the lens through which we see clinical research as one activity among many.

Second, I believe that while the various codes and regulations of research ethics reflect a plausible set of underlying values, the practical specification of those values has not always been wise. In particular, bioethicists have not adequately considered whether various policy recommendations are well-suited to non-ideal conditions. It is frequently argued, for example, that researchers may acquire obligations under non-ideal conditions that they would not acquire under more just or fortunate conditions. So it may be thought that researchers have an obligation to provide post-trial treatment in societies where such treatment is otherwise unavailable, but would not have such obligations in more affluent societies. Unfortunately, imposing such obligations on researchers increases the cost of doing such research and may have the effect of diverting research from precisely those societies in which people stand to benefit from participation.

Interestingly, whereas it is sometimes thought that researchers *should* treat some subjects differently in virtue of their different circumstances, it is sometimes argued that researchers should *not* treat subjects differently even though their circumstances are different. Some argue that if it would be unethical to conduct a placebo-controlled trial in a developed nation where effective treatments are available, then it is also unethical to conduct such a trial in a developing nation even though participation would not deprive participants of a treatment they would otherwise receive.[22] Such research may turn out to be unethical, but it certainly does not follow that just because it would be impermissible to conduct a placebo-controlled trial if subjects would otherwise have access to appropriate treatment that it is therefore impermissible to conduct a placebo-controlled trial under non-ideal conditions in which subjects do not have such access. Rhetorical appeals to notions of "double standards" will not resolve this and other issues.

Related to the previous point, a recurring theme throughout Chapters 4–6 is that it is of capital importance to distinguish between the moral status of interactions and the moral status of a person's background conditions. In some cases the distinction is intuitively clear. If someone is wrongfully injured and then seeks medical help, we do not think that the physician does anything wrong simply because he profits from treating the victim's wrongful injury. If someone is unjustly fired from a job, we do not think that another employer necessarily acts wrongly in hiring that person at a lower wage. We do not think the plumber does anything wrong in being paid to thaw frozen pipes. In these cases, the wrong or unfortunate background conditions do not contaminate our judgment of the transaction.

In other cases, however, the fact that people's background conditions are desperate or unjust (or desperate *and* unjust) appears to color the evaluation of interactions. Consider the controversy over selling live organs such as kidneys. Although there may ultimately be sound objections to the practice, I believe that much of the opposition to the practice wrongly conflates sensible concerns about the background conditions that would lead people to sell their kidneys with moral worries about the transactions themselves, given those background conditions. Assuming that it is wrong or unjust that anyone should be in a position where they must sell a kidney in order to support their family, it does not follow that such transactions are unethical given that some people are in such a position. This does *not* mean that one treats the *status quo* as morally acceptable. It means that whatever one's view of the moral status of people's background conditions, we must consider the ethical status of transactions that people undertake within that *status quo*.

And much the same is true for clinical research. Suppose it is easier for researchers to recruit subjects in less developed countries because their background conditions are miserable or unjust. It does not follow that there is anything problematic about the interaction between researchers and subjects. It would be a better moral world in which people were not so vulnerable, but given that they are vulnerable, it may not be wrong for researchers to take advantage of that vulnerability if participation renders those persons better off. That is not the end of the story, and there may well be important moral objections to the terms of a mutually advantageous interaction between researchers and subjects. But we must assess the ethical status of interactions on their own terms. Or so I will argue.

In his aptly titled book, Alan Blinder maintains that morally defensible economic policy requires a combination of hard heads and soft hearts.[23] (Readers can fill in the blanks as to how the left and the right may fall short). I aspire to think about research ethics in that way; although I no doubt fall short on both counts (the reader can decide where my deficiencies are greatest). I do not believe that bioethics suffers from an excess of hard heartedness, but, in my view, it is sometimes too conceptually sloppy and insufficiently empirical (soft-headed).

In saying that bioethics is insufficiently empirical, I do not mean that we can derive an "ought" from an "is." Rather, the point is that research ethics is a fundamentally practical endeavor. The point of the various codes, regulations, and most scholarship is to affect the practice of research so as to bring the practice (more) in line with the relevant values. In choosing among possible principles and policies, we must attend to the consequences of adopting or advocating those principles and policies in the world as we find it and as we can reasonably expect it to be. That requires empirical analysis. The present point is *not* that excessive concern for the welfare and autonomy of research subjects may impede research that would benefit a much larger number of people, although that might also be true and a cause for regret. The present point is *internal* to concern for the welfare and autonomy of subjects themselves. It is understandable that bioethics has been particularly concerned to protect vulnerable research subjects and to encourage more research on diseases that affect the poorest societies in the world. But in its concern to protect vulnerable subjects and their communities from allegedly exploitative research, bioethics may fail to serve the very ends which motivate its concerns. Or so I shall argue.

2 Facing up to Paternalism in Research Ethics[1]

Introduction

The reigning regulatory and ethical frameworks for human research emphasize the *protection* of research subjects. Although informed consent was given pride of place in the wake of the Nazi experiments and other infamous examples of nonconsensual research as a way for subjects to protect themselves, the current regulatory system—especially prospective risk-benefit assessment by independent ethics committees—is directed to protecting human subjects from protocols that pose undue risks of harm *before* subjects have the opportunity to consent to participate. Given that we do not provide people the opportunity to consent to participate in research that poses undue risks of harm, the question arises as to whether the standard protections for research subjects are inherently paternalistic and, if so, whether such paternalism is justified.

This question might be seen as motivated by the following thought experiment. Imagine that a research study recruits a group of prospective participants who have expert scientific and clinical knowledge and have exemplary skills of reasoning and judgment. Call them "ideal consenters." We should be perfectly comfortable relying on the consent of ideal consenters as the sole mechanism of subject protection, without any of the other standard safeguards. For, *ex hypothesi*, these individuals are fully competent to assess the social value of the research, the validity of its scientific methods, and completely understand the risks and potential personal benefits of participation.

By contrast with ideal consenters, most actual prospective subjects are vulnerable to a range of decisional deficiencies or impairments that render them unable to protect their own interests or advance their aims. This is not to impugn their general competence. They may simply lack the highly specialized information or training necessary to evaluate the risks and benefits of participation. And thus we are right not to rely exclusively on their consent as a mechanism to protect their interests.

In this chapter I defend a four-fold thesis. First, the regulatory system for human research is paternalistic at its core. Second, and more precisely, the regulatory system is best understood as a form of *group soft-paternalism*. Third, this type of paternalism may be perfectly justifiable. Fourth, and despite appearances to the contrary, this form of paternalism is compatible with the *values* that the principle of informed consent is designed to serve even though research regulation does not rely exclusively on the *mechanism* of informed consent.

Although these claims should not be particularly controversial, I believe that bioethics has not come to terms with the deeply and pervasively paternalistic character of research ethics and thus has failed to explore adequately the soundness and limitations of its view. It is somewhat surprising that bioethics has paid so little attention to paternalism in human subjects *research*. If we look at the literature on the ethics of *medical care*, we will encounter vigorous and (almost) unanimous arguments against paternalism. The dominant philosophical view has privileged respect for autonomy as a guiding principle and has challenged the Hippocratic tradition that the doctor is competent and entitled to decide what treatment is best for his patients. There is now a near universal consensus in the United States that competent adult patients have the right to refuse treatment even if the physician (rightly) thinks that the patient is mistaken and that physicians should not deceive or withhold information from patients just because they think it is in the patient's interests to do so. (I say United States because the paternalistic view is more dominant elsewhere). I suspect that bioethicists employ the word—paternalism—with respect to medical care precisely because the prevailing wisdom is anti-paternalistic.

When it comes to the ethics of research, however, things are different. To be sure, paternalism is implicitly recognized with respect to research involving children, incompetent adults, and other "vulnerable" populations, although the word "paternalism" is rarely used, even here. These groups receive special treatment in the U.S. Federal Regulations, known as the "Common Rule."[2] By contrast, it is not widely recognized that the current system of regulating human subjects research with competent adults is paternalistic at its core, by virtue of placing a variety of restrictions on permissible research beyond the requirement of obtaining informed consent. The theoretical justification of that practice does not come to terms with this paternalism or address why the ethics of medical research is sympathetic to paternalism, whereas the ethics of medical treatment is not. A well-known article by my colleagues at NIH—"What Makes Clinical Research Ethical?"— challenges the primacy of informed consent by regarding it as only one of seven criteria of ethical research and by placing it relatively low on the list.[3] But the authors do not explicitly acknowledge the paternalistic justification for some of those criteria or see the need to defend those criteria against the charge that they are paternalistic.

A cautionary note. It would be a mistake to claim that the current system is paternalistic just because it places restraints on permissible research beyond the requirement of obtaining informed consent. Some such constraints are not motivated by concern for the protection of subjects. For example, we may be concerned that scarce resources are not used for non-meritorious projects. We are legitimately concerned that researchers avoid conflicts of interest that would compromise the validity of research or public confidence in its value. Indeed, some constraints that appear to be motivated by the protection of subjects receive support from other values or goals. For example, we may not allow subjects to participate in risky research because it might undermine public confidence or trust in medical research—even if we were not concerned with protecting the subjects themselves. That said, "subject protection" is certainly the coin of the realm, and much of the concern for subject protection can best be explained by appeal to paternalism.[4]

Given the explicit rejection of paternalism in medical care, I suspect that paternalism has become so negatively-valenced that bioethicists prefer to avoid the word in research ethics, even if they are effectively supporting paternalism. Perhaps those who have developed and implemented the prevailing system of research protection do not want to confront the obvious tension between the avowed respect for autonomy and support for a system that might be thought to convey a lack of respect for the judgment of prospective subjects. So, as contrasted with the ethics of medical care, where there is less actual paternalism but more attention to the issue, there is little attention to paternalism in research ethics precisely because it is effectively endorsed and ubiquitous.

Whatever the explanation for this omission, it is time for bioethics to face up to paternalism in research ethics for both explanatory and normative reasons. First, it is necessary to face up to paternalism if we are to properly understand our practices. This is important in its own right. Second, we must face up to paternalism in order to thoughtfully consider whether and when those practices are justifiable. Contrary to the rhetoric of bioethics, there is no need to resist the view that paternalism *can* be justified. The hard task is to determine *when* paternalism is justified.

To accomplish these aims, my analysis proceeds along the following steps. It begins with an overview of the conceptual geography of paternalism. With several distinctions in hand, I will argue that the existing regulatory system is best understood as resting on what I will call *group soft paternalism*. In light of this conceptual framework, I illustrate the paternalistic character of the research regulation system. I then consider the limits of justifiable paternalism in research ethics by asking whether there should be a cap on the level of net risks to which competent adult subjects are exposed regardless of the potential social value of the research. Finally, I discuss the deeper theoretical connections between paternalism and the value of informed consent.

The Conceptual Geography of Paternalism

As a starting point, I adopt the general liberal presumption that people should be free to do what they wish with their lives, including the ability to enter into transactions or relationships to which they consent. Given this presumption, there are various possible justifications for limiting individual liberty, which is not to say that these are all *sound* justifications.[5] We may limit a person's liberty on the ground that it harms others (for example, rape) or that it offends others (for example, lewdness), or that it is intrinsically immoral (for example, prostitution). Of present interest, we may also limit a person's liberty on the paternalistic grounds that her behavior is likely to be harmful to herself (for example, seat belt laws).

There is considerable debate among philosophers as to how best to define paternalism. Although the standard cases are clear enough, there are disagreements at the margins. For example, it's not clear whether A is acting for paternalistic reasons if A prevents B from gambling for the sake of B's spouse.[6] We can ignore most of those controversies for present purposes. I do want to stress, however, that paternalism is best understood as a *justification, reason,* or *motivation* for an action or policy—not the action or policy itself. For example, the state is not acting for paternalistic *reasons* if it requires motorcyclists to wear helmets in order to protect *society* from excessive medical costs (thereby preventing harm to others), although I think that such arguments are often advanced precisely because they are perceived as more legitimate than paternalistic arguments.

Although the paradigmatic cases of paternalism involve interfering with someone's liberty of action, one can act for paternalistic reasons if one deceives or withholds information from another for her own good. One is acting for paternalistic reasons if one does not offer someone a job because one thinks accepting the position is not in her long-term interests. One can act for paternalistic reasons by manipulatively arranging the way choices are presented to people, as when an institution places the healthy food first on the cafeteria line.

Direct and Indirect Paternalism

In *direct* paternalism, we limit the liberty of the person whose interest we are trying to protect by requiring or prohibiting some action, as with seat belt laws or laws forbidding swimming in dangerous locations. In *indirect* paternalism, we seek to protect B by limiting the liberty of A, as when we prohibit psychotherapists from engaging in sexual relations with patients, forbid landlords from renting uninhabitable dwellings, or forbid manufacturers from marketing drugs without FDA approval. In these cases, we protect B by not allowing A to offer an opportunity to B or by treating B's consent as not rendering A's action permissible. Given this distinction, paternalism in research is mostly indirect, for the potential subjects are never given the opportunity to consent to participate in research that an institutional review board (IRB) is unwilling to approve.

Soft and Hard Paternalism

To use Joel Feinberg's terminology, a limitation of B's liberty is based on *soft* paternalism when it is justified on the grounds that B's decision-making is substantially impaired, when the agent lacks—or we have reason to suspect that she lacks—the information or capacity to protect her own interests.[7] Put slightly differently, soft paternalism operates to restrict conduct only when the agent's decision-making is judged to be substantially non-voluntary or non-autonomous. It is soft-paternalism when A stops B from drinking the liquid in a glass because A knows it is white vinegar but B believes it is water. In contrast, *hard* paternalism involves restricting the freedom of persons who are substantially autonomous, to protect them "from the harmful consequences even of their fully voluntary choices and undertakings."[8] It is hard paternalism if A prevents a competent and informed B from climbing Mt. Everest because A believes it to be too dangerous or if physicians require adult Jehovah's Witnesses to receive blood transfusions when medically indicated or if we require a motorcyclist to wear a helmet for his own good even if we concede that he fully understands the risks of not wearing one.

Given this distinction, we can raise two questions about a paternalistic intervention: (1) Is it a case of soft paternalism or hard paternalism? (2) Is the intervention justified or unjustified? To illustrate (1), consider Richard Arneson's example of the *Pouting Young Adult.*

> Tom is unreasonably distressed at some disappointment he has suffered. Perhaps he has been bested in competition for a job he coveted. . . . Whatever the cause of his distress, he is unhappy, and feels vaguely cheated by the world at large, and wants at the moment nothing more than to express his disappointment by committing suicide. He is not deceived, is aware that if he lives, he will come to forget his disappointment and go on with his life, but he right now has no interest in doing that. He wants above all to die. He is not mentally ill or incompetent, he just has unusual and unusually self-indulgent and immature preferences.[9]

Arneson thinks Tom is acting autonomously and that any interference would be a case of (perhaps justifiable) hard paternalism. I am less sure. It could be argued that Tom's failure to integrate his long term interests into his present decision betrays a serious impairment of judgment. If so, interference would be a case of soft paternalism.

With respect to (2), it is generally easier to justify soft paternalism than hard paternalism. Indeed, some scholars, such as Joel Feinberg, think that it is *never* justifiable to interfere with genuinely voluntary or autonomous conduct on the grounds that it is harmful to the actor himself. The problem with this absolute rejection of hard paternalism is that one must claim that conduct is not autonomous if one wants to justify interference. I prefer to think that hard paternalism can sometimes be justified even if it "expresses insufficient respect for the underlying valuable capacities, powers, and entitlements of the autonomous agent."[10] I do not see why respect for autonomy should trump all concern with an agent's welfare or interests or his future autonomy. So, even if we concede that Arneson's *Pouting Young Adult's* decision making is substantially autonomous (although I doubt it), it might be justifiable nonetheless to prevent him from committing suicide.

Feinberg's defense of soft paternalism builds on the classic work of John Stuart Mill. Mill says that some classes of people may need to be protected from harming themselves owing to their *general* decisional incapacities, as in the case of children and incompetent adults. As he puts it, the harm principle "is meant to apply only to human beings in the maturity of their faculties."[11] Call this *status* soft paternalism. Of greater relevance to our present concern, Mill thinks that we can justifiably interfere with the actions of generally competent adults if we have reason to think that *particular* decisions are substantially non-autonomous and clearly dangerous. Call this *decisional* soft paternalism. Mill endorses decisional soft paternalism in his famous bridge example: "If either a public officer or anyone else saw a person attempting to cross a bridge which had been ascertained to be unsafe, and there were no time to warn him of his danger, they might seize him and turn him back."[12] Mill says that we would not be interfering with the agent's liberty in this case "for liberty consists in doing what one desires, and he does not desire to fall into the river."[13] I think it more accurate to say that while we would be interfering with the agent's liberty, we would not be violating or failing to show respect for the agent's *autonomy* if he has not knowingly and voluntarily chosen to cross the unsafe bridge. As Feinberg puts it, "The defining purpose of the soft paternalist is to prevent people from suffering harm that they have not *truly chosen* to suffer or risk suffering."[14] And so even if one supports voluntary active euthanasia, it may not be permissible if the subject consents while in the grips of a temporary and treatable depressive episode. Similarly, it might not be permissible to tattoo someone if she consents while intoxicated.

A variety of defects in decision-making may make conduct substantially non-voluntary or non-autonomous and thus become the target for soft paternalistic intervention. These include:

- mistaken (or inadequate) factual beliefs (e.g., what one thinks is sugar is actually poison)
- inadequate information
- substantially impaired cognitive functioning
- gross defects in rationality
- impulsiveness
- lack of self-control or weakness of will
- distortions of judgment or appreciation relating to risks of harm; for example, the tendency to underestimate long-term risks or overweight short-term benefits
- vulnerability to power or authority.

I will not discuss these defects in any detail. The general point is that we can agree that soft paternalism is warranted *if* a person's judgment is substantially non-voluntary, even if we disagree as to *when* a person's judgment is substantially non-voluntary.

In this connection, it is of capital importance to distinguish between decisions that reflect genuine impairments or incapacities and those that are based on values or ends with which we may not agree. To prevent a person from climbing Mt. Everest because he mistakenly thinks it poses little risk to his life would be soft paternalism. But if he knows the risks and simply values the experience more than we think reasonable, then we must justify interference on grounds of hard paternalism or decide that interference is not justified at all. As Feinberg observes, "Reasonableness is one thing, and voluntariness is another." Although I think hard paternalism can sometimes be justified, it poses a higher ethical hurdle. So we should avoid an excessively expansive conception of "impairments," which risks collapsing the distinction between soft and hard paternalism and makes it possible to justify too much intervention under the umbrella of soft paternalism. It fails to show appropriate respect for an individual's right to determine the values by which she lives.

Before proceeding further, I take up a conceptual and a normative challenge to my view. It could be argued that if paternalism involves the violation of autonomy, and if soft paternalism is directed only at conduct that is substantially non-autonomous, then soft paternalism is not best described as paternalism in the first place. Although this is largely a linguistic matter, there are both conceptual and normative reasons for holding that we should continue to insist that soft paternalism is best regarded as a genuine form of paternalism.[15] First, soft paternalism should be regarded as paternalism because it typically involves interference with freedom for the agent's good even if it does not violate autonomy, and the label is useful for marking this reason for limiting liberty as contrasted with other reasons (for limiting liberty). After all, we do not deny that we act paternalistically towards children, even though children are not autonomous agents. Second, and more importantly, regarding soft paternalism as paternalism allows us to distinguish clearly between the *definitional* question as to what counts as paternalism and the *moral* question as to when paternalism is justified. If we say that soft paternalism is not genuine paternalism, then the justificatory work will be implicitly done behind the scenes by the process of classification. Once an intervention is described as a case of soft paternalism, there will be little left to say. I prefer to make the justification transparent.

Second, and as a normative proposition, it might be argued that interventions grounded in soft paternalism do not require much in the way of justification.[16] I disagree. I believe that interference with those that we have reason to think are non-autonomous does requires defense and referring to such interference as (soft) paternalism helps to avoid the question-begging position that it does not. First, if conduct is likely to expose decision-makers to little or no harm, it should be permitted even if it is not the optimal decision. We can allow children to choose the games they want to play or the musical instruments they want to learn even if they are doing so non-autonomously. Second, and as Mill argued at length, it is generally desirable for people to be able to learn from their mistakes even when their mistakes result from impaired judgment. So if a person would choose an option from which she would not suffer an irrevocable harm, we must certainly justify a decision to intervene even if her decision making is impaired. Third, people can choose autonomously to make what might otherwise be accurately described as nonautonomous choices. Fourth, even when a person's decision-making is impaired, his judgment about his interests may be better than anyone else's. If we are to justify paternalistic intervention, it is not enough that B's decision is impaired. We must have reason to believe that someone else's decision will be superior. People can make decisions as to whom to marry on the basis of relatively little information, but it does not follow that others are better positioned to choose for them. Fifth, even if an agent's *decision* is non-autonomous, it may be of moral importance to convey respect for the agent's general *capacity* for autonomous action. We should sometimes refuse to interfere with nonautonomous decisions of generally autonomous agents as a way of demonstrating respect for *them*.

Individual and Group Paternalism

Some soft-paternalistic interventions are targeted at individuals, as when we involuntarily commit a person to prevent him from committing suicide or stop Mill's uninformed person from crossing an unsafe bridge. Call this *individual soft paternalism*. By contrast, *policies* justified on soft paternalistic grounds are typically targeted at groups of individuals, some but not all of whom have impaired judgment. Call this *group soft paternalism*. Consider the regulation of prescription drugs. Some laypeople have the requisite knowledge and judgment to decide safely whether and how to consume a prescription medication. Yet under current policy, no one can obtain certain medications without a physician's prescription. Because many people lack the decisional capability to self-medicate effectively and safely and because it is not feasible or cost effective to differentiate between those who do and do not have the capacity to self-medicate, we adopt a policy under which the entire group of laypeople is required to get a prescription. The policy is *not* a form of hard paternalism with respect to those who can responsibly self-medicate, for the policy is not designed to advance *their* interests. Rather, competent decision-makers suffer restriction of their freedom as the unfortunate and unavoidable side-effect of a policy designed for the sake of those who are not capable of self-medicating.

It should be said that the requirement that one obtain a prescription before using certain drugs (and other forms of consumer protection) can be defended on non-paternalistic grounds, as a mechanism for liberating us from the need to become informed and make certain decisions.[17] Even those who have the cognitive capacity to self-medicate and could make an intelligent decision live in a world where their "cognitive budget" is limited and may prefer that others make certain choices for them so that they can use their time and energy on other matters.[18] Although this form of self-imposed paternalism may operate with respect to competent decision-makers, I suspect that the policy is best justified on group soft-paternalistic grounds with respect to those who are not well positioned to make competent decisions on such matters.

To further exemplify group soft-paternalism, consider the ban on sexual relations in psychotherapy. It is widely thought that the judgment of most psychotherapy patients who would consent to sexual relations with their therapist would also be distorted by the therapeutic process (transference) and that they are likely to be harmed by such encounters. Although it is also entirely possible that some subset of psychotherapy patients are capable of giving competent undistorted consent to sexual relations with their therapist and that such relations will be personally or even therapeutically beneficial, there is no reliable process by which the therapist or the patient or a third party can decide into which category they fall. And so we justifiably prohibit *all* sexual relations between psychotherapists and patients.

When is group soft-paternalism justified? What determines when it is justifiable to limit the freedom of those with no decision impairments in order to advance the interests of those whose decision-making is impaired? Obviously, the greater the proportion of impaired decision makers, the easier it is to justify intervention. The severity of the harm also matters. If impaired decision-makers were a clear minority but are likely to harm themselves severely if left to their own devices, then it may be possible to justify a policy that limits a majority's freedom if we can't reliably distinguish between the two groups. The degree of deprivation of freedom also matters. Consider the annoying child-resistant safety caps placed on medicine. A large majority of people endure a mild inconvenience in order to protect a small number of children because it isn't feasible or efficient to market products which can be sold exclusively to childless households.

Considerations of justice or equity are also relevant to the justification of group soft paternalism. Richard Arneson has argued that those who are less well off and less educated are likely to be poor decision makers by comparison with the affluent and well-educated.[19] If justice requires that we give priority to the interests of the least well off, then we should err on the side of protecting the poor decision makers from themselves, even if this works to the detriment of the better decision makers who might benefit from greater freedom.

There is certainly no algorithm by which to determine when group soft-paternalism is justifiable. Nonetheless, I hope to have established that we may be justified in limiting the freedom of an entire group of persons that includes a sub-group whose decision-making is not impaired or who would benefit from less intervention in order to protect the interests of the sub-group whose decision-making *is* impaired.

Paternalism in Research Regulation and Ethics

The basic contours of the research regulation system are well known and need not be elaborated here. For my purposes, the principal feature is that institutional review boards are charged to provide prospective review of protocols involving human subjects before potential subjects are given the opportunity to consent to participate. In designing and reviewing protocols, investigators and IRB members are guided by the relevant legal statutes ("The Common Rule") and established sets of standards or principles, including the Nuremberg Code, the Declaration of Helsinki, the Belmont Report, the CIOMS (Council for International Organizations of Medical Sciences) guidelines, and the literature on research ethics.[20]

The structure and operation of the research regulation system is best understood as being justified by group soft paternalism. I do not claim that IRBs are or should be consciously motivated by soft paternalism when they are making decisions. I am arguing that the structure of the system and many of the criteria that IRBs are asked to apply are best justified by group soft paternalism.

Unlike some paternalistic policies, the limitations on liberty of potential subjects that result from this process are largely indirect and invisible to the persons who are being protected. Whereas seat-belt laws impose a restriction directly on the persons whose interests the laws are designed to protect and who know that they do not have the option to ride in a car without a seatbelt, IRBs restrict the liberty of investigators in order to protect the interests of potential subjects who will typically not know that the options available to them have been limited in this way. Indeed, *no one* may know what options might otherwise have been available. In some cases, IRBs disapprove proposed protocols, and then we will know what opportunities for participation have been lost. In other cases, however, investigators do not propose protocols because they anticipate that they would not be approved. We do not and probably cannot know what protocols would be available in the counterfactual world in which the regulatory structure did not operate. The important point is that the research regulation system serves to restrict the opportunities available to potential research subjects. For example, if researchers are not permitted to recruit prisoners as subjects because it is thought that incarceration affects "their ability to make a truly voluntary and uncoerced decision," then the prisoners are denied the opportunity to participate and the benefits they might be offered in exchange for their participation.[21] I do not claim that this policy is unwise (although some prisoners seem to think so). I do claim that it is a limitation of the liberty of prisoners that is best understood as protecting them from choices that do not advance their interests.

The research regulation system affects the liberty of prospective subjects with respect to both the availability of a study and the *terms* on which it is conducted. For example, the research regulation system constrains the sorts of medical and financial benefits that might be otherwise available to participants. IRBs typically permit financial incentives to be offered to healthy volunteers in Phase I trials and other forms of "non-therapeutic" research. But they may place restrictions on the level of financial compensation that researchers can offer or refuse to approve any compensation at all to patients owing to concerns about coercion or "undue inducement." Moreover, even if IRBs do not actually enforce any particular set of restrictions, investigators may share the worry about undue inducement or be reluctant to propose financial inducements that they think will be rejected. I suspect that the overall effect of these worries is huge.

For ease of explication, my argument proceeds by examining the seven ethical requirements for clinical research explicated by Emanuel and colleagues, which is synthesized from the U.S. Federal Regulations, established sources of ethical guidance, and the research ethics literature.[22] I call this the "NIH canon." These requirements, some of which overlap, include social value, scientific validity, fair subject selection, favorable risk-benefit ratio, independent review, informed consent, and respect for enrolled subjects. Although Emanuel et al do not use the word "paternalism" in explaining or justifying *any* of these ethical requirements, I believe that many (although not all) are best understood as justified—at least in part—by group soft paternalism.

Social Value and Scientific Validity

The first two criteria of the "NIH canon" are not the best examples of my thesis. Evaluating protocols for "social value and scientific validity" is no doubt partly justified by the goal of making good use of scarce resources devoted to biomedical research and ensuring that the study design will generate findings that will advance the standard of care for future patients.[23] But this has little to do with subject protection. After all, to the extent that people participate for self-interested reasons, the social value and scientific validity of the study is irrelevant to *them*. A poorly designed study might still be a "good choice" from the subject's perspective, if the expected personal benefits are greater than the expected personal risks and burdens. The study may not advance the goals of clinical research, but the subjects themselves are not harmed any more than construction workers are harmed if they are hired to build a condominium that goes belly-up (assuming they are paid).

That said, these criteria receive some support from concerns for the protection of subjects. People sometimes participate in research—at least in part—for altruistic reasons, because they want to contribute to the development of generalizable knowledge. But altruistically motivated subjects are often not in a position to know whether the risks to them are adequately compensated by the potential benefits to *others*. And so IRBs are charged with reviewing the social value and scientific validity of research protocols in their stead. In these cases, the IRB is not protecting subjects from harm or burdens, per se. Rather, the IRB is protecting subjects from harm or burdens that do not serve their altruistic ends. Thus the application of these criteria serves what we might call altruistic paternalism.

Fair Subject Selection

Fair subject selection serves multiple values, some of which are orthogonal to concerns about the protection of subjects. Nonetheless, when this principle is invoked to argue that research should not exploit the most vulnerable groups in society, it implicitly appeals to soft paternalism. Tom Beauchamp and colleagues have argued, for example, that we must be particularly careful when the homeless are asked to participate in pharmaceutical research.[24] But why? If the homeless were capable of deciding when their long-term interests or aims are best served by participation, there would be no need for heightened protection. The authors advocate placing limits on the incentives that may be offered to the homeless because they might be tempted by the "irresistible inducements" of payments to participate in research that does not advance their interests.

Risk-Benefit Assessment

Risk-benefit assessment of a research protocol involves determining that the risks to subjects have been minimized, in view of what is necessary to answer the scientific question, and that the remaining risks are justified by the prospect of benefits to the subject or the potential value of the knowledge to be gained. The fact that IRBs are charged with risk-benefit assessment of protocols before prospective subjects can be given the opportunity to enroll in research signifies that the subject's consent is not adequate to protect her interests. On its face, prospective risk/benefit assessment can best be justified by appeal to group soft-paternalism.

Henry Beecher maintained that "[o]rdinary patients will not knowingly risk their health or life for the sake of science."[25] To the extent that Beecher is right about patient motivations, it is easy to see why otherwise competent adults may find it difficult to protect their own interests in assessing the risks and benefits of research. First, they lack the requisite scientific and clinical knowledge. Few subjects are in a position to determine whether risks have been minimized in a study that uses imaging procedures involving ionizing radiation to probe the understanding of a given disease. Risk-benefit assessment also requires comparative consideration of alternative study designs: Can the study question in this case be answered by using an imaging procedure without radiation, such as MRI? Few subjects have this sort of knowledge.

Second, and technical knowledge aside, patient-subjects are vulnerable to distortions of judgment. Prospective subjects who are suffering from a disease under investigation are particularly vulnerable to "the therapeutic misconception," that is, the tendency of patient-subjects to mistakenly assume that research interventions are designed to benefit them. In addition, patient-subjects who are desperate for the chance of medical benefit from access to experimental treatment may overestimate the benefits and underestimate the risks of research participation. Moreover, even if some people are willing to altruistically incur *some* risk to their health or life for the sake of science, they may need soft-paternalistic protection from risks that are *greater* than they are prepared to incur.

Independent Review

The principal procedural mechanism for protecting research subjects is prospective review and approval by an independent committee. The IRB is charged with implementing the substantive requirements of ethical research, which (as we have argued) are justified to a large extent on soft paternalistic grounds. If research subjects were able to adequately protect themselves by means of informed consent, there would be much less need for independent review.

To put the point in different terms, I believe there is an unacknowledged but important structural parallel between the IRB/subject relationship and the parent/child relationship with respect to consent. Pediatric research typically requires the *informed consent* of the parents and the *assent* of children of sufficient age.[26] In both cases, however, the consent (or assent) of the subject is (ordinarily) necessary but not sufficient to render the research permissible. The consent of the parents is required because we assume that the child does not have the decisional capacity to make such decisions. The assent of the child is required because we think it is generally wrong to impose research without the prospect of direct medical benefit on an unwilling child. Similarly, the consent of the IRB to a subject's participation is required before subjects are permitted to give the functional equivalent of a child's assent, albeit at a higher level of information and competence and with fewer restrictions as to acceptable risks.[27] The present point is that both children and parents need the approval of at least one "higher" decision-maker before they have the opportunity to consent.

I do not want to exaggerate the explanatory power of soft-paternalism. As with other criteria we have (and will) consider, the need for independent review receives support from several values. Because there is a deep ethical tension at the heart of research ethics between the interests of participants and the ends of society, we may need independent review to ensure that clinical research advances serve those social goals and that (at least in the case of publicly funded research) scarce social resources are being used appropriately. In addition, it is important that the research enterprise includes mechanisms for maintaining social trust about the way it treats participants— not for the sake of the participants themselves, but so that research can continue to fulfill its social function. Scandals such as the Tuskegee study not only harmed the subjects, they also harm the research enterprise to the extent that others are more reluctant to participate or support funding for medical research. Although this justification of independent review is not directly paternalistic, paternalism is lurking in the background nonetheless. After all, if we thought that people can and should protect themselves by refusing to consent to excessively risky or inappropriate research, we would have less need to reassure society that subject protection mechanisms are in place.

Informed Consent

And that takes us to informed consent. The requirement to obtain the informed consent of competent research subjects would appear to be one requirement of ethical research that is decidedly *non*-paternalistic, for the purpose of informed consent is to enable individuals to judge for themselves whether research participation is consistent with their preferences and values. Even here, appearances are deceiving. By requiring investigators to positively disclose the character and risks of participation, rather than allowing subjects to determine what information they want, it is arguable that the very principle of *informed* consent is at least somewhat paternalistic. After all, there are many areas of life where people are responsible for obtaining the information they need to make a decision. *Caveat emptor* or something close to that. Those who rent boats do not need to disclose the risk of capsizing in bad weather or being hit by lightning. We allow people to consent to employment without being informed of the occupational risks. We allow people to consent to sex, marriage, and gamble without much information as to the risks of these decisions. In contrast, we do not allow subjects to say "If the study is being conducted by the University of Michigan School of Medicine, that's all the information I need." The paternalistic dimension of informed consent is heightened when the consent process include procedures to test the comprehension of prospective subjects before permitting them to enroll. For example, in a sham-controlled trial of arthroscopic surgery for osteoarthritis of the knee, prospective subjects were required to write in their own hand that they understood that they might receive a fake operation which would not benefit them.[28] I do not say this policy is unjustified. I say that it is paternalistic to require subjects to comply with the policy.

Respect for Enrolled Subjects

This general requirement contains a variety of norms not all of which involve the *protection* of subjects from harm, such as the communication of study results at the conclusion of research. However, some requirements ordinarily placed under the rubric of respect for subjects are directed at the protection of subjects and are arguably best justified by soft paternalism. For example, it is universally held that subjects have an inalienable right to withdraw from research at any time (assuming it is safe to do so). But why can't subjects make a (relatively) binding commitment to remain in a protocol particularly if they are paid more to do so? After all, everyday life contains numerous contexts in which people can (indeed, have the right to) make commitments from which it is difficult to withdraw (marriage) or in which they subject themselves to penalties for non-compliance (contracts). It is not entirely clear why we do not allow research subjects to make similar sorts of commitments, but it is presumably because we believe that they do not have the information or judgment to properly anticipate the situations in which they might want to withdraw.

Alternative Explanations

I have argued that group soft paternalism is a plausible explanation for the research regulation system and prevailing ethical guidelines. Of course, a given policy can be justified by more than one principle or value. Can other ethical considerations adequately explain the structure and operation of research regulation to protect subjects without appeal to paternalism?

When one looks at research regulation and ethics from the perspective of the history of abusive human experimentation, it may appear that the principal rationale for guidelines to protect research subjects is to prevent them from being harmed by unscrupulous investigators. On this view, the operative principle is *nonmaleficence* rather than paternalism.

Appearances can be deceiving. Properly understood, the principle of nonmaleficence does not prohibit A from harming B, full stop. After all, A is generally permitted to harm B if B consents to be harmed or assumes the risk of being harmed, as when A sells cigarettes to B or engages in a prizefight with B. As the legal expression puts it—*volenti non fit injuria* (to one who consents, no wrong is done). If the principle of nonmaleficence were to adequately ground research regulation, then it might have sufficed to prohibit experimentation without consent, sanctioned by criminal and civil penalties. Indeed, this is the primary way in which human experimentation was regulated in the U.S. before 1966. And if it were thought that prior review and ongoing supervision were desirable, then the purview of IRBs arguably would, and should, be confined to making sure that consent documents accurately and intelligibly reflect study protocols and, perhaps, by supervision of the informed consent process itself. Thus the principle of nonmaleficence cannot provide an independent non-paternalistic basis for risk/benefit assessment and a process that does not permit subjects to decide for themselves what research risks they are prepared to assume.

Some have argued that preventing *exploitation* is perhaps the central rationale of research ethics and the regulation of research.[29] Would "avoiding exploitation" constitute a non-paternalistic rationale? Here we must be careful. To (over) simplify a complex matter, it is useful to distinguish between two types of exploitation: (1) harmful and non-consensual exploitation where persons are harmed by the transaction and do not consent at all (as in the Nazi experiments) or do not give morally transformative consent (as in the Tuskegee study); (2) mutually advantageous and consensual exploitation (as, say, when vineyard owners employ immigrants to pick grapes for low wages). In the latter case, exploited persons benefit from the exploitative transaction and give voluntary, competent, and informed consent to the transaction.

Given this distinction, the goal of preventing harmful nonconsensual exploitation does not do any moral work that is not accomplished by the principle of informed consent. If subjects do not give the semblance of consent, then it is obvious that appeal to the principle of informed consent should be sufficient. When research subjects are vulnerable to a variety of decisional defects, they need soft paternalistic protections to prevent them from being exploited without their morally transformative consent. But avoiding exploitation adds nothing to the argument. On the other hand, if we focus on mutually advantageous and genuinely consensual exploitation, then it is true that the goal of avoiding exploitation cannot be justified by soft paternalism, for interference will not benefit the subject. But then it is also not clear whether the non-exploitation principle should be accepted. Why *should* we prevent the grape pickers or research subjects from being exploited *if such work is their best option?* It might be thought that we should prevent mutually advantageous and consensual exploitation because exploitation is wrong even when people consent to and benefit from being exploited. That may be correct, but it has little to do with the protection of subjects that underlies the concern with exploitation.

In arguing that the research regulation system is *best* justified by group soft paternalism, I do not assume that any particular research regulations or ethical guidelines *are* actually justified by group soft paternalism. It is at least partially an empirical question as to whether and how many subjects are capable of protecting their own interests or whether their decision-making is substantially impaired. It is a normative question as to whether the impairment justifies intervention. As I argued above, there may be good reasons to allow people to make impaired decisions rather than to attempt to decide for them. Moreover, if it is feasible to mitigate such impairments, then it is arguable that we should strive to enable subjects to make autonomous decisions rather than rely on prior review to protect them. I do not seek to resolve those issues here. My aim here is to lay bare the justificatory structure of research ethics, not to say what features of that system are actually justified at the end of the day.

The Limits of Paternalism in Research Ethics

I have argued that appeal to group soft paternalism for research subjects does not necessarily conflict with the liberal values of respect for individual autonomy. If an individual or her decision is not autonomous, then we do not violate autonomy when we fail to respect that decision. This is particularly so when research subjects are not intending to put themselves at risk for the sake of science or society and mistakenly believe that they will personally benefit from participation.

But now consider research in which it is clear to all concerned that the subjects would be altruistically assuming risks in order to contribute to socially valuable research, and where there is no reason, *a priori*, to think that the subjects are not competent. There are two views about the permissibility of such research. The first view is exemplified by the U.S. Federal Regulations which, strictly speaking, place no upper limit on approvable research involving adults capable of giving informed consent. The Common Rule states that "Risks to subjects are reasonable in relation to anticipated benefits, if any, *to subjects, and the importance of the knowledge that may reasonably be expected to result*"[30] (emphasis added). So, if the last mentioned variable is great enough, even very risky research may be reasonable "in relation to anticipated benefits." The second view, exemplified by the Nuremberg Code, stipulates that "No experiment should be conducted where there is an *a priori* reason to believe that death or disabling injury will occur; except, perhaps, in those experiments where the experimental physicians also serve as subjects."[31] Although the Nuremberg Code appears to forbid (very) high risk research regardless of the expected social benefits, its exception was introduced with an eye to the famous experiment led by Walter Reed, in which one of the investigators died after being exposed to yellow-fever-carrying mosquitoes.[32] It is not clear why this exemption should be endorsed. Certainly, the fact that an experimenter is willing to sacrifice *himself* for a social cause does not entail that it is permissible to sacrifice *others*—even if those others consent to join the experiment. The exemption could be understood as evidentiary. If the authors of the Nuremberg Code accept the possibility that extremely high risk research is permissible if the expected social benefits are sufficiently great, then an experimenter's willingness to serve as a subject might serve as *evidence* that they believe this is so.

But whatever the laws and codes suggest, there remains the question: should there be limits on the risks to which competent adult subjects are exposed? Suppose that a contemporary analogue of Walter Reed and his colleagues seek to enroll subjects (but not themselves) in research of great public value but posing high risks. Should they be allowed to do so? Provided that stringent measures are put in place to assure that the decisions of subjects are not impaired and that they give robust consent, there can be *no* justification on soft paternalistic grounds for such a limitation, unless we assume that anyone (or, at least most) who would consent to such risks must suffer from impairments that have not been identified. And that seems unreasonable. We do not assume that people are impaired when they take considerable risks with their own lives and health for the sake of a personal challenge, and we do not prevent people from climbing Mount Everest on hard paternalistic grounds even though by 2003 179 persons had died attempting to do so. We do not assume that people are impaired when they take morally admirable risks for the sake of others, as when they serve as fire fighters or soldiers and we certainly do not prevent them from doing so on hard paternalistic grounds. We do not think that we should stop people from acts of heroism. Although Mill was prepared to stop someone from unknowingly crossing an unsafe bridge, his principles would not support stopping Wesley Autrey from jumping onto New York City subway tracks in front of an oncoming train in order to lie on top of a man who had accidentally fallen onto the tracks (both survived).[33] Given this, I find it hard to argue that it would be irrational for someone to altruistically take grave risks to their life or health for the sake of research with extraordinary public health potential.

A Nuremberg-type prohibition of high risk research might be justified on non-paternalistic grounds. It might be argued that high risk research should be prohibited in order to protect the professional integrity of physician-investigators even if the subjects themselves are fully prepared to accept such risks. On this view, because physicians have obligations qua physicians— "Do no harm"—it would be wrong for *them* to engage in imposing serious risks on subjects even if it were not a wrong *to* the consenting subjects, and even if accepting such risks were an act of admirable altruism.

This argument moves much too quickly. First, it is questionable to what extent "Do no harm" is an inviolable principle for medical care. We do allow physicians to take a kidney from one person for the sake of another, a procedure that—like research—is justified on grounds of beneficence, not to mention that physicians perform cosmetic surgery which may pose medical risks to patients without any compensating *medical* benefit. On the other hand, physicians will not remove a vital organ, such as a heart, from a parent who is willing to die so that her child might live and not, I think, because it is assumed that such consent is of dubious validity. So causing limited "harm" seems acceptable, but causing death is not.

But even if we think that the "Do no harm" principle should be accepted as a *prima facie* norm for *medical care*, it does not follow that the principle applies in the same way to *research* activities.[34] Whereas physicians generally are justified in exposing patients to the risk of interventions only when they have reason to believe that they offer a compensating prospect of medical benefit, I assume that investigators are justified in performing research procedures (such as blood draws) that carry risks or burdens (sometimes quite small) without any medical benefits to subjects. If physician-investigators and IRBs are justifiably convinced that the potential value of the knowledge to be gained from a study justifies the risks to subjects, and if subjects are willing to accept such risks, it is arguable that there should be no bar to proceeding based on an appeal to the professional integrity of researchers. For what is at stake is the professional integrity of researchers, not physicians practicing clinical medicine.

The previous point aside, it can't be wrong to perform an act *because* doing so will compromise one's integrity. For performing an act can't compromise one's integrity unless it is (already) wrong. Compromising one's integrity is not an *independent* reason not to perform some act. As Thomas Nagel has written, "it is a confusion to suggest that the need to preserve one's moral purity might be the *source* of an obligation."[35] And so it must be shown that it is wrong for investigators to enroll subjects in high risk research that meets all other ethical requirements, including uncontroversially robust consent, save for the fact that it is high risk.

It remains possible that high-risk research might be ruled out for the sake of protecting the research enterprise from loss of public confidence. The death or grave illness of subjects caused by research participation might produce a public outcry which threatens support for the conduct of valuable research and the willingness of people to participate. And this might be so even if the research itself were (otherwise) ethically justifiable and even if the subjects themselves have no genuine moral complaints. This argument for prohibiting high risk research is coherent and plausible. However, and as with all consequentialist arguments, we would need to determine if the negative consequences of allowing high risk research ultimately outweigh the social value it produces. And in calculating such consequences, we must be on guard against the tendency to stress the harmful but visible effects of allowing high risk research while underestimating the beneficial but less visible opportunities that will be lost by foregoing such research.

Paternalism and Consent

I have argued that much of the prevailing system of research regulation is best explained by appeal to group soft paternalism. I have also argued that there is a fundamental connection between soft paternalism and the *values* that underlie informed consent. If subjects were ideal consenters, there would be no need for much of the subject protection framework. When IRBs apply the various criteria of ethical research, they can be understood as attempting to replicate the judgments that ideal consenters would make. In this section, I want to pursue the connection between soft paternalism and consent in a little more detail.

There is a tendency to see informed consent as being motivated solely by the value of the agent's autonomy as contrasted with the agent's welfare or interests. But people want to be in control of their lives not just to protect some abstract value of autonomy or right to self determination, but also to protect their interests from those who would harm them. Moreover, people want to be able to enter into transactions and relationships that advance their interests and allow them to pursue their aims by authorizing others (through consent) to do things that it would otherwise be impermissible for others to do. Consent is the process through which mutual gains from interactions and relationships become possible.

The protection and promotion of an agent's autonomy and the protection and promotion of one's interests ordinarily converge, in part because one's interests reflect one's preferences and in part because people have a distinct interest in and obtain satisfaction from having their lives go according to their choices. The protection and promotion of an agent's autonomy and the protection and promotion of her interests are not identical, however, because an agent can autonomously decide not to advance her interests, say, for moral or altruistic reasons. Such cases aside, if an agent consents to another's action it is typically because the agent *believes* it is in her interest to do so. Indeed, it cannot be completely coincidental that the very factors that are thought to compromise the *validity* of consent to another's action, such as lack of information, deception, coercion, and incompetence, are factors that reduce the likelihood that another's action will not advance her interests or welfare.

If I am right, the values that underlie independent risk-benefit assessment and informed consent—the two pillars of protecting research subjects— are linked by the goal of protecting the interests of subjects. If we could rely on the subject's consent as a mechanism by which to adequately protect her interests, there would be little need for independent risk-benefit assessment. But since subjects are not in a position to make the necessary judgments, we need independent risk-benefit assessment on soft paternalistic grounds. From a *chronological* perspective, risk-benefit assessment comes first: investigators solicit consent only after an IRB determines that the risks of the research are reasonable in relation to the anticipated benefits. From a theoretical perspective, however, it is actually the values that underlie consent that motivate the need for risk-benefit assessment.

At a higher theoretical level, the primacy of the values served by consent might also be seen as reflected in a contractualist justification of the central features of a group soft paternalist approach to research ethics. The regulatory policies for protecting research subjects can be understood as the policies that that rational persons would hypothetically endorse in a suitably-designed choice situation because rational persons recognize their own decisional deficiencies. As Rawls puts it,

> [T]he principles of paternalism are those that the parties would acknowledge in the original position to protect themselves against the weakness and infirmities of their reason and will in society. Others are authorized and sometimes required to act on our behalf and to do what we would do for ourselves if we were rational, this authorization coming into effect only when we cannot look after our own good.[36]

On this view, a major—not the only—point of the regulatory apparatus of research is to increase the probability that subjects give their somewhat deficient actual consent to participate in research only when they would consent to participate if they were in a position to give ideal consent to participate.

Conclusion

I have argued that much of the reigning regulatory and ethical frameworks for human research can be seen as receiving much of its justificatory support from considerations of soft paternalism. Understanding research ethics in this way may have implications that are not obvious and may not yet be accepted.

Here is one example. Investigators, IRBs, the legal and quasi-legal guidelines, and bioethics scholars have all displayed considerable concern about the use of financial payment to recruit research subjects. There is considerable support for the view that such incentives may constitute "undue inducements" that distort the judgment of prospective subjects and that the size of such inducements should be restricted so as not to cause such distortion. Although I consider this issue in more detail in Chapter 4, here I will simply say that a soft paternalist justification for intervention only works if the agent's judgment is distorted, and it is far from clear that financial incentives typically have that effect. If financial incentives do not distort the judgment of prospective subjects, then restrictions on payment to research subjects that investigators would otherwise be prepared to offer cannot be justified on grounds of subject protection.

The general and more important point is that we must face up to the paternalistic character of the regulation of research. Protecting potential research subjects may justifiably limit their choices, but limit their choices it does. When we face up to this paternalism, we can then go on to ask when such paternalism is justified and when it is not. The answers are by no means obvious.

3 Preface to a Theory of Consent Transactions in Research: Beyond Valid Consent[1]

Introduction

In the previous chapter, I argued that the reigning regulatory and ethical frameworks for research with human subjects is directed at protecting subjects from undue risks of harm before they are given the opportunity to consent to participate. That said, the principle of informed consent remains at the epicenter of medical ethics and research ethics. It is central to *all* of the established codes or canonical statements. As the Nuremberg Code puts it, "The voluntary consent of the human subject is absolutely essential."[2] Informed consent has been no less prominent in the scholarship of bioethics.[3] Although the centrality of informed consent is unquestioned, it is actually regarded as neither sufficient nor necessary for ethical research.[4] We have seen in Chapter 2 that informed consent is not sufficient, in part for reasons unconnected to the protection of subjects, but also because prospective subjects are not capable of protecting themselves through the mechanism of informed consent. In addition, and as we shall see below, some believe that informed consent is not sufficient to assure that research is ethical because informed consent does not—by itself—block the charge that research wrongfully uses subjects "merely as means" for the benefit of society.

It is also commonly accepted that informed consent is not strictly necessary for ethical research. Even if we set aside cases in which surrogates consent for the subject, there are special circumstances, such as emergency research in which subjects are unconscious, where research may be justified but where no sort of consent is possible.[5] Research without *any* kind of consent may also be justifiable when it involves collection of data from health records or in cluster randomized trials where it is impractical or impossible to seek everyone's consent, or, perhaps, more controversially, when a randomized controlled trial compares two established, proven effective drugs for a given condition.[6] Research without *informed* consent may also be justifiable where subjects must be deceived if research is to produce scientifically valid data. Still, all that said, there remains a wide spectrum of cases in which it is now uncontroversial that informed consent must be obtained. In those cases, the question is not whether informed consent is necessary, but *what is required by informed consent*. The principal task of this chapter is to recast the way in which this question is approached and answered.

Now it might be thought that if consent is not a necessary feature of ethical research, then we need not worry so much as to what is required by informed consent. Not so. Consider this analogy. It is permissible for the police to search a person's home without the owner's consent—if the police have obtained a warrant or if some special exception exists, such as the imminent destruction of evidence. The police can also search a location without a warrant if the owner consents to the search. But the fact that nonconsent searches are permissible does not diminish the importance of determining what counts as the sort of consent that renders it permissible for the police to conduct a "consent search" without a warrant or weaken the requirements for such consent.

Before turning to the main task of the chapter, I want to consider two challenges to the principle of informed consent. The first challenge, as advanced by Hans Jonas, claims that informed consent is *not sufficient* for ethical research if people consent for the wrong reasons. The second challenge claims that informed consent is *not necessary as a general principle* beyond the exceptional cases noted above. So whereas Jonas claims that even soliciting participants is ethically dubious because it amounts to a form of "conscription," the second challenge bites Jonas's bullet and maintains that if conscription of labor or the use of people's bodies *is* justifiable in other contexts, it may be similarly justifiable in the context of research.

Both challenges can be understood as testing the implications of the Kantian Formula of Humanity: "So act that you use humanity, whether in your own person or in the person of any other, always at the same time as an end, never merely as a means."[7] For present (non-Kantian) purposes, call this the *never merely as a means principle* (NMMP). Assuming we accept NMMP (and it is not self-evident that we should), the question arises as to whether using people who have given ordinary competent, voluntary, and informed consent is sufficient or necessary to satisfy NMMP.

Merely as a Means

Although elucidating Kant is a task that is beyond my pay grade, I would not defend an extreme form of that principle as it might be ordinarily understood. As Amartya Sen has suggested, if one can prevent a heinous rape by taking B's car without B's consent and against B's well-informed objections, one arguably violates NMMP, but any principle that would condemn such a "use" should be rejected.[8] At the same time, because NMMP seems to capture something of moral importance and has become a virtual mantra in bioethics, it is worth asking what it might imply with respect to the recruitment and use of research subjects.

As is often and correctly pointed out, no sensible moral principle could prohibit using people as a means. NMMP prohibits using people *merely* as a means—whatever that is. If I take a taxi, the taxi driver uses me as a means to earn an income and I use him to get to my destination. There is nothing remotely problematic here if we both give valid consent to the terms of the transaction—he does not deceive me about the fare and I do not make what Kant calls a "false promise" to pay him. It is not clear whether robust consent is always sufficient to satisfy NMMP, but it must go much of the way towards doing so.

Yet, actual robust consent is surely not necessary to satisfy NMMP. Consider Derek Parfit's example of the scientific use of animals.

> One scientist . . . does her experiments in the ways that are most
> effective, regardless of the pain she causes her animals. This
> scientist treats her animals merely as a means. Another scientist
> does her experiments only in ways that cause her animals no pain,
> though she knows these methods to be less effective.[9]

Parfit claims that the second scientist is not treating the animals *merely* as a means because her "use of them is restricted by her concern for their well-being."

If concern for well-being is sufficient to satisfy NMMP with respect to animals, what does it mean not to use a *person* merely as a means? Parfit says that we treat someone "*merely* as a means if we . . . regard this person as a mere instrument or tool: someone whose well-being *and moral claims* we ignore, and whom we would treat in whatever ways would best achieve our aims."[10] On this view, it's not that doing X to B is wrong because doing X violates NMMP. Rather, doing X violates NMMP because doing X is wrong. A person's moral claims may include respect for their rationality or autonomy or rights as well as concern for their well-being, but the specification of those claims is the relevant task. As Richard Arneson has argued, if NMMP is interpreted as the injunction not to use people "in ways that are unacceptable according to correct moral principles," everything turns on the content of those principles, a matter on which NMMP is silent.[11]

It is sometimes argued that NMMP requires that we never treat people in ways to which they could not possibly give *rational* consent. Kant thought that false promising violated NMMP precisely because one could not consent to be deceived in that way. But NMMP does not require that people always give actual consent as a prerequisite of ethical interaction. Kant thought that we do not violate NMMP when criminals are given their just deserts. On his view, we can justifiably punish people without their consent perhaps because they could give rational consent to the system under which they are punished. We do not violate NMMP when we treat unconscious people without their actual consent because they could give rational consent to such treatment.

It might be thought that the possible consent view is too permissive because it allows A to use B without B's actual consent so long as B *could* rationally consent to such use. And that is clearly false. Certainly, the fact that B could rationally consent to have sexual relations with A does not render it permissible for A to have sexual relations with B without B's actual consent. But this is compatible with the rational consent view, because whereas we could give rational consent to some acts without our actual consent, there are other cases—such as sexual relations—in which we could not give rational consent to be treated or used in that way without our actual consent.

Is research like sex? If we say that it is *prima facie* acceptable to use someone in a way to which they could give rational consent, the question now arises as to whether we could rationally consent to a research system (1) only if it requires more than voluntary informed consent or (2) if it requires no more or less than ordinary voluntary informed consent. Or could we also consent to a system (3) that does not require actual consent at all?

Jonas's view

Jonas defends (1) although he does not defend it by appeal to the principle of possible consent. On his view, experimenting "on" human subjects involves what John Arras calls an "ontological fall from grace" and the participant's status as an agent is degraded to that of a mere thing.[12] Jonas says that while ordinary voluntary informed consent (2) is surely a "non-negotiable minimum requirement, [it] is not the full answer" to the justifiability of using people as research subjects. Jonas claims that soliciting research subjects is morally suspect because ". . . the mere issuing of the appeal, the calling for volunteers, with the moral and social pressures it inevitably generates, amounts even under the most meticulous rules of consent to a sort of *conscripting*."[13] It is not clear why Jonas thinks "moral pressure" amounts to wrongful conscription. After all, Kant argued that an act has true moral worth only if it is done out of a sense of obligation. But Jonas clearly thinks that some motivations for consent do not justify including the subjects in research even though they give what would otherwise constitute voluntary informed consent.

Jonas has an ambivalent view of the moral force of a *patient's* consent. On the one hand, he says that sick patients need special protection because their "consent is marred by lower resistance or captive circumstance, and so on."[14] On the other hand, because patients may gain direct medical benefit from participation or from the knowledge obtained from research, the "appeal for volunteers can be properly made on the basis of the subject's self-interest."[15] In those cases, it seems that a patient's consent would meet with Jonas's approval. But when patients do not stand to benefit from participation or when research uses healthy volunteers, it is not enough that consent be competent, informed, and voluntary as those terms are ordinarily understood. No, if research is to pass ethical muster, subjects should *identify* with the ends of research—". . . the appeal for volunteers should seek this free and generous endorsement, the appropriation of the research purposes into the person's own scheme of ends. Thus, the appeal is in truth addressed to the one, mysterious, and sacred source of any such generosity of the will – 'devotion'" . . .[16] In Jonas's view, "all experimentation, even when it is non-harmful, treats the experimental subject as a passive 'token' . . . and thereby threatens the dignity of the person as a unique individual." And any attempt to appeal to people's sense of social obligation "would certainly be a way to pressure people and so would endanger the moral validity of the act of consent."[17]

A full treatment of this argument would take us too far afield. For present purposes, it is important to note that Jonas believes that participation in research is always supererogatory; neither patients nor healthy volunteers have an obligation to participate in even minimal risk clinical research. He may be wrong. If, as I have argued elsewhere, people have a *prima facie* obligation to do their "fair share" of participation, there is no violation of the Kantian principle when people voluntarily do what they have an obligation to do.[18]

Setting the issue of obligation aside, Louis Jaffe has criticized what he regards as Jonas's "excessive ethical fastidiousness" with respect to motivations.[19] I would put it differently. The view that participants must strongly identify with the goals of the research fails to respect what prospective subjects regard as good reasons to participate, be it to help others or to get better medical care or to receive financial compensation or out of curiosity. Jonas assumes a form of medical exceptionalism. We do not think that a construction worker must "identify" with the aims of the project in order to justify the risks he incurs. It is enough that workers are treated fairly and consent to the employment. Autonomous agents have different reasons for doing things and Jonas's "identification" view is unfair to those subjects whose reasons for participating stray from the preferred road.

Is consent necessary?

Although Jonas denies that ordinary consent is sufficient for ethical research, he regards it as a "non-negotiable minimum." Is he right? There are some special contexts where we might think that the benefits of abandoning consent justify the violation of that ethical principle. The cost of adhering to the informed consent criterion is perhaps most clear in contexts where it is impossible to obtain consent or where surrogates are or should be reluctant to consent for the subjects. It is—and arguably should be—difficult to recruit children to participate in pediatric research. After all, it is one thing for an adult to consent to bad choice research for altruistic reasons or because she is compensated for doing so. It is quite another for an adult to consent to research on her infant child, for the child cannot be compensated and parents have obligations to protect their children's interests that they do not have towards their own interests. At the same time, the difficulty of securing parental consent for testing drugs on children has severely compromised the quality of pediatric care, for we cannot easily extrapolate from what we know about the efficacy and safety of a drug when used with adults to its safety and efficacy with children.[20] Or consider emergency research. It is critically important to evaluate the efficacy and safety of emergency interventions, but those patients who might be used for such research are often *not* in a position to consent and surrogates may be unavailable. Moreover, it may be feared—not without reason—that some minority groups may be over-represented in the potential pool of subjects for such research. Some think that we should therefore be reluctant to do such research, and if this means that the class of emergency patients will suffer, so be it.[21]

Setting aside such special contexts and also setting aside questions about the use of data about people or the use of their stored tissues, should we accept the principle that consent is a *sine qua non* of ethical research? Put more crudely, would it be legitimate to *conscript* people to serve as subjects? Alan Donagan has observed that Robert Servatius, a German lawyer who defended Nazi physicians at Nuremberg, argued that if we accept the legitimacy of military conscription, then we must endorse the legitimacy of the Nazi experiments.[22] But that would be preposterous. The Nazi experiments were horrific on so many grounds that it would be a mistake to assume that they were wrong simply because the subjects were forced to participate. Unless "the Nazis made that argument" is accepted as conclusive grounds for rejection of any moral proposition, the argument for the moral legitimacy of conscripting research subjects should be considered on its own merits, say, if the research served an important purpose, if conscription were fair, if subjects were treated as well as possible, etc.

I say "moral legitimacy," not "moral justifiability." Here I follow Joel Feinberg's discussion of liberty-limiting principles.[23] In his four-volume series on the moral limits of the criminal law, Feinberg aims to identify the principles that it is legitimate for the state to use in criminalizing behavior, such as "harm to others" and "offense to others," and those that it is not legitimate for the state to use, such as "harm to self" or "harmless wrongdoing." Feinberg observes that there is an important distinction between policies that are "*legitimized*" by valid moral principles and those that are *justified* on balance as being both legitimate *and* useful, wise, economical, popular, etc."[24] Even if it is legitimate for the state to criminalize some offensive behavior, it does not follow that the state is justified in doing so in a particular case. On the other hand, even if it would be socially beneficial to criminalize some self-harmful behavior, it is wrong for the state to do so because it does not pass the test of moral legitimacy.

Could people give possible rational consent to the conscription of research subjects? To consider this question, it will be useful to distinguish between policies that take a person's *external resources* that include both his financial and non-financial property, and policies that take a person's *internal resources*, i.e., her body and labor. In considering such issues, it is commonly thought or simply assumed that we should accept what Kasper Lippert-Rasmussen calls *The Asymmetry Thesis* (AT)—namely, that ownership of external resources such as financial and non-financial assets is intrinsically different, morally, from ownership of one's mind, body, and labor."[25] Interestingly, both the statist and the libertarian may reject AT. The statist will argue that if the state can take a person's external resources without her consent, it can also take her internal resources without her consent. The libertarian will argue that since the state *cannot* take a person's internal resources (e.g. her organs) without her consent, it cannot take her external resources without her consent. By contrast, the "liberal" will accept AT and argue that it is legitimate for the state to take a person's external resources (say through taxation) without her consent, but it is not legitimate for the state to take a person's internal resources (conscripting organs for redistribution).

Should we accept AT? I will assume but not argue here for the proposition that it is justifiable to take a person's external resources for the benefit of other individuals (education, welfare, medical care, etc). I will also assert but will not defend the view that the "separateness of persons" or respect for individual rights does not entail that taxation for purposes of redistribution is illegitimate. I have a similar view about taking internal resources. Some policies that involve taking internal resources without consent may turn out to be illegitimate or unjustifiable, but appeals to doctrines such as "separateness of persons" or "rights" won't get us there. As James Griffin puts it:

> Human rights are best seen, I think, as grounded in, as being
> protections of, our personhood — that is, our choosing our own
> course through life and then acting to realize it. So we have a right
> to *some sort* of bodily integrity; protection of body is part of the

protection of agency. But exactly what protection does the right require? Does it, for instance, prohibit a state from demanding a pint of my blood or to up the stakes, one of my kidneys? *We shall not get answers to these questions simply out of the key moral notion of protecting our personhood.*[26]

As Cecile Fabre observes, one can be under an enforceable duty to provide some personal services or labor and some invasions of one's body without ceasing to be a person.[27] If, as I argued above, we violate NMMP when a person's interests and moral claims have not been afforded appropriate weight and respect, then we cannot use NMMP to support AT, since the soundness of AT as a moral principle is precisely what is at issue.

Defenders of AT typically appeal to widely and deeply held intuitions about the moral distinctiveness of the body rather than a straightforward argument. Charles Fethe says

> "Tax me but don't test me," seems a perfectly sensible view.
> Taxation . . . represents a standard procedure for exacting social
> obligations; but introducing a social duty to volunteer for medical
> experiments presents a claim for a different kind of sacrifice: here
> my body rather than my fungible resources is being used, and so
> the sacrifice is more personal, deeper within that sphere which we
> normally like to think of as protected from social encroachment.[28]

Ronald Dworkin takes a similar view.

> Would it be outrageous to require blood donations according to
> some fair lottery? Kidney donations? Eye donations? We might well
> wish to resist this chain of questions by adopting a prophylactic
> line that comes close to making the body inviolate . . . We might
> justify this by appealing to the importance of protecting the person,
> and the danger in adopting any line less bright.[29]

Also along similar lines, Nir Eyal writes: "it is very problematic to ignore the "prophylactic membrane" that surrounds our bodies within deep and widespread perceptions about disrespect."[30] Although neither Dworkin nor Eyal defend AT as a deep moral truth, both argue that adopting a reasonably bright line around the body is a useful guide in moral, political, and legal analysis. In Dworkin's case, this prophylactic line has the benefit of stopping the slippery slope from relatively minor and assumedly acceptable bodily invasions to those that we would regard as impermissible. For Eyal, the pro-phylactic "membrane" responds to our deep *perceptions* about the impor-tance of the body.

Of course, we can accept Eyal's advice not to "*ignore* the 'prophylactic membrane' that surrounds our bodies," without taking that membrane as dispositive or impenetrable (emphasis added). And while Dworkin may be right that there is a danger that acceptable invasions or uses of the body will lead to unacceptable invasions and uses of the body, it is also possible that the slope is not as slippery as Dworkin fears. Just as accepting the paternal-ism of seat belt laws did not lead us to ban Ben and Jerry's high-fat ice cream, we may not need to deny ourselves the benefits of compelling minor inva-sions of the body in clinical research as the price for avoiding unjustifiable major invasions.

One might try to defend AT by appeal to a principle of *self-ownership*. It might be thought that we "own" our internal resources in ways that do not apply to external resources, such that the burden on the conscription of internal resources is *much* greater than the burden on taking external resources—even if that burden can sometimes be overcome. As a contingent matter, it is probably more difficult to justify conscription of internal resources than external resources, but Lippert-Rasmussen has argued convincingly that there are no "fact-insensitive" ownership rights over one's body. One can argue that control of one's body is of great moral significance because it is crucial to one's agency or to one's life's plan or one's needs, but then the importance of control of one's body will depend upon whether such control is, in fact, essential to one's agency or to one's life plan or needs.

Lippert-Rasmussen uses his argument to defend positive rights against the libertarian challenge. After all, if my right to control my body derives not from self-ownership but from the contingent fact that one needs one's body or the fact that it is important to one's agency, then the fact that one also needs some external resource or possessing an external resource is important to my agency may ground a right to that external resource as well.[31] Of greater relevance to our present concern, if the degree to which one "needs" some part of oneself (one's blood or one's kidney) in order to pursue one's plan of life determines "the stringency of [one's] self-ownership rights," then one can't say "you can't take my blood" simply because it's bodily tissue. Rather, one would have to show that one's right to control one's blood is protecting "something important in one's life."[32] And it may not.

Once the issue is put this way, it seems that the moral issue is not whether a resource is external or internal, but whether having control of some internal or external resource is necessary to whatever it is that is morally important. From this perspective, it is *not* true that external resources are all fungible or relatively unimportant. It is one thing to take my money without my consent (through taxation). It is quite another to take my house through the process of eminent domain—even if I receive "just compensation" as required by the Fifth Amendment. Because people often come to have deep personal attachment to their homes, such takings are held to a higher standard. At the same time, it is not true that all internal resources are of equal moral importance.[33] It is one thing to take a kidney without consent. It's quite another to compel people to provide a unit of blood. Indeed, I suspect that many people would find it more important to protect their house from appropriation by the state than to protect a unit of their blood from state appropriation.

Given this, could we possibly consent to a system that would compel people to participate in research? Because participation in research involves both a form of labor and invasions of the body, consider a range of cases in which the state is at least arguably justified in coercing people to engage in labor for the benefit of society or to being subject to invasions of their body without consent. Let's start with the body. We require that people be vaccinated against certain diseases for paternalistic reasons and for the good of society. Some states require premarital testing for certain diseases. We may sometimes require that people undergo a DNA test of paternity. The justice system frequently requires bodily invasions. It may require blood samples or breathalyzer tests from those suspected of driving while intoxicated. We may require a blood sample from those suspected of criminal activity. The Fifth Amendment provision that no person "shall be compelled in any criminal case to be a witness against himself" does not extend to providing *evidence* against oneself. One can't be required to speak, but one can be required to provide blood.

With respect to labor, we do well to recall that while Mill defended individual liberty and self-determination against paternalistic or moralistic intervention by the state, he supported several forms of compulsory service to the society: "There are also many positive acts for the benefit of others, which he may rightfully be compelled to perform; such as, to give evidence in a court of justice; to bear his fair share in the common defence, or in any other joint work necessary to the interest of the society of which he enjoys the protection."[34] As we have already noted, the state is prepared to conscript people for military service. Moreover, it is commonly argued that it would be desirable to require all citizens of a certain age to devote a period (perhaps six months to two years) engaged in civilian service to the society. It would be unjustifiable to require that people be assigned to an entire *career* that they do not choose. That would render one's life deeply non-autonomous. But to be required to serve society for a limited time is another thing altogether.

Consider other forms of "forced labor." On a mundane level, observe that many communities require that people recycle various goods. True, this is a relatively trivial imposition and it would be more than hyperbolic to call it "involuntary servitude." But that is the point. Participation in much research is not much riskier and—over time—is less burdensome than the weekly or daily task of recycling, given that participation in research may be a short-term affair. But we do *not* say that it's permissible to take my fungible money for environmental protection but not permissible to require me to sort my garbage, place it in the appropriate receptacle, and move it to the curb in front of my home. And it would surely be churlish (to say the least) to refuse to help build a dike to stem a flood by appeal to a principle of "no forced labor."

The justice system requires various forms of service, including some that may put people at considerable risk. We may require people to testify as witnesses in both civil and criminal cases, even though they may reasonably fear retaliation against themselves or their families. We have a witness protection program for a reason. We may require victims of crime to testify in court, sometimes against their very strong desire not do so. Perhaps more analogous to participation in research, we require people to serve on juries at considerable inconvenience and perhaps loss of income. And while sequestration is rare, the fact remains that we think it justifiable for the state to require citizens to live away from home and without contact with the external world for an extended period.

Finally, and to beat one more dead horse, we may think it justifiable to follow Mill, who thought that the state could legitimately require people to perform "certain acts of individual beneficence, such as saving a fellow-creature's life"[35] Although one can defend bad Samaritan laws without accepting Mill's claim that failing to make such rescues constitutes a harm to others, the general point is that it is commonly thought that society is justified in conscripting our labor for such purposes, at least if the burden is not excessive.[36] So whereas Nozick opposed welfare-state type policies by arguing that

"taxation of earnings from labor is on a par with forced labor," Arthur Ripstein runs the argument the other way: "[T]the forced labour involved in
making an easy rescue is on a par with taxation."[37]

I do not want to justify the case for each of these examples from the
ground up. Let us simply assume for the sake of argument that it is legitimate
for the state to compel the use of internal resources without consent in some
of these cases. We may certainly quarrel about what constitutes "joint work
necessary to the interest of . . . society (emphasis added)." After all, Jonas
regarded the pursuit of medical progress as an optional goal. But if we accept
the general structure of Mill's principle, it would seem that there is a *prima
facie* case for adopting a similar position with respect to participation in
research. I said *prima facie*. Even if it is in principle *legitimate* for the state to
require that people participate in research, it does not follow that it would be
wise or morally justifiable to recruit subjects without their consent. That
depends on the weight of the reasons for and against such a policy.

Before considering the reasons for resisting the argument for rejecting
consent as a necessary condition of ethical research, we must ask to whom
the argument might apply. At first glance, it would seem that the argument is
easier to sustain with respect to healthy volunteers than to patients. In principle, healthy volunteers could be conscripted by a process similar to the
lottery that was used for military service or jury service. We don't need everyone to serve, but all suitable persons would be deemed eligible to contribute
their fair share of participation.

By contrast, it may be thought more problematic to coerce sick patients
into participating in research. Jonas says that "the afflicted should not be
called upon to bear additional burden and risk [because] . . . they are society's
special trust and the physician's particular trust."[38] Along similar lines, Howard
Trachtman has argued that whereas military service falls on a "well defined
segment of the population . . . disease . . . strikes randomly and indiscrimi-
nately in all people regardless of age, gender, or ethnicity,"[39] and so the analogy does not hold. In addition, David Wasserman and Robert Wachbroit
have argued that if researchers need subjects "with particular conditions,"
then an enforceable "universal duty of research participation would do little
to meet their needs."[40]

These objections are not persuasive. It is unfortunate but true that the
sick are often in a unique position to be used in the search for generalizable
knowledge that will contribute to the health of other patients (or prevent
them from becoming sick). A diabetes drug can only be tested on patients

with diabetes. It is similarly unfortunate but true that victims of crime are in a unique position to contribute to the pursuit of justice. We do not say that an assault or rape victim need not testify simply because she has already suffered a horrendous burden. If we need her to serve as a witness to obtain a conviction, so be it. I see no reason—in principle—to think that we have less reason to burden the sick. It is true, as Trachtman suggests, that disease strikes randomly, but the unpredictability of obligations is a familiar feature of our moral lives. Some obligations drop on us out of the blue. We pass by a person in need. We witness a crime. The randomness of such events is not a reason to avoid the imposition of such obligations.

We should also not confuse the universality of a duty with its specific instantiations. There is a universal duty to "give evidence in a court of justice" and a universal duty to save "a fellow-creature's life," but some will never be in a position where these duties apply. *Pace* Wachbroit and Wasserman, a universal enforceable duty can supply the subjects with particular conditions, if that duty is activated when subjects have the relevant conditions.

In suggesting that it may be legitimate for society to place rescue-like enforceable obligations on healthy volunteers or the sick to participate in research, I am not claiming that it would be legitimate to put them at great risk. Just as a bad Samaritan statute may demand that people come to the aid of another person only when they can do so at relatively little risk, we may think that we may demand that the sick participate in research only when the risks are minimal or moderate, as when two interventions are in genuine equipoise.

As I noted above, although it is important to establish plausibility of view that consent is not a "non-negotiable minimum," it does not follow that it would be wise or even morally permissible to abandon the principle of informed consent. Mill argued that just because "harm to others" can "alone justify the interference of society," it does not follow that "it always does justify such interference."[41] Similarly, even if there are no claims of autonomy or rights or self-ownership or personhood that would preclude the conscription of research subjects without consent, the moral reasons for opposing conscription of research subjects may well outweigh those that support it. Such a policy may be legitimate but unjustifiable.

I take the need for bright lines and rules quite seriously even when they do not capture the underlying moral complexity.[42] On the view I prefer, it may ultimately be wise to draw a relatively (although only relatively) inviolable prophylactic barrier around a person's body or labor such that the burden that must be overcome before the state can take a person's external resources is *much* lower than the burden that must be overcome before the state can take a person's internal resources, just as the burden the state must overcome before using race or religion (a "suspect classification" that requires a "compelling state interest") as a regulatory category is much greater than the burden the state must overcome before using a category such as age (a non-suspect classification that requires only a rational basis). Given the considerations I discuss below, it might well be rational to insist on informed consent as a general requirement of participation in research even if conscription is morally legitimate.

Although the following list is by no means exhaustive, here are several reasons for adopting such a rule. First, conscription may be unnecessary. Even if we do not view medical progress as "optional" a la Jonas, there is no reason to crank up the coercive powers of the state if an adequate supply of subjects can be obtained in other ways. Just as we may obtain enough volunteer soldiers by increasing the financial incentives for military service, we may be able to recruit an adequate number of research subjects if we relax some of the constraints on payment (see Chapter 4).

Second, the use of coercion and the consequent limitations of freedom are a genuine moral cost. It is true that a system that requires that everyone do their share may result in a more equitable distribution of the burden, but there is much to be said for trying to maximize the opportunities for people to live according to their own lights even if it permits some unjust free-riding.

Third, there are good consequentialist reasons for resisting conscription of research subjects. Even if the conscription of research subjects was done fairly and was otherwise justifiable, and even if the intuitive support of AT is not well founded, those sentiments are real and should not be discounted by any sensible view about public policy. A policy of conscripting research subjects would generate considerable anxiety and would likely be met with considerable resistance. The game may not be worth the candle. Whereas the public does not think that we wrongly "use" people when we require them to testify or serve on a jury, the fact remains that people may have a different view about the use of "guinea pigs" for medical research.

Fourth, and related to the previous point, the medical system relies on trust. Much of the apparatus of contemporary research regulation is a response to the legacy of the Nazi experiments and the Tuskegee study, and the other scandals discussed in Henry Beecher's famous article.[43] Our reaction to these historical events stems not just from the fact that people were treated horrifically. It stems from the fact that the experiments were performed by *doctors* engaged in *research*. Just as we react more intensely when innocent people are punished by the state than when innocent people are victimized by crime, we react more intensely when people are wrongfully used as research subjects than when patients suffer from mistaken medical practice that is not supported by the evidence. And while more people die because they are treated wrongly by physicians (including treatments not supported by adequate research) than because they participate in medical research, wrongful treatment at the hands of well-meaning physicians does not seem to compromise our trust in the medical profession as much as ethically dubious medical research.

David Schmidtz has highlighted the importance of trust in the medical profession by contrasting two famous philosophical hypotheticals. In *Transplant* we ask whether it would be permissible to kill one healthy person who is in a hospital and transplant his organs to save five persons who would otherwise die (two kidneys, one heart, one liver, one lung). One dies; five live. In *Trolley*, we ask whether we can switch the trolley from a track on which it is destined to kill five persons to a track where it will kill only one. One dies; five live. Although it may appear that the problem posed in *Transplant* is identical to the problem posed in *Trolley* "in a surgical mask," the cases are actually quite different.[44] Whereas *Trolley* is about one versus five, *Transplant* is "about trust."

> We can't trust people who assume a right to harvest our liver
> whenever we stray too close to a hospital . . . hospitals cannot
> serve their purpose unless people can trust hospitals to treat
> people as rights-bearers. Institutions have utility by creating
> conditions under which people can trust each other *not* to operate
> in an act-utilitarian way. . . . [W]e need constraints that enable
> patients and doctors to trust each other. If those constraints also
> stop doctors from killing one patient to save five, that is good,
> because doctors who can be trusted to respect that constraint will
> save more lives than doctors who cannot.[45]

So to the extent that even a fair system of conscription of research subjects would undermine that trust, there is good reason to avoid it and even better reason if we're not confident that the system would be fair.

Fifth, and on democratic grounds, it would be *prima facie* wrong to use state coercion without public support even if a policy is meritorious. By way of analogy, Aaron Spital argues that a policy of confiscating cadaveric organs for transplantation would save lives without imposing any harm on the deceased. (People may be prospectively bothered by a policy that would authorize such confiscations post-mortem and family and friends may be aversely affected as well). But while he thinks this "stimulating idea" has substantial merit, he also believes its "time has not yet come." Whatever its merits, a large majority oppose such a policy.[46] Even if the majority's view is wrong on its merit, a commitment to democracy implies that there are second-order moral reasons not to adopt policies that are supported by first-order moral reasons.

Much more could be said on both sides of this issue and it is not my purpose to resolve it. I have argued that it is far from obvious that the principle of informed consent should enjoy its exalted status as a *sine qua non* of ethical research. There is a plausible case for the moral legitimacy of the conscription of research participants, but justifiability is another matter altogether. At the end of the day, there may be compelling reasons to continue to think that research with human subjects is typically justifiable only if the subjects give the sort of informed consent of which they are capable (subject to the limitations described in Chapter 2). And so we must ask what that requires. And if abandoning informed consent is morally illegitimate, then we certainly must ask what informed consent requires. It is to that task that we now turn.

Widening the Lens

Although the current consensus presupposes a rather expansive conception of informed consent, the paradigmatic examples of unethical research are ones in which there was not even the semblance of the expression of consent or where there was egregious deception or non-disclosure of basic information. A stripped-down version of informed consent would have been sufficient to bar Nazi experimentation, the Tuskegee study, or the Jewish Chronic Disease Hospital study in which subjects were not told that they were being injected with live (but probably harmless) cancer cells for research purposes.[47] With the core of the principle now unquestionably secured, the issue becomes just how far it should be extended.

The expansion of the principle of informed consent follows a pattern common to the development of many moral principles. The pattern begins with a minimal demand that eventually becomes widely accepted and then progressively extended, engendering debate about its proper scope. The pursuit of racial equality moved from the abolition of slavery to the end of segregation to worries about stereotyping and to the call for affirmative action. The pursuit of sexual equality moved from eliminating the outright exclusion of women from the voting booth, educational institutions, and professions to the need for role models to the demand for maternity benefits. The rights of homosexuals moved from abolishing prohibitions on consensual sexual relations to non-discrimination in the work-place to the provision of benefits for same-sex partners to the legalization of same-sex marriages. We begin with a "core" principle to defeat the most severe transgressions and then press outward towards the margin where issues that were once entirely off the radar screen (e.g., same-sex marriage) are now the subject of extensive discussion and increasing acceptance.

So, too, with informed consent. Current ethical debates about informed consent do not focus on egregious violations of the principle, but rather with cases in which subjects express consent, where they are not physically coerced (unlike the Nazi cases) and are provided with adequate information (unlike the Tuskegee study), but where their consent may still be regarded as importantly deficient. We now debate whether informed consent is satisfied if information is not fully understood or if subjects are excessively optimistic that they will benefit from research or whether the promise of medical care (for the uninsured) or financial incentives constitutes coercion or "undue influence."[48]

Consider the problems posed by the "therapeutic misconception."[49] Assuming that subjects are told that they will be participating in a randomized controlled trial, do they give informed consent if they wrongly believe that they will be receiving personalized medical care? According to Gopal Sreenivasan, the reigning view is that such subjects do not give informed consent and that it would be unethical to enroll such subjects, thereby threatening to bring many (otherwise) ethical clinical trials "to a near standstill."[50] Baruch Brody suggests that we may need to face up to this possibility. He describes a placebo-controlled study of the benefits of arthroscopic surgery in which subjects were required to write by hand that they understood that they might be receiving "sham surgery."[51] Although this procedure generated a "significant refusal rate," Brody maintains that this is "the price you may have to pay if you increase potential subjects' understanding." No one said that ethics comes cheap.

Although it is possible that the price of informed consent is too high if it would seriously hamper valuable medical research, we cannot assume that we must choose between informed consent and the viability of clinical research until we have a satisfactory understanding of the principle of informed consent itself. Is it actually compromised by the therapeutic misconception? By inducements? By excessive optimism? By exploitation?

Despite all that has been written, I believe a new tack is necessary. In my view, much of the literature has tried to make progress by looking more and more closely at an ideal of consent and asking what sorts of mental states it requires. But to use a motif of the book, we need a wide angle lens as well as a microscope. Because bioethics has been in the grip of a specific historical legacy and an associated set of canonical statements and legal doctrines, it has failed to locate the principle of informed consent within the more general terrain of contexts in which people regularly alter their moral and legal status by consent. As soon as one looks at other social contexts, one realizes that the principle of informed consent so familiar to bioethics is actually quite atypical. We usually speak of consent—not informed consent—in most of the other realms in which people make mundane as well as life changing decisions, such as sexual relations, contracts, jobs, and marriage. It's not merely that we don't use the *term* "informed" in these contexts. We think that the provision of information is not morally required.

Faden and Beauchamp acknowledge that their analysis of informed consent could be regarded as excessively narrow when seen against this backdrop, although they do not see this as a compelling reason to broaden their approach.

> A wide variety of consents have nothing to do with medicine or research . . . informed consent . . . could be applied to autonomously authorizing appliance repairs, withdrawing money from a checking account, hiring an agent, and hundreds of other daily activities. . . . We do not deny, of course, that the concept of informed consent could be broadened to mean *any* authorization that is substantially autonomous. *But we do deny that this is a plausible reading of what the term has meant in any significant document on the subject of informed consent.* (Emphasis added)[52]

If my task were primarily exegetical, it would indeed not make sense to worry about appliance repairs and checking accounts. But if the task is to develop a theoretically defensible account of informed consent for clinical research, then we need to look beyond the history, documents, and interpretive literature that have shaped its meaning. An adequate conception of informed consent to research should be rooted in an approach that is adequate for the full range of contexts in which consent plays an important role.

I title this chapter "A Preface to a Theory of Consent Transactions: Beyond Valid Consent" because I seek to recast the way in which bioethics thinks about consent. First, I seek to change the focus of the analysis of consent from a preoccupation with the characteristics of the participant's mental states to a focus on the *bilateral* transaction between the consenter and the recipient of consent. Second, and despite all that others and I have previously suggested, the crucial question is *not* whether the consenter gives *valid* consent as contrasted with (mere) consent, although the concept of valid consent is eminently serviceable in most cases.[53] Rather, the crucial question is whether the consent *transaction*—considered as a whole—is *morally transformative,* whether it renders it *permissible* for the (putative) recipient of consent to proceed.

Two Approaches; Two Models

An attractive theory of informed consent to participate in research should be but one instantiation of a more general theory of consent. We need to step back before we go forward. Before we can arrive at the best understanding of consent, we need to determine how we should approach that task. Broadly speaking, one can take an internal approach or an external approach to the development of such an account.

On an *internal approach,* we take the concept of consent as more or less given and we look to the internal logic of the concept. We ask, in effect, what consent or informed consent "really means." If a proper analysis of the concept of consent combined with the relevant facts entails that valid consent has not been given, then we have three options: (1) we can conclude that the consent is not morally transformative; (2) we can overtly or covertly weaken the criteria for morally transformative consent in the name of practicability; (3) we can retain a stronger conception of valid consent but treat it as a *prima facie*, but not necessary, requirement of permissible action. In any case, on the internal approach, informed consent means what it means.

By contrast, an *external* approach to a theory of consent maintains that judgments of moral transformation within consent transactions are the *output* of moral reasoning rather than logic or conceptual analysis. Rather than looking inside the concept of consent, we begin by inquiring into the moral work that consent transactions are meant to perform, bearing in mind the constraints of interpersonal understanding and communication. We must examine what values consent transactions are meant to serve, and how we should adjudicate among possible tensions among those values, and we must then ask what construction of consent transactions fits best with these moral considerations. For reasons that will emerge, I believe that the external approach is more likely to yield a satisfactory account of consent transactions.

In addition to the contrast between the internal and external approach to developing a theory of informed consent, I will contrast two models or conceptions of consent transactions. The internal approach is perhaps best exemplified by what I referred to as the *lock and key/autonomous authorization* model (LK/AA) of consent transactions. The LK/AA model has two components: (1) *the lock and key*—the claim that valid consent is necessary (the lock) and sufficient (the key) for moral transformation; (2) a conception (AA) as to what constitutes valid consent. In principle, LK could be combined with different conceptions of valid consent, but the prevailing theory, best developed by Faden and Beauchamp, is that valid consent should be regarded as equivalent to *autonomous authorization* (AA).[54] In other words, A is permitted to proceed in doing X in response to B's consent token if, and only if, B has autonomously authorized A to do X. Although autonomy is a nebulous concept, the general outlines of AA are quite familiar. On AA, B's consent is valid if and only if B's consent reflects her autonomous will; that is, only if B understands that to which she is consenting and intends to give consent, B's consent is substantially voluntary (i.e., it is free from "controlling influence"), only if B is competent to make such choices, only if B's judgment is not distorted by excessive optimism, and so forth. The main point is that AA emphasizes the *authenticity* of B's choice or what T.M. Scanlon has called the "quality of will."[55]

Although there are several possible alternatives to LK/AA, I will defend what I will call the *fair transaction* model (FT) of consent transactions. Simply put, FT claims that A is permitted to proceed on the basis of a consent transaction if A has treated B fairly and responds in a reasonable manner to B's apparent or actual token of consent. The emphasis on fairness may mislead, because fairness can be both *procedural* and *substantive*. It can refer to the process by which consent is attained and to the terms of the transaction. For present purposes, FT focuses on the procedural dimension of a transaction, although it is an open question as to whether this distinction can be sustained.

It is important to forestall another possible misunderstanding of FT. It might be thought that LK/AA represents the best *ideal* conception of informed consent, but that LK/AA is simply impractical in clinical research, and we should therefore adopt some weaker non-ideal version of informed consent so as not to jeopardize the research enterprise. That is *not* my view. I believe that FT is a superior *moral* conception of consent transactions, in part because LK/AA presumes an excessively narrow conception of the values at stake.

First, a morally defensible theory of consent transactions needs to account for the interests of consenters in both their well-being and their autonomy, and this includes their interest in being able to generate a moral transformation when their consent is less than fully autonomous. There is both a negative and positive dimension of autonomy itself. The *negative* dimension of a person's autonomy encompasses an agent's interest in *not* undergoing interventions or *not* acquiring commitments unless such interventions are the result of her autonomous choice. The *positive* dimension of a person's autonomy refers to her interest in being able to facilitate interactions with others in order to bring about a desired result. The LK/AA model tends to focus on the negative dimension of autonomy. The FT model is sensitive to both dimensions.

Second, consent transactions are bilateral. A morally defensible theory of consent transactions also needs to account for the interests of those who solicit and receive consent (and society at large) in having clear, practicable, and fair standards by which recipients can determine when they are entitled to proceed with cooperative or transactional activities. The LK/AA model is silent on this matter. The FT model provides a more complete account.

My Plan

In an effort to widen the angle of vision, I will consider informed consent to participate in research as one species of the more general category of consent transactions. A relatively complete theory of consent transactions should elucidate a number of related elements. I will first examine the *logic* of consent transactions. Here I will describe the ways in which consent is *morally transformative*. Given my purposes, I will emphasize one form of moral transformation: B's consent renders it permissible for A to do X when, as a rule, it would be impermissible for A to do X without B's consent. I will then examine the *values* that underlie consent transactions. I will argue that consent transactions serve to protect and promote the consenter's well-being (or interests) as well as autonomy, or, put slightly differently, that autonomy has instrumental as well as intrinsic value. I will also argue that consent transactions serve both to protect the agent's negative autonomy or control over herself and, quite crucially, to serve her positive autonomy by facilitating mutually beneficial and altruistic interactions with others. I then consider the *ontology* of consent. Is consent a *mental state,* an *action* (or performative), or a hybrid of these components? If consent has a behavioral component, what constitutes a token of consent? I then turn to the *criteria of moral transformation* (CMT). When is a consent transaction morally transformative? When does a consent transaction between A and B render it permissible for A to proceed?

Before considering the CMT for research, I pause to examine the way in which CMT seem to operate in a range of contexts, such as sexual consent, commercial consent, employment, and the like. I will argue that CMT for one context may be importantly different from CMT for other contexts, or, perhaps more accurately, that a given criterion such as fairness will have different implications when applied in different contexts. To be fair to one's opponents in golf is to penalize oneself for unobserved infractions (such as inadvertently moving the ball). By contrast, although it would be unfair if a basketball team tried to take advantage of a referee's confusion and pretend that its best foul shooter was fouled (or at least I think people would regard this as unfair), many do not regard it as unfair when basketball players feign being knocked down. Whereas fairness in business negotiation allows for considerable deception, this may not be true in recruiting research subjects. Based on this review of various consent contexts I argue that the CMT are better accounted for by FT than LK/AA. Finally, and to explore the practical punch of this theoretical analysis, I examine four issues. Can subjects give morally transformative consent if they are in the grip of a *therapeutic misconception* (TM)? Can subjects give morally transformative consent under unfair background conditions where they face a severely restricted range of options? Can subjects give morally transformative consent if they have been deceived? Can subjects give morally transformative consent if they are exploited?

A plea for patience. Some readers may be frustrated with my approach because I devote considerable space to other contexts of consent. I believe that the circuitous route will pay interest (we can quarrel about the rate). Indeed, if I am correct that a sound theory of informed consent in research must be consistent with a sound general theory of consent, we can't arrive at a sound understanding of informed consent to participate in research by attempting to go there directly.

The Logic of Consent Transactions

The purpose of consent is to produce moral transformation in our interactions with others: "Consent . . . is an act in which one person alters the normative relations in which others stand with respect to what they may do."[56] There are several different kinds of transformations. B's consent may give A permission to do X if it would otherwise be wrong for A to do X.[57] In some contexts, we may say that B's consent authorizes A to do X. In still other contexts, B's consent may constitute a promise, as when B consents to review a manuscript or pay a fee to A in exchange for A's services or goods, or when one agrees to abide by the rules of an organization. In addition, B's consent may transfer ownership of some resource to another person.

In the present context, the principal moral transformation of consent transactions is to render it morally permissible for the researcher to proceed— to administer experimental interventions and conduct research procedures that would otherwise be impermissible for the researcher to perform. Although consent to participate in research could conceivably also involve a morally binding promise to remain in a protocol, the reigning view is that participants have an inalienable right to withdraw at any time and so the obligation-creating dimension of consent appears to be inoperative.

Now the phrase "permissible to proceed" can be understood in at least three different ways: (1) it is *morally* permissible for A to proceed; (2) it *should* be *legally* or *institutionally* permissible for A to proceed; (3) as a matter of positive law or institutional rules, it *is* permissible for A. Thus, as a matter of positive law (3), it is not a crime in any state for A to have sexual relations with B if A deceives B about A's marital intentions before B tokens consent. At the same time, it may not be morally permissible (1) for A to take advantage of B's deception-induced consent. There is also an important distinction between (1) and (2). Given that the criminal law is a blunt instrument, it is arguable that even if it is not morally permissible (1) for A to take advantage of consent produced by his own deception about his marital intentions, it should not be a *crime* for A to do so.

Second, to say that B's consent to A's doing X renders A's doing X morally permissible is a *limited* form of moral transformation. It is to say, among other things, that A does not violate B's rights if A does X. It might also entail that third parties are not entitled to interfere with A's doing X to B. At the same time, to say that B's consent renders it *permissible* for A to do X does not imply a positive moral assessment of A's action. For example, it may be permissible for A to perform breast enlargement surgery on B if B gives morally transformative consent, but it does not follow that it is good for A to do so. In addition, B's consent may render A's action morally permissible with respect to B's rights, but it may not render it morally permissible, *tout court*. It may be morally impermissible for A to have sex with prostitute B even if B gives robust consent. Nonetheless, B's consent is morally transformative because it negates *one* reason for regarding A's action as morally impermissible. A does not violate B's rights. Whatever else we think, A has not raped B.

The Value of Consent Transactions

Consent is a mechanism or process—not a value. Roughly speaking, consent serves two primary values: (1) autonomy or self-determination or respect for persons and (2) well-being. Although bioethicists tend to see the value of consent in terms of autonomy and respect for persons, the Nuremberg Code's insistence on the primacy of consent was primarily designed to protect subjects from harm and not to protect something as abstract as autonomy. Buchanan and Brock state that there are two different reasons why people have an interest in "making significant decisions about their lives for themselves."[58] First, self-determination "is instrumentally valuable in promoting a person's well-being," particularly if we assume that a person's well-being at least partly depends on "the particular aims and values of that person." In addition, people want to make decisions for themselves and the simple satisfaction of this desire is also a component of their well-being apart from the intrinsic value (considered below) of making decisions for oneself.[59]

Second, consent transactions serve the non-instrumental values of self-determination, respect for autonomy, or rights. We generally believe that we have some reason to respect a person's decisions, even when doing so does not advance her well-being or interests. Thus we may respect an adult Jehovah's Witness's refusal of a life-saving blood transfusion.

As the previous example illustrates, the two values served by consent sometimes conflict. Although I do not attempt to determine how that tension should be resolved, I think the degree of that tension is sometimes overstated.

If people consistently made choices that did not advance their interests, it is hard to imagine that we would come to value what we call their autonomy or their right to make such decisions. It cannot be entirely coincidental that the very conditions that are thought to render an agent less than fully autonomous—coercion, deception, incompetence—are also conditions that reduce the likelihood that her decisions advance her well-being. Bad choices are (non-dispositive) evidence of non-autonomous decision-making. If an infirm widow were to sign a contract to sell a $100,000 farm for $10,000, we would not say, "Ah, this doesn't advance her interests, but we need to respect her autonomous choice." Rather, we would say, "This wasn't an autonomous choice; she didn't know what she was doing."

As I noted above, the moral transformative power of consent transactions serves both autonomy and well-being through a *protective* or negative function and a *facilitative* or positive function. Jeremy Waldron puts it this way:

> Why does my consent make it permissible for someone to do
> something to me that would otherwise be impermissible? The
> reason lies first in our need for control over what happens to us, as
> part of our general interest in controlling the course of our lives;
> and second, in the fact that as social beings we can help, assist,
> and enjoy one another in various ways. Giving individuals the
> power of consensual legitimation helps to reconcile these two
> important elements—our individual need for control and the
> desirability of our interactions with others.[60]

If our legal and social practices did not allow us to render it permissible for others to act in ways that would otherwise be impermissible, then our ability to advance our well-being and aims would be seriously compromised. In addition, having the capacity to effect a moral transformation is as central to one's capacity for self-determination as one's ability to block another's actions. For example, respecting a person's autonomy requires that she has the power to bind herself or to acquire an obligation, for if she cannot bind herself to perform some act (for example, pay a debt), then she cannot achieve the control of her life that she desires, in part because others will not cooperate with her to her advantage unless she can undertake a commitment to them and we fail to treat her as a responsible agent.

Even if we focus on the value of autonomy, it is not clear what we should do when an agent's decision is less than robustly autonomous or rational, say, because the subject is not fully informed or competent. To overemphasize the negative or protective function of consent by not allowing a person to enter into transactions unless her consent is robustly autonomous or authentic is, in effect, to compromise the facilitative function of consent transactions by disabling her from entering into transactions and relationships that she seeks and that may promote her well-being.

Consider a moderately competent elderly patient with a fatal disease who has not completed an advance directive. Should we honor her request that medical interventions be withdrawn? We can make two different sorts of errors: (1) We could erroneously allow her to consent to the withdrawal of life-sustaining interventions when doing so does not advance her interests or aims because her decision-making is less than fully autonomous; (2) we could erroneously refuse to treat her consent as transformative on the grounds that her decision-making is less than fully autonomous when allowing her to authorize withdrawal of intervention actually advances her interests or aims and represents an important exercise of her limited capacities. We cannot simultaneously minimize both types of errors and it is not clear how to strike the right balance.

In some contexts, the positive dimension of autonomy looms large. Consider sexual relations. It is, of course, of great moral importance that people be protected from sexual relations to which they do not consent. But as the ugly story of prohibitions on homosexual sexual relations makes clear, it is of importance that people be able to render it permissible for others to have sexual relations with them. Because the focus of research ethics has been with the *protection* of subjects *from* participation in research, its discourse on consent has focused on the negative or protective dimension of autonomy. For example, there is great concern that a subject's decision not be distorted by financial incentives. By contrast, there is much less concern to insure that subjects not be denied the opportunity to receive the medical benefits of participation or financial payment or, for that matter, to participate in research for altruistic reasons. The emphasis may be right, but its rightness cannot be defended simply by appeal to the value of negative autonomy. An adequate theory of consent must attend to both dimensions of autonomy.

The Ontology of Consent

There are two principal questions that we can ask about consent transactions: (1) Does B consent (at all)? (2) Does B give morally transformative consent?

The first (1), is a question about the ontology or fact of consent; (2) is a moral question. Roughly speaking, there are three principal accounts of what we might call the "ontology" or fact of consent. A *subjective* view argues that consent is a psychological phenomenon: B consents if and only if she has the relevant mental state. A behavioral view defines consent in terms of observable behavior: B consents if and only if she tokens or expresses consent in an appropriate way. A hybrid view maintains that the appropriate mental state and the appropriate behavior are both requirements of factual consent.

As with most moral issues, an appeal to ordinary language is of little help. The issue is not what consent "means" but which understanding of the ontology of consent explains how a consent transaction between B and A could render it permissible for A to do what would otherwise be wrong for A to do. From this perspective, most (but not all) scholars reject the pure subjective view. As John Kleinig puts it, "Consent is *an act* in which one person alters the normative relations in which others stand with respect to what they may do"[61] (emphasis added). A. John Simmons acknowledges that there are senses of the word "consent" that signify a (subjective) attitude of approval, but argues that this sense of consent is irrelevant to the sort of consent that generates an obligation or renders another's action permissible.[62] That requires behavior. After all, if we ask what could change the moral status of *A's* action, it is hard to see how B's mental state—by itself—can do the job. Although secret consent would be perfectly possible on a subjective view of consent, it would be odd to think that it was morally permissible for a physician to proceed because the patient consented to the surgery, but didn't tell anyone.

The pure subjective view has been endorsed by some scholars, and seems to have been at least partially incorporated in many statutes on sexual relations.[63] Heidi Hurd argues that "if autonomy resides in the ability to will the alteration of moral rights and duties, and if consent is normatively significant precisely because it constitutes an expression of autonomy," then consent must constitute the "exercise of the will." Hurd concedes that there may well be *prudential* reasons for the law to require observable behavior" that provides evidence of B's mental state before according a defender a legal defense of consent. Nonetheless, she insists that observable behavior is *morally* irrelevant—"as a moral matter, a person *can* consent to another's actions without manifesting her consent in any manner whatsoever."[64] I disagree. If the moral point of consent is to render it permissible for A to proceed, it is of the utmost *moral* relevance—not just legal or prudential relevance—whether B has *given* A reason to think that B wants or is willing

for him to proceed. I readily grant that tokens of consent are morally significant precisely because they are generally reliable *indicators* of the consenter's desires, intentions, choices, and the like. But if the point of consent is to
actually alter one's normative relations with others, then some observable
indication of one's will is required.

Assuming that morally transformative consent requires some behavioral
component, it is not clear what sort of behavior is required. To some extent,
this is largely conventional. B's behavior is a token of consent if it is so understood (nodding one's head at an auction). Still, there is considerable room for
disagreement. Does one consent to obey the law by not leaving one's country (as Socrates says) or traveling freely on the highway (as Locke suggests)?
I doubt it. Does one consent to pay the bill for one's meal simply by ordering? I think so. Does one consent to sex by silently not resisting (if one
smiles)? I think so. By inviting someone up for coffee? No, although it may be
an indicator that one is likely to subsequently consent. Does one agree not to
bring outside food into the movie theatre when one buys a ticket (in full view
of the "no outside food" sign)? I think so, but many disagree.

There may be situations where B does not intend or believe that her
behavior constitutes a token of consent but where others reasonably believe
that it does.

> *Department Meeting.* A, a department chair, says: "I'm going to
> appoint C to our new position unless anyone objects."
> B is daydreaming, and says nothing. A assumes that B has
> authorized him to appoint C.

I do not think that B has tokened consent in this case, although it could be
argued that she has. Either way, we can still ask whether the consent process
is morally transformative. Whether or not one says that B has consented, it is
plausible to think that B's silence renders it permissible for A to proceed in
Department Meeting. Why? Because B is responsible for his inattention and it
may be unreasonable to expect A to determine the reason for B's silence.
This is not a genuine case of tacit consent, where the parties understand and
intend that silence constitutes consent. But it does illustrate an important
point, namely, that a consent *transaction* can be morally transformative without valid consent.

Consent is content specific. If B consents to A's doing X, it seems that
B must consent to A's doing X as opposed to some other action that A might
perform.

> *Lawn Blower.* A asks B whether he can borrow B's lawn blower.
> B mistakenly thinks that A has asked to borrow his lawn
> mower. B says "Sure, it's in my garage; help yourself when
> you need it."

In *Lawn Blower*, B understands that she is consenting to allow A to borrow something (as opposed, say, to being kissed). Given these sorts of mistakes and misunderstandings, it will sometimes be questionable as to what B consented. Linguistic intuitions go both ways. B might say: (1) "I didn't realize I was agreeing to let you take the lawn blower, but I guess I did." Or (2) "I didn't agree to let you take the lawn blower, but, given the misunderstanding, you didn't do anything wrong." In my view, the important moral question is not whether (1) or (2) is linguistically more felicitous, but whether A acts wrongly or is justified in proceeding. This is an irreducibly normative question, not a question about the concept of consent. And it is a question that is better answered by FT than LK/AA. For on LK/AA, it would seem that if B did not consent to A's borrowing his lawn blower, then A has acted wrongly in taking B's lawn blower without permission, although A might be excused for such wrongdoing. That is an upshot that I reject.

Criteria of Moral Transformation

In most contexts, we assume that "no means no." Period. If a person refuses to token consent to an intervention that is rendered permissible only with (valid) consent, then the other party is not entitled to proceed whether or not the refusal to consent is non-autonomous. We would never say, "B was drunk when she refused to have sex with A, and so we should regard her "no" as a transformative "yes." I do not deny that it is sometimes permissible for A to *disregard* B's no, as when we justifiably intervene on paternalistic grounds in the face of an agent's refusal. But that is not because we treat her refusal as transformative. By contrast, and much more commonly, we do not always assume that "yes means yes." We might well say, "B was drunk when she agreed to have sex with A, and so A should disregard B's yes." And so assuming that B unambiguously tokens consent, we must still determine if B's token of consent is morally transformative.

The distinction between a consent token and morally transformative consent can be put in different ways. Peter Westen distinguishes between "descriptive consent" and "prescriptive consent."[65] In bioethics, the distinction between (mere) consent (or a token of consent) and "valid consent" has become the coin of the realm. But however the distinction is put, the criteria of moral transformation is the site of the most important theoretical action about consent transactions. To see some of the difficulties, consider these cases.

> *Condom.* Elizabeth Wilson was awakened at 3:00 a.m. by Joel Valdez, who was approaching her with a knife. He ordered her to take off his pants. Ms. Wilson, fearing that Valdez would stab her if she resisted and that he would infect her with HIV if she submitted, agreed to submit to sexual intercourse with Valdez if he put on a condom.[66]
>
> *Biopsy.* A mammogram reveals suspicious areas in B's breast. A tells B that he wants to do a biopsy under general anesthesia and, if positive, perform a lumpectomy. B listens, but her anxiety overwhelms her thought processes. A asks her to sign a consent form authorizing both procedures (if necessary). B reads the form, but does not process its content. B thinks that A will only be doing a biopsy. She signs.
>
> *Illiterate Contractor.* A presents B a contract to sign. Because B is embarrassed that he cannot read, he pretends to read the contract and signs.
>
> *Infatuated Patient.* B is infatuated with her psychotherapist, A. She proposes that they have sexual relations. A accepts.
>
> *Sitter.* B is a fourteen-year-old who baby-sits for A's child. B has an enormous adolescent crush on A, who is thirty-four. When A is driving B home one evening, B says "I'm a virgin, but they say older men are better. Would you teach me about sex?"
>
> *Intoxicated Tattoo.* B goes out drinking with his buddies, becomes severely intoxicated and enters A's tattoo parlor. B asks A to put a tattoo on his arm, and signs a consent form.
>
> *Leaky Roof.* B is proposing to buy A's home. B does not ask about the condition of the roof, but A's disclosure form fails to note that the roof leaks. B signs a contract to purchase.
>
> *Single.* A and B meet in a night class, and have several dates. B makes it clear that she refuses to have sex with married men. When asked, A lies and says that he is single.

Sister. A has had a sexual relationship with B's sister. B does not
   know this. A proposes that A and B have sex. B agrees.

Rental Car Speeding. B rents a car from A's company. The fine
   print of the rental contract contains a clause stating that
   vehicles driven in excess of the 75 miles per hour will be
   charged $150 per occurrence and that this will be billed to the
   renter's credit card. A uses a GPS system to track B's driving.
   The system finds that B is driving over 80 miles per hour and
   charges $150 to B's credit card.

Teenage Abortion. B (from *Sitter*) is pregnant. She does not want to
   inform her parents, and goes to an abortion clinic where she
   seeks an abortion and consents to the procedure.

Inhibitions. A and B have dated. B has said that she is not ready
   for sex. Without thinking much about it, B consumes several
   drinks at a party. When A proposes that they have sex, she
   feels much less inhibited than usual and says "there has to be
   a first time."

Trust. A tells B that she needs surgery for breast cancer.
   As A begins to explain the options, B says, "I trust you;
   do whatever you think is best."

Dinner. A invites B to dinner, asking for a firm commitment.
   A does not disclose the other invitees and B does not ask.
   B accepts.

B tokens consent in all of these cases, but B has certainly not given morally transformative or valid consent in all of them. In some cases, such as
Condom or *Leaky Roof,* it is clear that B has clearly not given morally transformative consent. People may disagree about other cases, such as *Single.*
Some cases illustrate the distinction between claiming that A is *morally* permitted to proceed and claiming that *it should be legal* for A to proceed. We
might think that it should be legally permissible for A to proceed in *Single,* or
Inhibitions, or *Sister,* but that A is not *morally* permitted to proceed in these
cases. Interestingly, some might think that B's consent in *Sitter* should not
render it legally permissible for A to have sex with B, but that B's consent in
Teenage Abortion should render it legally permissible for A to perform an
abortion. The puzzle is to explain why this might be so.

These cases illustrate a more general point. Whether we are discussing
sex, contracts, tattoos, abortions, medical care, or participation in research,

the interesting question is not whether B merely tokens consent but whether the consent transaction is morally transformative. Here the contrast between LK/AA and FT has some practical importance. On LK/AA, it would seem that A is *not* permitted to proceed (or B may not acquire an obligation) in cases such as *Biopsy, Illiterate Contractor, Sitter, Teenage Abortion, Rental Car Speeding,* and *Dinner.* By contrast, it is an open question as to whether B's consent is morally transformative on FT in these cases. I say open. To say when the transaction is morally transformative on FT requires a more complete theory of fair transactions than I am prepared to offer. I am, however, inclined to think that it is permissible for A to proceed in *Trust* and that B has made a morally binding commitment in *Dinner,* even though neither consent was fully informed. Why? Because B has tokened consent in a context in which A has treated B fairly and because a contrary view would be unfair to A.

Although Faden and Beauchamp endorse AA as an ideal of informed consent, it is not entirely clear whether they endorse LK/AA as a framework for moral transformation.

> It is a separate issue whether this criterion of substantial autonomy should be the only source for distinguishing consents or refusals that are "valid" from those treated as "invalid." There may be compelling policy or moral justification in some contexts for adopting consent requirements that establish a threshold below the level of substantial autonomy, in effect treating *less than substantially* autonomous consents as *valid* or, more precisely, *effective* consents.[67]

Faden and Beauchamp distinguish between what they call sense$_1$ informed consent, which corresponds to AA, and sense$_2$ informed consent, which in a bow to reality represents the consent that we should regard as sufficient to render it permissible for A to proceed.

> By contrast to sense$_1$, sense$_2$, or *effective* consent, is a policy-oriented sense whose conditions are not derivable solely from analyses of autonomy and authorization, or even from broad notions of respect for autonomy. "Informed consent" in this second sense does not refer to *autonomous* authorization, but to a legally or institutionally *effective* (sometimes misleadingly called *valid)* authorization from a patient or a subject. Such an authorization is

"effective" because it has been obtained through procedures that satisfy the rules and requirements defining a specific institutional practice in health care or research.[68]

Faden and Beauchamp say that it is "misleading" to refer to "effective" consent as "valid" consent because they regard "valid consent" as equivalent to AA. Rather, they argue that we can regard non-valid consent as "effective" consent if it has been obtained through certain procedures.

But this does not resolve the question as to whether non-AA consent can be morally transformative "on its own." I think it can be. It's not merely that less than fully autonomous sense$_2$ consent might satisfy "the rules and requirements defining a specific institutional practice." After all, those rules and requirements might treat consent as morally transformative when they should not. Rather, if we reject LK/AA and adopt FT, we can see how it may be morally justifiable for A to proceed in the absence of valid consent, rules and regulations to the side.

In a recent essay, Beauchamp has slightly revised his view. He does not back away from the emphasis on autonomy, but he argues that we need to be flexible as to what counts as autonomous authorization. He says that any theory that "declares *nonautonomous* the acts of average persons in opening a bank account, writing a will, selling a house, or refusing an offered surgical procedure . . . is unacceptable." It is true that autonomy is a "range concept," that one's decisions can be more or less autonomous and that we need to draw a line somewhere in saying that a decision is properly characterized as autonomous. And it is possible that most cases in which people open a bank account or write a will or sell a house actually do qualify as falling within the range that deserves to be called autonomous. Still, we shouldn't fudge with our account of autonomy in order to reach the desired conclusion about the transaction. Rather than treat some marginally autonomous consent as sufficiently autonomous to generate a moral transformation, it is better to argue that it may be morally transformative even though it may fall short on grounds of autonomous authorization.

Beauchamp also worries that if we "declare such choices nonautonomous," we wrongly imply that "another person may legitimately serve as guardian and decision maker" and thus "a will could be invalidated or a surgical procedure authorized against the person's wishes."[69] This is not a serious cause for worry. First, there are some cases in which a person's wishes *should* be overridden for paternalistic reasons (see Chapter 2). Second, to declare B's choice to be nonautonomous does *not* automatically entail that someone *else* may legitimately serve as a surrogate decision-maker. For even if B's choices are less than sufficiently autonomous, she may be better positioned than anyone else to make such decisions.

Although I believe that we should ultimately reject LK/AA and adopt FT, I need to more fully explain why we should do so. Once again, it will prove useful to step back and broaden our perspective. When we look at non-medical contexts of consent transactions, we often find that the law and prevalent moral beliefs requires nothing approximating AA as necessary for moral transformation. Of course, existing laws and prevalent moral beliefs may not reflect the best moral view. Nonetheless, it will prove useful to examine the way in which our views of the criteria vary from context to context. In some contexts, AA and FT will be close to extensionally equivalent. In other contexts, they will have rather different implications.

Consent to Sexual Relations

Unlike consent to participate in research, where we typically require written tokens of consent, one can token consent to sexual relations verbally or by one's behavior. Although the (in)famous Antioch College Code required that one receive explicit verbal consent to every new level of sexual contact ("May I kiss you?"), few would deny that B has tokened consent to sex if A says, "Would you like to go into my bedroom," and B says nothing, but smiles, follows A, takes off her clothes, and responds positively to A's advances.

Assuming a clear token of consent, there is still the question as to when B's token of consent renders it permissible for A to proceed. There is no lack of clarity as to whether B tokens consent in *Sitter, Sister,* or *Infatuated Patient.* The question is whether B's consent is morally transformative. The standard view is that morally transformative consent must be voluntary, informed, and competent. This is fine as far as it goes, but each of these general criteria must be interpreted. B is clearly coerced if she has been subject to the use or threat of physical force, as in *Condom.* It is another question as to what forms of non-violent pressure count as coercion or compromising voluntariness, as when A says "If you don't agree to sex, I'll stop dating you."

As a matter of social convention, the informational requirements for morally transformative consent to sex are not particularly high. Not only do we not require the positive disclosure of information in sexual relationships (save for sexual diseases), we have generally been quite permissive with respect to some forms of deception. The *law* would not charge A with a sexual offense in *Single* or *Sister*, although we might think that it is not permissible for A to proceed because B's consent was based on deception in *Single* or a failure to disclose information that would be relevant to B's decision in *Sister*. We might think A is sleazy if he falsely tells B that he loves her, but we would hardly claim that A was not permitted to proceed simply because B is in the grips of a "romantic misconception." Indeed, sexual relations is a context in which people may expect and even desire some deception. Our criteria of moral transformation reflect this.

With respect to competence, we allow people to have sex at younger ages than we allow them to sign contracts or purchase alcohol. We also allow people to grant permission to others to have sex with them after they have become quite intoxicated, as in *Inhibitions*, although many states do not allow people to get a tattoo under similar circumstances. We treat the patient's consent in *Infatuated Patient* as non-transformative because the process of psychotherapy often distorts a patient's judgment and a sexual relationship is likely to be harmful in ways that she may not anticipate. Consent by the mentally retarded illustrates the tension between the negative and positive dimensions of consent. We could protect the negative autonomy of the mentally retarded from sexual predators by claiming that they are simply not capable of giving valid consent to sexual relations, but doing so would come at the price of compromising their positive autonomy, by disabling them from an important dimension of human life.

Commerce

Consent in the commercial context ranges over a wide range of activities, and there is no univocal standard as to what counts as giving the sort of consent that results in a valid or enforceable agreement. Many commercial transactions require a token in writing, but one can agree to pay for a meal simply by ordering it (even if one is not told the price), and one can authorize an auto repair ("you need a new transmission") or the sale of stocks over the phone. We no longer endorse *caveat emptor*. But with the exception of some products, such as drugs, alcohol, and cigarettes, or the sale of a house, there is no assumption that a seller must provide a prospective purchaser with information about the risks or defects of a product. Think bicycle, baseball bats, and soccer balls.

With respect to voluntariness, note that contracts can be regarded as valid or binding even when made in the face of considerable pressure or very hard bargaining. The Godfather's offer to the bandleader who hired Johnny Fontaine ("either your brains or your signature will be on the contract") would invalidate a contract on grounds of duress (if the bandleader were ever in a position to seek a remedy), but if McDonald's threatens one of its suppliers to take its business elsewhere unless the supplier agrees to a reduction in price, the supplier's agreement would probably be regarded as valid. For unlike Don Corleone, McDonald's does not propose to violate the supplier's rights if the supplier refuses, and a contract is ordinarily voidable on grounds of duress only if A proposes to violate B's rights if B does not acquiesce.[70]

What about misunderstandings? If B believes he is agreeing to X (say, teach 3 courses per year), whereas he signs an agreement to do Y (say, teach 4 courses per year), the law does *not* rely on a version of *LK/AA*. It does not say, "B is not bound by the contract because he was mistaken about the terms of the agreement." The law will make a judgment as to who should bear the liability for the mistake. If B had a fair opportunity to understand the terms of the agreement, the law may side with A. On the other hand, if A was trying to sneak something by B, or if the penalties are regarded as excessive, perhaps as in *Rental Car Speeding,* the law might side with B.

Gambling

Gambling is an interesting analogue to participation in research because it may involve considerable risks. The person who makes a wager is, in effect, consenting to allow the other party to keep his money if he loses. When is such consent transformative as a matter of law? Almost always. There are few if any legal requirements with respect to disclosure of information. Race tracks do not openly announce that they return only $.82 on every dollar bet. Casinos do not announce the "house take" on slot machines or the roulette wheel. States do not openly disclose that the "expected value" of a lottery ticket (the proportion of the amount wagered that is returned to the wagerers) is about $.50 for each $1. Instead, they engage in manipulative techniques to get people to participate. And whereas we worry as to whether the therapeutic misconception (TM) compromises the validity of consent to research, we do not worry about those who suffer from the "gambler's fallacy."[71]

With respect to competence, states establish minimal age requirements, but that's about all. Whereas one cannot get a tattoo in many states if one is intoxicated, we allow people to make significant wagers while severely intoxicated and even allow casinos to ply gamblers with "free" drinks that distort their judgment and reduce their inhibitions.

Jobs

We allow people to consent to employment under considerable strain and on the basis of relatively little information about the responsibilities and risks involved. We might think that consent by the employee has little force since they are generally able to opt out of employment at will. Nonetheless, a person's agreement to take a job may shield the employer from (some) complaints and liabilities concerning the terms of employment. Moreover, taking a particular job often involves significant opportunity costs, such as relocation. One cannot typically receive compensation if things work out badly. And even if an employer can be held liable, *ex post*, for some forms of harm to the employee, there is no functional equivalent of an IRB that must prospectively approve the terms or risks of employment or the level of information that must be provided to the employee.

How much understanding is required? I suspect that the specific responsibilities and benefits of employment are often not well understood. More importantly, employers do not typically have an obligation to inform prospective employees of the risks of employment. Some risks are reasonably transparent. People understand that timber cutting, coal mining, and military service (in time of war) are risky, although I suspect that many workers seriously underestimate occupational risks. But some occupational risks are much less transparent. Do 7-11 clerks understand the risks of being victimized by armed robbery? Do pizza deliverers understand the risks of driving? Do (or did) professional football players understand the risks of concussions?[72]

Although people have long been coerced into employment via slavery, involuntary servitude, or military conscription, we do not say that people are coerced into taking jobs because they would otherwise be poor or unemployed. Moreover, whereas many worry as to whether financial incentives compromise the validity of consent to participate in research (see Chapter 4) we obviously have no such worries with respect to ordinary employment. Moreover, and unlike participation in research, we have few objections to paying people additional compensation for taking special risks, as when structural steel workers are paid more than jobs that require similar skills.

Marriage

The decision to marry is one of life's momentous choices, but the standards of morally transformative consent are not particularly high. We do set minimal age standards, but one can give legally valid consent to marry on the basis of relatively little information about the other party and with minimal competence to understand the long term implications of one's decision. It is also worth noting that while (literal) "shot gun marriages" were always regarded as voidable on grounds of duress, we have never worried as to whether financial incentives (such as being supported for life) or the opportunity to have children (with appropriate financial support) compromise the voluntariness of consent to marry.

Gifts and Donations

Given that participation in research is at least sometimes motivated by altruism, note that we allow people to give small and large amounts of their resources to *charity* on the basis of very little information. Charities are under no positive obligation to disclose the uses to which their money will be put or their efficacy in using its funds. In addition, we make no effort to assess the competence of the donor. We allow people to give away their assets without anything approaching the standards of "autonomous authorization." Moreover, we allow organizations to aggressively solicit donations, to put people "on the spot," and to manipulatively appeal to the emotions of the prospective donors in ways that we would not dream of permitting in the recruitment of research participants.

Medical Care

Here I want to make two simple points and one extended point. First, the explicitness of consent to treatment varies considerably with the nature of the treatment and is premised on the assumption that physicians have a fiduciary obligation to promote the interests of their patients. We do not worry all that much about consent to specific procedures required by ordinary medical care in part because a patient arguably consents to the "package" of treatment and because a patient's explicit informed consent to specific procedures is generally not necessary to protect or advance her interests and aims. Although researchers must frequently seek consent for procedures such as blood draws and lumbar punctures precisely, physicians need not explain the risks and benefits of taking a patient's blood-pressure or the insertion of a device into the vagina.

Interestingly, virtually all of the concern in the literature on informed consent to *treatment* (as opposed to *research*) focuses on information rather than voluntariness. Given the looseness with which some argue that financial incentives can undermine the voluntariness of participation in *research*, it is worth noting that we do *not* regard the much greater pressure exerted by illness itself as undermining the voluntariness of the patient's consent to *treatment*. Surprisingly, Arthur Caplan, a prominent bioethicist, argued that the parents of infants could not give voluntary consent to have their child included in a gene transfer study because parents of dying infants are "coerced by the disease of their child."[73] This is puzzling, given that we would *not* say this with respect to consent to life-saving treatment. If a patient must choose between death and surgery, we do *not* say that she cannot make a voluntary choice because there is only one reasonable option for the patient to choose. Although it is difficult to explain why the prospect of death does not compromise voluntariness on AA, it is relatively easy to explain on FT. On FT, A coerces B to do X only if A proposes to treat B unfairly (or violate B's rights) if B does not do X. Don Corleone's famous "offer that can't be refused" ("Either your brains or your signature will be on the contract") is coercive not because it gives the target only one reasonable alternative but because he proposes to violate the target's rights if he does not acquiesce. By contrast, the surgeon's proposal ("Either surgery or you will die") is not coercive because the surgeon does not propose to violate the patient's right if she refuses.

What Have We Learned?

I am not attempting to derive an ought from an is. Although it is clear that the reigning moral consensus is that consent that falls far short of autonomous authorization is still transformative in many contexts, it is possible that it would be better to apply a strong version of AA throughout. Possible, but not likely. Although the current legal regime may reflect the power of casinos and employers rather than a defensible moral view, I think it improbable that we would want to insist on AA in all of these contexts even after serious moral reflection. If we adopt AA as our model, the standards for valid consent could not vary (quite) so much. Whether one were authorizing the repair of one's car or selling land to a developer or agreeing to a "one night stand," we would insist that consent is morally transformative only if the consenter has the competence and requisite understanding to make the relevant decision. But if we are right to adopt the external approach to the specification of the criteria of moral transformation as dependent upon context, we are likely to adopt something like FT, in which case we may demand something close to AA in some contexts, but not in others.

When one surveys the range of consent contexts, it is clear that there is considerable variation as to what counts as tokening consent. It is doubtful that we would want to require written consent to sexual relations or to many ordinary commercial activities, for example, buying and selling groceries, ordering a meal, or taking a taxi. Whatever advantages greater explicitness might yield would clearly be outweighed by the consequent changes in the nature of the activity and the increased costs—to all—in consummating transactions. We have also observed very different standards with respect to information, ranging from contexts in which non-disclosure or even deception is somewhat permissible to those in which there is a positive obligation to disclose.

What would justify such variability in the criteria for moral transformation? The answer lies in the values that consent transactions serve. As we have argued, we are not interested in consent for its own sake. We want to be able to give or withhold consent when doing so protects our interests and values or allows us to advance our interests and aims. If we were to think about the criteria that we would hypothetically choose *ex ante* in an original position, I suspect that we would prefer that some things not happen to us without our contemporary autonomous authorization (as in *Infatuated Patient*), but we might also prefer that we can make other things happen when our decision making is less than fully or substantially autonomous (as in *Trust* or *Inhibitions*). FT can be sensitive to such differences while reflecting a stable ethical principle; AA does not have the resources to allow such variability.

Informed Consent, The Lock and Key Model and the Criteria of Moral Transformation

I have suggested that the specification of CMT for a given context is the output of moral reasoning and cannot be "read off" of a conceptual or linguistic analysis of consent. We always have to ask: what do we *want* from consent in a given context, given the values served by the possibility of morally transformative transactions? From that perspective, there are several reasons to think that LK/AA should be rejected as a general model of moral transformation, although we may want to approximate its demands in some contexts. First, any acceptable moral principle must be responsive to the basic facts about human beings and social life. Our competence, information, and knowledge are always imperfect. And we often find ourselves under considerable strain. Second, we are and should be sensitive to the costs in time, energy, and resources in obtaining something like AA consent. We don't want our doctors to spend their time or ours explaining very low risk procedures before gaining our consent. We want some transformations to be quick, easy, and cheap even at some risk that we will make a choice that we will regret. Third, to the extent that we value consent because it advances the consenter's well-being and self-determination, we may want the consenter to be able to trigger transformations even when her decision is less than fully autonomous. Fourth, we don't want our concern to assure autonomous authorization to undermine the object of choice. To insist on informational disclosure and written consent for sexual relations would thoroughly distort the activity to which consent is being given. Fifth, CMT must always balance the costs of wrongly precluding a moral transformation against the costs of wrongly permitting a moral transformation. In some cases, it is reasonable not to worry excessively that we may wrongly preclude a moral transformation. If we do not allow a fourteen year old to authorize sex with a 30-year-old male, they may lose an opportunity for a pleasurable experience, but no great harm has been done. By contrast, the costs of wrongly permitting such a transformation can be grave. On the other hand, there are contexts in which a decision *not* to allow someone to engage in morally transformative consent can be a very serious matter indeed. Permitting consensual assisted suicide or active euthanasia risks ending the lives of people when their choices, driven by suffering or despair, are not fully autonomous. But prohibiting these practices risks condemning people to live with intolerable suffering when they choose to end their lives. Fifth, the criteria of moral transformation must also reflect a comparative judgment about the competence of potential decision-makers. Someone has to make a decision. Before we decide not to recognize B's consent as morally transformative, we need to conclude that someone else is better positioned to consent or to refuse to consent on B's behalf or be satisfied with the default position in which no transformation occurs.

An additional reason to reject the demand for contemporaneous autonomous authorization concerns the acquisition of information. A prospective consenter may have an interest in foregoing information or the effort to understand that information even though it is relevant to the decision at hand. The acquisition and understanding of information is costly in terms of time, mental energy, psychic stress, and money. It is not irrational for a woman who wants to have an abortion not to want to know any details about the status of the fetus or to see a sonogram or for a traveler not to want to read the details of the rental car contract. Moreover, if, as in many cases of medical research, a prospective subject can have confidence that participation does not involve significant risks or has the prospect of direct medical benefit, then it is perfectly rational—from *her* perspective—to think that the benefits from further information and comprehension do not justify the costs of acquiring and processing that information.[74]

As a general principle, the criteria of moral transformation must accommodate the tension between the consenter's interest in being protected from the consequences of her "moderately autonomous" consent and her interest in having her "moderately autonomous" consent be treated as morally transformative. Consider cases in which women become voluntarily intoxicated and subsequently token consent to sexual relations. (I am *not* referring to cases in which a woman is unconscious). Some people want to engage in drunken sex and would prefer, *ex ante*, a regime in which their intoxicated consent is transformative, even though they realize that they may, on occasion, regret their actions *ex post*. Others might benefit from and prefer a regime in which their intoxicated consent is not regarded as transformative, even though this regime may deny them opportunities they would have enjoyed. Given these differences, it's not clear whether we should regard such consent as transformative. The best approach may depend, in part, on the proportion of people in each group and the magnitude of the regret as compared with the magnitude of the foregone benefit.[75]

Or consider consent that is allegedly given under desperate circumstances such as poverty. Although we may think that we are offering agents *more* protection when we refuse to treat their consent as transformative, we may effectively prohibit them from moving from a very bad state of affairs to a less (but still) bad state of affairs, and this is inconsistent with a fundamental values that consent is meant to serve; namely, to allow people to advance their well-being.

Note that the present point does *not* concern the balance between society's interest and the interest of individuals. It is true that we must balance the interest of society (and future patients) in the research enterprise against the prospective subject's interest in being protected by rigorous standards for morally transformative consent. My present point is that when we evaluate the criteria of moral transformation from the prospective consenter's *own* perspective, we see that LK/AA does not represent a compelling moral vision.

Diachronic Authorization and Hierarchical Preferences

Advocates of LK/AA might respond to these concerns by modifying AA along two related lines. First, it might be claimed that AA does not require *contemporary* autonomous authorization if there is a prior autonomous authorization for a subsequent non-autonomous authorization, as when B, who is seeking an abortion, decides at Time-1 that she does not want full information about the status of the fetus at Time-2. Such cases strike me as relatively unproblematic even on LK/AA, although some defenders of LK/AA might insist that one should not be able to waive one's right to make an autonomous decision at Time-2.

Second, AA might be construed as encompassing second-order or higher preferences rather than first-order or lower preferences. Along lines developed by Harry Frankfurt, ". . . autonomy is conceived of as a second-order capacity of persons to reflect critically upon their first-order preferences, desires, wishes, and so forth and the capacity to accept or attempt to change these in light of higher-order preferences and values."[76] And so a drug addict's decision to consume a drug is not autonomous even if it is informed, rational (under the circumstances), and uncoerced, if she has a higher-order preference not to consume drugs. By the same token, consent that appears not to be autonomous because the agent lacks sufficient understanding could be considered autonomous in so far as it is consistent with her second-order reflective preferences about her desire for information as in *Trust*.

I do not think this move is likely to save AA. I am doubtful that most cases of arguably non-autonomous consent that we are inclined to regard as morally transformative are consistent with articulated reflective, second-order preferences. More importantly, this approach poses serious practical difficulties. As a bilateral transaction that morally transforms the relationship between B and A, it is vital that A, who receives consent, is in a position to assess whether B's consent renders it permissible for him to proceed. As a general matter, how is A to know that B's consent token is consistent with her (dispositional) second-order preferences? In some cases, this can be done. In *Trust*, the doctor might ask the patient whether she is sure that she is not interested in understanding the risks and benefits of surgery as contrasted with the alternatives. If the patient indicates that she does not want additional information, we do not have a second-order preference. We have a specific autonomous waiver. By contrast, in *Biopsy*, the patient is giving signs of adequate understanding and an intention to authorize the lumpectomy if indicated, though she has not autonomously authorized this procedure. Although the consent token may not be consistent with the patient's second-order preferences, it is difficult to see why the doctor is not entitled to proceed.

The Fair Transaction View

The fair transaction view states that B's consent token is morally transformative if B tokens consent or appears to token consent under conditions in which A has acted fairly towards B in obtaining B's consent. The emphasis here is on the process by which A obtains B's consent and not (necessarily) the terms of the agreement between A and B or the fairness of A's behavior towards B, *tout court*. The transformative power of B's consent (or behavior) is a function of the *circumstances* under which B chooses (including the behavior of A) rather than the specific mental states that characterize or motivate B's choice. Although FT acknowledges that minimal comprehension and intention are necessary for *valid* consent, FT rejects the LK linkage between valid consent and moral transformation.

The FT model is closely related to what might be called the *fair opportunity* view of moral transformation (FO). Fair opportunity maintains that B's consent is morally transformative if B has had a fair *opportunity* to make an informed and competent choice whether or not B's choice is fully competent or informed. But FT and FO are not identical. On FT, a consent transaction may be morally transformative if A has acted fairly towards B even if B's background circumstances are such that B does *not* have a fair opportunity not to consent. The FT model's conception of fairness is *bilateral* or *transaction specific*, whereas FO's conception of fairness may be global. It remains an open question as to what it means for A to act fairly towards

B within a transaction. That will depend upon the context and a more fully developed theory of fairness in transactions. After all, whereas hard bargaining between business negotiators may not be unfair, hard bargaining between a physician and a patient or between an investigator and a prospective subject is another matter altogether. It is a virtue of FT that it can give different answers in different contexts.

One advantage of the fair transaction approach is that it offers a theoretically attractive *unifying* account of the various criteria of morally transformative consent that are central to AA—voluntariness, information, and competence—that is consistent with our intuitions about moral transformation across a range of contexts and which does not involve the difficulties associated with LK/AA. If A threatens to harm B unless B agrees to some transaction or interaction, then A has obviously not acted fairly towards B and thus B's consent token would not be morally transformative. As a general rule, it is unfair for A to deceive B and such deception would render non-transformative. And thus the researcher's deception about the injection of live cancer cells in The Jewish Chronic Disease Hospital case would render the subjects' consent non-transformative on both FT and AA.[77] Interestingly, however, there are some cases in which consent is morally transformative in the face of deception, and one advantage of FT over LK/AA is that it can explain why that is so. If A and B are negotiating the sale of a home, and A falsely states that he will not pay more than $400,000 (he would actually pay $425,000), then B's consent to sell at $400,000 is morally transformative if, as I suspect, fairness in negotiations does not require that one be truthful about such matters.

There are cases in which fairness requires truthfulness but not a positive disclosure of information. If the information is relatively accessible to all, then it may be more fair to let B decide how much information he wants. By contrast, if the information is deeply asymmetrical, then fairness may require that the more knowledgeable party make the information available to the less knowledgeable party. The seller of a house is under a positive obligation to disclose defects because it is difficult for a buyer to acquire such information. Even if it were possible for the buyer to acquire such information (one can hire an inspector), it may be much cheaper (in the long run for all parties) to assign the burden to the seller. Much the same could be said about the provision of information by researchers. Here too, FT can explain the differences, whereas AA does not have the resources to differentiate between these cases. I should say that I am not operating here with a well-developed theory of fairness. At this point, I am prepared to travel light and appeal to our ordinary intuitions. The present task is to argue that FT provides a defensible and superior framework for determining when consent is morally transformative and not to fill in all the details.

Interestingly, there are contexts of asymmetrical information in which fairness does not require the more knowledgeable party to share his information with the less knowledgeable party. Consider *Painting*.

> *Painting.* A has spent years studying art history and has done
> considerable research on a painting owned by B. A estimates
> that the painting has a market value of $100,000. A offers to
> buy the painting from B for $50,000. B accepts.

If A has made significant investments in acquiring general knowledge about art and particular information about B's painting, then fairness may not require that he share such information with B. After all, if A were morally required to disclose his estimate prior to reaching an agreement, then A would have little incentive to acquire the information in the first place. So, *ex ante*, it is in *B's* interest that A not be under an obligation to disclose information, even though it is in B's interest, *ex post,* that the information be disclosed once A has acquired the information. I am not wedded to a particular answer to whether the transaction in *Painting* is transformative. The point is that FT provides a sensible framework for coming to that answer.

Defects in competence are a bit trickier, but, here too, FT has advantages over LK/AA. There may not be a large gap between LK and FT with respect to permanent deficiencies in competence. The (relatively) permanent noncompetent are not capable of autonomous authorization and A does not act fairly towards B if A takes advantage of B's deficiencies. By contrast, LK/AA and FT may have different implications with respect to temporary and self-inflicted deficiencies in competence. Recall *Inhibitions*. Although it is arguable that AA *must* treat such deficiencies as invalidating consent, the transformative power of B's consent remains an open question on FT, as it should be. On the one hand, it might be thought that it is not unfair for A to take advantage of B's incompetence, given that B has had a fair opportunity to avoid it. On the other hand, it may be unfair for A to take advantage of B's self-inflicted incompetence nonetheless and, if so, B's consent token would not render it morally permissible for A to proceed. I readily concede that FT does not provide a unique view as to whether B's consent is transformative. That requires a more well-developed account of fair transactions than I have supplied (or will supply). But I do not regard that as a defect of the approach, since I believe that it *is* an open question as to what to say in this case and that it would be a mistake to assume that the answer dictated by AA is correct.

As I just noted, a principal virtue of FT is that it explicitly acknowledges that there are at least *two* parties to a consensual transaction, both of which have interests at stake. It is, of course, important that B is able to make a decision that reflects her preferences and aims. But it is also of moral importance that A is able to know whether he can proceed with the transaction or interaction. Fairness is bilateral. It's not just that B must be fair to A, but that *we* must be fair to A in determining whether it is permissible for him to proceed given that we hold A accountable for transacting with B without B's consent or with respect to the costs we impose on A in securing B's consent before allowing A to proceed.

Consider the problem of mistakes again.

> *Rock Star.* B consents to sexual relations with A because she falsely believes A to be a rock star, although A has made no such representation and has no reason to think that this is what motivates B's consent.

Given B's mistake about A's identity, it seems that she has not given valid consent on AA. In my view, it is a virtue of FT that it could go one of two ways. Assuming that A has acted in good faith in relying on B's token of consent, it would be unfair to A to refuse to treat B's consent token as morally transformative. Why should A be saddled with the burden of ascertaining B's beliefs before he can reasonably rely on the permission he has received? On the other hand, if A knows that B consents to sex with him because she confuses him with a rock star, then it is arguably not morally permissible for him to proceed on FT. FT gives us the right answer for the right reason.

I have argued that FT's conception of fairness is bilateral or transaction specific, not global. This perspective enables us to accommodate cases in which B's background conditions or circumstances are unfair or desperate, but where A has acted fairly towards B within the framework of those conditions. Consider "third party coercion." If B can give morally transformative consent to A when she is coerced by C, then it is relatively easy to show that

B can give morally transformative consent when her background conditions are unfair but not the result of coercion.

> *Pimp*. C tells B that he will beat her up unless she earns $500 this
> evening. B proposes to A that they have sexual relations for
> $100. A accepts.

It may be thought that if B is coerced into having sex, then her consent cannot be morally transformative. But that is too quick. B is coerced by C, not A. If A and B live in a jurisdiction in which it is a felony to engage in nonconsensual sexual relations, I think it would be wrong to prosecute A for violating such a statute. It is easy to see why this is so on FT. For whereas C is treating B unfairly in coercing her into having sex for money, it by no means follows that A is treating B unfairly. B is coerced in the "larger moral world" that she occupies. But there is a "smaller moral world" in which the issue is between A and B, and B is not coerced in that world, or, perhaps more accurately, she is not coerced in a way that would render her consent non-transformative vis a vis A.[78]

It might be objected that the transformative power of B's consent turns, in part, on whether A knows (or should believe) that B is coerced by (some) C. It is not that simple. For given B's objective condition—that she will be beaten by C if she does not earn enough—B *wants* A to accept her proposal. Indeed, B may well solicit A. A does B no favor if he says, in effect, "I know you're only doing this because you're coerced. I don't want to rape you." It is possible that, in the long run, B (or others similarly situated) will be better off if A is prohibited from interacting with B because this will give the likes of C less incentive to coerce B. But this strategic justification for prohibiting the transaction would not be based on the view that B's interaction with A was nonconsensual.

How might third party coercion be treated on LK/AA? Faden and Beauchamp do not explicitly consider third party coercion although they imply that any coercion "deprives the person of autonomous choice, and thus is incompatible with informed consent."[79] It is possible that a modified version of *AA* could regard her relationship with C as part of her objective situation and, within that situation, B's decision to have sex with A might be regarded as autonomous. Although AA *could* be reconfigured to accommodate this case, it could do so only under considerable strain. By contrast, it is relatively easy for FT.

If specific third-party coercion (as between C and B) does not necessarily negate the transformative power of B's consent, then, *a fortiori*, the general background unfairness of B's situation does not necessarily undermine the transformative power of B's consent. Consider:

> *Desperate Mother.* B becomes a prostitute because she believes it is the only way she can earn enough to pay for her child's expensive medical care. B solicits A. A accepts.
>
> *Unjust Firing.* C has unjustly fired B from her previous job as a well-paid lawyer. B accepts A's offer to teach business law at the local community college at a much lower salary than she had been receiving.
>
> *Battery.* C has intentionally injured B. B seeks medical care from A and authorizes A to perform a procedure and agrees to pay A's fee.

It is not clear how AA would handle these cases. On FT, B's consent is morally transformative. Because A has acted fairly towards B within the framework of B's background conditions even though those background conditions are unfair. Assuming that A is not taking unfair advantage of B's (unfair) background conditions, it seems unfair to ask A to rectify conditions for which he is not responsible as a basis for a mutually advantageous transaction.

In addition, to regard B's consent as not transformative is unfair to *B.* For if we say that B can give valid morally transformative consent only when her background conditions are "globally" fair, and if we assume that A cannot be expected to rectify those background conditions, then to refuse to treat B's consent as transformative is to deprive B of the opportunity to improve her condition by transacting with A. Indeed, we do well to remember that many normal and unproblematic transactions would not occur were it not for injustice in B's background conditions.

I have argued that FT provides an attractive and comprehensively applicable account of the criteria of moral transformation. As I argued above, on the external approach to a theory of consent, the criteria of morally transformative consent are the output of moral theorizing. We don't start with the principle of consent and ask what it requires. Rather, we ask what we have moral reason to require of consent. On this view, the question as to whether LK/AA or FT or some other view provides the best account of moral transformation will depend upon the question as to what constitutes the best moral theory. Not surprisingly, I hardly have the answer to that question. Nonetheless, I believe that the general outline of FT is attractive on its face, is compatible with our intuitions, and is also consistent with two major non-consequentialist approaches to moral theory which might be used to support a theory of morally transformative consent. Although consistency with these non-consequentialist theories does not constitute a positive argument for FT, I would have less confidence in FT if it were clearly incompatible with a plausible moral theory. I think it is not.

Why *non*-consequentialist? If consequentialism is the right moral view, then the correct view about morally transformative consent is, in principle, an empirical matter: what view of moral transformation has the best consequences? Autonomy would have no independent or intrinsic value, and there would be no deep principles to debate. It is possible but doubtful that consequentialism would lead us to adopt something close to LK/AA given that LK/AA is not sensitive to the wide range of interests a person has in transacting with others and is also not sensitive to the interests of all the parties to the transaction.

If we set consequentialism aside, we can first note that FT is consistent with a deontological commitment to respect for persons. We often show respect by refusing to hold persons accountable for choices that they did not have a fair opportunity to avoid, but we also show respect for them— *including their choice to decide carelessly or imprudently*—when we honor those choices that they make under reasonably favorable conditions and, I would add, under desperate or unfair conditions that are not caused by the party with whom they are transacting. It might be thought that a Kantian version of a deontological approach would require autonomous authorization for moral transformation. I disagree. First, and however NMMP is unpacked, it is arguable that A does *not* treat B merely as a means when he acts fairly towards B, and responds to what he—in good faith—regards as B's autonomous consent, even when he is mistaken about this. Recall *lawn blower*. It seems that A does not treat B merely as a means to gaining use of B's lawn blower in this case even if B has not given AA consent. Second, a Kantian commitment to justice would have to be sensitive to the rights and obligations of *both* parties to a consent transaction. From that perspective, there is no reason to think that a deontological approach would be more likely to support LK/AA than FT.

One could also argue for FT from a contractualist perspective. Along Rawlsian lines, we could think of the criteria of moral transformation as those that individuals would choose in an original position from behind the veil of ignorance, where the criteria they choose would have to take account of cases involving less than fully autonomous decisions, unfair background conditions, flawed consent transactions, and the like.[80] From that perspective, they would opt for a perspective that is sensitive to the interests of *both* parties to a consent transaction rather than focusing exclusively on the authenticity of the consenter's decision.

T.M. Scanlon's version of contractualism argues that we can think of the principles of morality as those that "no one could reasonably reject as a basis for informed, unforced general agreement."[81] Although Scanlon does not endorse FT in so many words, he specifically rejects what he calls the "quality of will" approach that underlies LK/AA. On Scanlon's view, it is the objective conditions under which a person chooses that determine whether we can treat a person as responsible for her choice—"the fact that an outcome resulted from a person's choice under good conditions shows that he was given the choice and provided with good conditions for making it, and it is these facts (not the authenticity of B's will) which make it the case that he alone is responsible."[82] Although Scanlon does not press the question as to how contractualism would handle choices made under unfair or desperate conditions, I suspect he would arrive at a position close to the one I have defended.

I have not argued that all plausible moral theories would opt for FT over LK/AA. I hope to have shown that FT is consistent with several prominent non-consequentialist theories.[83] Given that it is just those Kantian-inspired theories which are thought to provide the strongest support for LK/AA, this gives me more confidence that I am on the right track.

Validity, Permissibility, and Moral Transformation

At various points, I have suggested that a consent transaction can be morally transformative, even if B does not intend to give consent at all or is mistaken as to what she is consenting. In other words, I have rejected what I call the "lock and key" approach, in which permissibility or moral transformation tracks valid consent. On FT, there may be cases in which it is permissible for A to proceed in the face of what I will call a *flawed consent transaction*; for example, where B has not tokened consent (*Department Meeting*) or where B is mistaken as to what she is consenting (*Lawn Blower*). Moreover, and as I shall explain below, there may also be cases where it is *not* permissible for A to proceed even though B *has* given consent that is valid on AA.

Recall *Department Meeting*. If B is unaware that his silence was understood as indicating agreement to A's proposal, it is difficult to claim that

B is *consenting* to A's proposal. Nonetheless, it is arguably reasonable for A to *construe* B's silence as a token of consent and to let the burden of B's daydreaming fall on B. So here is a case where there is a morally transformative consent transaction without B's consent, much less B's valid consent. Suppose, however, that A is aware that B is likely to reject his proposal and is attempting to take advantage of B's propensity to daydream to get his way. Then it is arguable that it is not justifiable for A to proceed. Here, too, FT gives the right answer.

By contrast, it would seem that LK/AA must say that A is not entitled to proceed in *Department Meeting*. The advocate of LK/AA might claim that whereas there is no consent in this case, it *is* permissible for A to proceed *as if* there were. He might say that AA is meant to provide an account of valid consent, and not a full account of moral transformation. I grant that AA could respond in this way, but then its account of consent does much less work than advertised, for a major task of a theory of consent is to identify the conditions under which A's consent renders it permissible for B to proceed.

I suspect that it is difficult to get an accurate picture of the relationship between valid consent and moral transformation because something like LK underlies our linguistic intuitions about consent. We are inclined to say that if B does not give valid consent, then A is not permitted to proceed and so if as a substantive moral judgment, we believe that A *is* permitted to proceed, we think we had better say that B *has* given valid consent. Consider three versions of *Lawn Blower*.

1. A asks to borrow B's lawn blower. B understands this and says, "Sure."
2. A asks to borrow B's lawn blower. B mistakenly believes that A has asked to borrow B's lawn mower, and says, "Sure."
3. B is not home, but in view of the history and character of their relationship, A assumes that it would be permissible to borrow B's lawn blower, and so just takes it.

Now it may well be permissible for A to take B's lawn blower in all three cases. Scenario (1) is a case where B has given valid consent and this renders A's action permissible. Scenario (3) is a case in which it may be permissible for A to take B's lawn blower without B's consent.

The present issue concerns a flawed consent transaction, such as (2), in which A reasonably regards B's consent as justifying his proceeding, but where A and B have different understandings as to what B has consented.

First, it might be said that there is no valid consent in (2), but that it is permissible for A to act because he *attempted* to generate a moral transformation in good faith. On a second view, B actually gives valid consent to A's taking the lawn blower in (2) although B did not *intend* to do so. Both views are linguistically plausible. On the first view, B might say "I didn't give you permission to take my lawn blower, but, given the misunderstanding, you were justified in taking it." On the second view, B might say "I didn't *intend* to give you permission to take my lawn blower, but I guess I did."

It might be objected that B's utterance in (2) can play no role in justifying A's action, given that B does not understand that to which A believes she is consenting. Along these lines, Monica Cowart argues that "Consenting can only occur if both participants in the conversation understand what X is. When [A] proposes X to [B], [A] must have the same understanding as [B] of what X is."[84] Given that consenting did not occur, Cowart seems committed to the view that it is impermissible for A to take B's lawn blower.

I have two responses to this objection. First, I believe that people can plausibly say that they unwittingly consented to X—"I didn't think I was agreeing to let you take my lawn blower, but I guess I did. My error." Second, and more importantly, I believe that Cowart's "speech act" analysis does absolutely nothing to resolve the moral issue at stake. For assuming that B has *not* consented to A's taking her lawn blower, we *still* have to decide whether the flawed consent transaction renders it permissible for A to take the lawn blower. And it seems highly dubious to insist that A has acted wrongly when he innocently acted on what he reasonably believed was B's consent.

Just as B may be mistaken about the nature of the activity to which she is giving consent, she could also be mistaken about the consequences of her refusal to give consent.

> *Fear.* B falsely believes that A has implicitly threatened her with
> a refusal to continue to treat her illness if she does not
> participate in a research protocol. A has done nothing to
> motivate such a belief. B agrees to participate

Is B's consent morally transformative? On LK/AA, probably not. To the extent that AA focuses on B's mental state, it is difficult to claim that B has given voluntary consent. On FT, however, there may or may not be a moral transformation. If A realizes or should realize that B is or might be laboring under a misimpression about his intentions, then it may be unfair for him to take advantage of B's (false) belief without attempting to clarify the issue.

But if A has no reason to believe that B is motivated by this false belief, then there is no unfairness that renders the consent non-transformative.

I have argued that it may be permissible for A to proceed even though B has not given valid consent. Interestingly, although less commonly, it may *not* be permissible for A to proceed to do X even though B *has* given valid consent to A's doing X.

> *Nondisclosure.* A intentionally fails to disclose information about the risks of a surgical procedure because he believes that B will wrongly overestimate the importance of those risks. Unbeknownst to A, B has consulted with another physician and has a full grasp of the risks. B signs the consent form because she wants A to perform the surgery.

A does not know that B's consent is fully informed. Indeed, A has attempted to prevent B from making an informed decision. In this case, FT would imply that A is *not* permitted to proceed because A has treated B unfairly even though B has given valid consent on AA.

The distinction between valid consent and moral transformation can be illustrated by the following table in which I ask two questions: (1) whether a given example constitutes valid consent and (2) whether there is moral transformation. In addition to *Lawn Blower* and *Non-Disclosure,* consider these two cases:

> *Business Bluffing.* A tells B that he will not accept less than $25,000 for the car that B wishes to purchase. A is actually prepared to accept $24,000. B agrees to pay $25,000.
> *MRI.* B has been experiencing back pain. A (B's physician) recommends an MRI because he profits from each procedure. A does not actually believe that an MRI is necessary. B agrees to have an MRI.

If my intuitions about these cases are correct, then moral transformation does not always track the validity of consent. In *Lawn Blower,* we have moral transformation without valid consent. In *Nondisclosure,* we have valid consent without moral transformation. The table also illustrates how fairness varies with the context of moral transformation. It is not clear whether B's consent is valid in *Business Bluffing,* given that A deceived B. Nonetheless, the deception in *Business Bluffing* is compatible with moral transformation, whereas this is clearly not so in MRI. Why? Because this sort of deception

Table 3.1

	Valid Consent?	Moral Transformation?
Business Bluffing	(?)	Y
MRI	N	N
Lawn Blower	N	Y
Nondisclosure	Y	N

may be regarded as fair in business where A has no fiduciary obligation to protect B's interest, but it is clearly unfair in medicine. Finally, and most importantly, the table illustrates that, for moral purposes, the second column is the key, not the first.

Now, in saying that it is permissible for A to proceed in cases of "mistaken" (or non-) consent, such as *Lawn Blower* and *Department Meeting*, it may be argued that I have confused the claim (1) A is justified in proceeding because the consent transaction is morally transformative and (2) A is not *justified* in proceeding because there is no valid consent, but A's action can be *excused*, given that A has a reasonable belief that B has given consent. Although I think that (1) is more accurate, I do not think much turns on the distinction between excuse (1) and justification (2) in the present context. If, as seems evident, the truth of (2) turns on the *reasonableness* of A's belief rather than the bare fact of the belief itself, then excusability involves a decidedly moral judgment about the justifiability of A's action in (2). This is, perhaps, clearest in *Department Meeting,* where A might say "What do you mean I'm *excused?* Give me a break. I was perfectly justified in proceeding." If A is permitted to proceed in *Lawn Blower* and *Department Meeting*, then the interesting theoretical conclusion follows that valid consent is not a *necessary* condition for a morally transformative consent transaction. If my account of *Nondisclosure* is correct, then valid consent is not *sufficient* for moral transformation. Instead, we need to focus on the fairness of the bilateral consent transaction.

Does this mean that the canon should be revised? If it is moral transformation that matters, not the presence of valid consent, does this mean that we should remove "informed consent" as a normal requirement of ethical medical care and ethical medical research and put moral transformation in its place? I think not. The framework of informed consent or valid consent is well entrenched and serves the relevant values reasonably well. The contingent linkage between valid consent and moral transformative consent transactions is sufficiently strong so as not to justify a linguistic transplant, not to mention that "morally transformative consent transaction" is a clumsy expression. If we can continue to say that "the sun rises" even though it is the earth that turns, we can certainly continue to talk about the presence or absence of valid consent so long as we are able to keep the point of the previous analysis in mind.

Application of The Fair Transaction View to Research: Four Issues

I have described, albeit in quite general terms, what I take to be an attractive approach to consent. Working out the details of this approach is a long-term project, but I now want to show how it can shed light on four current controversies about consent to participate in research.

Therapeutic Misconception

Many canonical documents and bioethicists implicitly or explicitly assume that "understanding is a requirement of informed consent."[85] The Nuremberg Code states that voluntary consent requires that the prospective participant "should have sufficient knowledge and comprehension of the elements of the subject matter involved as to enable him to make an understanding and enlightened decision."[86] The Declaration of Helsinki states that the researcher should obtain the prospective participant's consent only "after ensuring that the subject has understood the information" that has been provided.[87] The Belmont Report states:

> Investigators are responsible for ascertaining that the subject has comprehended the information. While there is always an obligation to ascertain that the information about risk to subjects is complete and adequately comprehended, when the risks are more serious, that obligation increases. On occasion, it may be suitable to give some oral or written tests of comprehension.[88]

> Faden and Beauchamp echo these views.

> An autonomous person who signs a consent form without reading or understanding it is *qualified* to give an informed consent, but has failed to do so. Similarly, if an autonomous person acts in a

way he or she did not intend—for example, by accidentally signing form x when he or she meant to sign form y—then the act of signing x is not autonomous, although it is the act of an autonomous person.[89]

It is not clear whether the views stated here regard comprehension as a requirement for the permissibility of *research* as opposed to being a requirement for *informed consent*. If we assume that autonomous authorization is a prerequisite for valid consent, then there is no valid consent if subjects are in the grips of TM. But Faden and Beauchamp could argue that whereas a person cannot give valid consent without comprehension, we can (sometimes) justifiably treat nonvalid consent *as if it were* valid or regard research as permissible without valid consent.

On FT, the question is not whether participants can give "valid consent" if they are in the grips of TM. Perhaps they cannot. Rather, we should ask whether it can be permissible for investigators to proceed if subjects wrongly believe that they will be receiving personalized medical care. The general outline of my view should now be clear, as should the relevance of a case such as *Lawn Blower*. Although bioethicists often treat TM as a problem of consent that is special to research, the failure to comprehend the content or meaning of a transaction is a potential problem for a wide range of consent contexts. And I think FT provides a better solution to these problems than AA. In the research context, FT would endorse an affirmative obligation of investigators to disclose pertinent information to prospective subjects, because the asymmetry of information about risks and benefits makes it fairer to assign the informational burden to investigators. But, for several reasons, FT does not *require* comprehension as a *sine qua non* of moral transformation. First, any observation of the subject or test of comprehension will not be fail-safe. Second, even if prospective subjects comprehended the information on a cognitive level, they may fail to appreciate its meaning for them. Denial and (excessive) optimism can be powerful forces. Third, the cost to researchers of requiring comprehension may be excessive. Fourth, requiring comprehension may be unfair to the subjects themselves.

Interestingly, the Belmont Report can be read as endorsing something like FT. Although the just cited Belmont passage says that comprehension is required, another passage says that "Respect for persons requires that subjects . . . *be given the opportunity* to choose what shall or shall not happen to them" (emphasis added). Belmont does not state what should happen if subjects are given a fair opportunity to make an informed choice but do not take advantage of that opportunity and thus comprehend some of the relevant information. Fairness may require that the information be provided in understandable form and may even require some effort to assess comprehension. But to require comprehension is not only impossible and impractical. It is also unfair.

There are, then, a number of reasons to think that prospective subjects can give morally transformative consent to participate in research even if they are in the grips of TM. First, and somewhat ironically, a requirement of comprehension places a greater burden on *subjects* than they desire. A prospective subject will reasonably want an opportunity to comprehend, but may understandably resent being *required* to comprehend in part because it may be perfectly rational for a person to forego the acquisition of information or the effort to understand it. Second, and relatedly, the comprehension requirement unduly restricts the freedom of choice of prospective subjects when research offers them a personally favorable risk-benefit ratio or presents no more than minimal risks and does not threaten the values that motivate the demand for consent. Third, a comprehension requirement places excessive obligations on researchers.

Interestingly, although Horng and Grady say that understanding is a requirement of informed consent, they also say that a "high prospect of personal benefit from the trial may support *tolerating* a subject's TM, since significant health benefits are most likely to be consistent with the subject's overarching goals." It is not clear whether they are arguing (1) research is ethical without valid consent when there is a positive risk/benefit ratio or (2) the criteria for morally transformative consent are lower when there is a positive risk/benefit ratio. If we follow LK/AA, then it seems that TM must compromise the agent's autonomy even when the risk/benefit ratio is clearly positive and thus consent cannot be morally transformative in such cases. But if, as FT claims, the investigator's fundamental obligation is to treat the potential participant fairly and with respect for the full range of values served by consent, it seems plausible to suppose that he owes more to the potential participant in efforts to assure comprehension when there is greater risk.

To further explore the implications of FT, consider this case.

> *Depression Trial.* B is clinically depressed, but cannot afford
> psychotherapy or drug treatment. She enrolls in a randomized
> controlled trial where some participants are randomized into

> short-term psychotherapy and some receive medication.
> Although the investigators explain the randomization process,
> B mistakenly believes that she will receive the treatment that
> the investigators believe is best for her. The investigators
> believe that B will be better off in either arm of the trial than
> if she were excluded.

On LK/AA, B's therapeutic misconception renders it impermissible to enroll her. On FT, it may be permissible to enroll B because participation is predictably advantageous to B.

The FT model brings into focus an important safeguard for valid consent that is obscured by the AA model. Institutional protections for consenters often operate in the background to assure confidence that the values served by consent are being satisfied in consent transactions despite the possibility (or probability) of consent that falls short of autonomous authorization, owing to defects in comprehension. By way of analogy, consider the ordinary purchase of goods and services or employment, where consent transactions occur within the context of consumer regulations. I can give morally transformative consent to order and pay for my meal in a restaurant without being informed about or comprehending the hygienic status of methods of food preparation in the kitchen. Public health regulations and surveillance (should) make this unnecessary. When people rent automobiles, or take out mortgages, they are asked to sign lengthy boilerplate contracts, which few people bother to read. Consumers who sign such contracts are, and should be, adequately protected by regulatory guidelines and judicial review on equitable grounds, and, therefore, we don't deem such consent to be invalid despite their uncomprehending consent.

In the case of research, prior review and approval and ongoing monitoring by research ethics committees in accordance with detailed regulations (should) provide comparable safeguards. These institutional protections are part of the fair conditions for cooperation that make consent transactions morally transformative and serve the values of consent. Given this institutional context, the interests of consenters will often be adequately protected despite consent that is defective in comprehension and serving those interests is one of the principal aims of requiring consent. Lack of autonomous authorization does not leave subjects in the lurch when trials, vetted by research ethics committees, offer them a personally favorable risk-benefit profile. Thus the FT model relies, in part, on the sort of regulatory safeguards discussed in Chapter 2. This vital institutional background to the validity of consent plays no role in the AA model because it focuses exclusively on the quality of authorization given by consenters. The package of protections afforded by the IRB's screening before the consent process seems fair to the prospective subject even if they are in the grips of TM.

All that said, whereas TM does not automatically render research impermissible on FT, a fully developed account of FT will probably require that investigators take affirmative steps to counteract TMs by clarifying the differences between research participation and medical care in their disclosures to prospective subjects, by avoiding language that conflates these two activities, by taking appropriate steps to ascertain whether key features of the research have been understood, and perhaps by signaling the distinction between research and treatment by paying patient-subjects at least a nominal fee for volunteering as a symbol that they are undertaking an activity different from medical care. While there is no guarantee that these steps will prevent TMs, researchers should be particularly rigorous when research presents subjects with predictable and substantial disadvantages as compared with standard medical care, as in placebo-controlled trials that withhold proven effective treatment and those that involve invasive procedures for research purposes, such as sham surgery controls or biopsies to measure study outcomes. For here the values served by consent may well be undermined unless we have good reason to believe that the subject is intentionally and knowingly engaged in an altruistic endeavor in which she accepts risks for the benefit of generating knowledge that can help future patients.

While it may be unfair to demand comprehension that is free of TMs in research with a personally favorable risk-benefit ratio, I am not ready to endorse Truog's view that there is no obligation at all to inform prospective subjects that they are participating in a randomized trial that evaluates two medically indicated treatments for their condition, either of which might reasonably be recommended by their physician.[90] For even if this approach does not compromise the subject's medical well-being, people may have a legitimate interest in knowing the purposes for which they are being used. Consider this case.

> *Blood.* The Red Cross has data that indicates that many blood
> donors falsely believe that their blood will be used locally.
> In fact, the blood will be shipped to any location that needs it.

The Red Cross decides not to explicitly disclose its policy
because it does not want to deter donations. B gives blood
because she wants to help people in her community but
would otherwise not donate.

Although the Red Cross's failure to disclose its policy does not cause any
palpable harm to B, B's "donor misconception" undermines her ability to
control the terms on which she donates. Similarly, although patients may not
be medically disadvantaged by being unwittingly enrolled in a randomized
trial comparing two medically indicated treatments, they are not offered a fair
opportunity to choose whether to participate in research, and it does not
seem unduly burdensome on physician-investigators to require such
disclosure.

Background Unfairness

I argued above that, on FT, a person can give morally transformative consent
to do X even if she would not consent to do X but for her unfair background
conditions or, for that matter, because she is coerced by a third party. Some
prospective subjects token consent to participate in research because it provides medical services (such as a physical examination) or treatment for a
known condition that would otherwise be unavailable or because they are
offered financial incentives that renders participation more attractive than
their other alternatives, given their background economic situation. Let us
assume the following for the sake of argument:

(1) B's background conditions are the result of unfairness.
(2) a just society would provide universal access to medical care
   such that B would not have to participate in research in order
   to receive medical care.
(3) B's society does not provide universal access to medical care.
(4) it is rational for B to participate in research in order to receive
   basic medical care.

Given these conditions, does B give morally transformative consent to participate? Although B does not have a fair opportunity to withhold her consent, given (1) – (3), FT would hold that B's consent may be morally
transformative so long as A is treating B fairly in obtaining B's consent *within*
the framework of these unfair conditions.

Consider this case:

> *Vasectomy research.* B and C are married. C has an adverse
> reaction to oral contraceptives. C tells B that unless he gets a
> vasectomy, she will not agree to sexual relations. B is unable
> to pay for the procedure but finds a protocol that evaluates
> two different methods of vasectomy. B goes to A, a
> urologist-investigator, and consents to enter A's study.

It is not clear whether C's proposal is a coercive threat on the rights-violating view I have defended. On FT, it does not matter. B may have a complaint against C (who may have had other options) or against the society (if society should be paying for this procedure), but he has no complaint that A is treating him unfairly in the way his consent has been obtained.

LK/AA might well regard B's consent as not valid. On FT, however, the simple fact that B has no reasonable alternative but to consent to participate in research does *not* entail that his consent to participate in research is not transformative. Contrary to loose talk about such cases, there is no coercion here; nor is there necessarily any unfairness on the part of investigators that calls into question the permissibility of their actions. Indeed, it clearly would be unfair to exclude prospective research subjects facing background injustice, such as lack of health insurance, who are attempting to advance their interests via research participation simply because their background conditions are unfair.

Deception

As a general principle, it would seem that consent induced by deception would not be morally transformative under either LK/AA or FT. But we have also seen that deception is problematic in some contexts but not others. Why is bluffing permissible in poker? There are two related answers. First, deception is intrinsic to the game. Second, the poker player gives non-deceptive consent to participate in the game full well expecting that others will attempt to deceive him within the game.

Note that there is an important distinction between *expecting* to be deceived in a negotiation and *consenting* to the practice in which the deception occurs, as in poker. If I am buying a car, I expect that the salesman may be deceiving me when he says that he can't sell the car for less than $25,000. But even if one's expectation of deception removes ignorance as a defect in one's consent, it does not follow that the practice of deception is legitimate or that one has "consented to a regime permitting deception."[91] We can't imagine the game of poker without deception, but we can imagine the game of buying and selling cars without negotiation even if negotiation requires deception.

How should we think about deception in research? We should distinguish between deception about the palpable risks and benefits of participation, which renders consent non-transformative on both LK/AA and FT, and deception about the purposes of a study that could not be conducted without deception. Deception is a common practice in behavioral and neuroscience research, as it would often be otherwise impossible to achieve valid experimental data about beliefs, attitudes, expectations, and other psychological dispositions. Although placebo controlled trials do not involve deception, since subjects are told that they may be receiving a placebo, it may be necessary to use deception to do scientifically valid research on the placebo effect itself.

In principle, there are two ways of justifying deceptive research. The first approach looks to a non-deceptive mechanism of consent. The second approach is based on a waiver of consent. The practice of "authorized deception" exemplifies the first approach. If prospective research subjects consent to participate after having been informed that some aspects of the research will be deceptive, then the use of deception would seem to be compatible with morally transformative consent on both LK/AA and FT. In that case, prospective subjects could freely decide whether or not they are prepared to volunteer for research that employs deception just as one freely decides whether to play poker. And so it is also arguable that B can give morally transformative consent to deceptive research if she has been given a fair opportunity to decide whether she wishes to volunteer for research that uses deception. There remains an issue as to how much specificity is required for authorized deception. The U.S. Federal Regulations state that informed consent requires that investigators provide "an explanation of the purposes of the research" and "a description of the procedures to be followed."[92] Yet both of these typically are not described truthfully even in those cases of deceptive research that inform subjects that *some* aspects of the disclosure about the research are deceptive. In some cases, such information probably cannot be provided without compromising the goals of the research itself.

Authorized deception is not commonly employed in deceptive medical research.[93] And without authorized deception, it would seem that consent to participate in deceptive research is not transformative on either LK/AA or FT.

On LK/AA, the use of deception interferes with adequate comprehension of the nature of the research and with the intention to authorize the actual study that is being proposed to the prospective subject. On FT, the subject lacks a fair opportunity to decline participation because he or she has not been accurately informed about the nature of the research and has no reason to expect deception. The use of "debriefing" to explain and justify the use of deception at the end of study participation may be an ethically important corrective procedure for deceptive research, but it cannot work to render consent morally transformative.

The second approach to justifying deceptive research involves waiving or bypassing the requirement of consent. I noted at the outset that informed consent is not a necessary condition of ethical research, as in some cases of emergency research or research with medical records. As theories of moral transformation, neither LK/AA nor FT is positioned to determine whether deceptive research can be ethical, all things considered, in the absence of morally transformative consent. It could be argued that a transformative consent process should be viewed as a *prima facie* requirement that can be overridden by other moral considerations or simply ignored in some contexts. Perhaps the relatively minor harms or wrongs of some deceptive research are outweighed by the social value of studies that require deception. Indeed, the Common Rule specifically allows for a *waiver of consent* if "the research involves no more than minimal risk to the subjects" and, among other things, if "the research could not practicably be carried out without the waiver or alteration."[94] The alternative of authorized deception places this position in some doubt, but there may be studies in which authorized deception might bias the responses of research subjects, and thus we must ask whether such studies can pass ethical muster.

Consider two studies.

Placebo Research-1. A wishes to study the placebo effect in depression. He designs a 3-arm study: (1) some receive an antidepressant drug; (2) some are told that they are receiving the drug but are actually given a placebo; (3) some take no pill at all. The point of the study is not to compare (1) and (2), but to compare (2) and (3). The participants are misled about the purposes of the study. They are told that they will be randomized as between (1) and (3), when they are actually randomized as between (1), (2), and (3).

> *Placebo Research-2.* A wishes to study the placebo effect in
> depression. Without telling any patients, he conducts a
> two-arm study: (4) some patients are told they will be
> receiving an anti-depressant, but actually receive a placebo;
> (5) some patients are given nothing.

There is clearly no consent to participate in research in *Placebo Research-2.* What should we say about *Placebo Research-1?* It is possible that FT could yield the conclusion that participants give morally transformative consent. Alternatively (and more honestly), one might claim that the research is ethical notwithstanding the fact that there is no morally transformative consent process. It might also be thought that some research is ethical if there is *some* semblance of consent, but it need not be morally transformative consent. What does partial consent accomplish? On this view, it is one thing to deceive potential participants about the protocol design as in *Placebo Research-1* if participation carries little risk. At least they know that they would be participating in *research.* It is quite another to deceive subjects with respect to the fact that they are participating in research as in *Placebo Research-2.*

Exploring the implications of FT for deceptive research is a long-term project. For present, I would suggest that to the extent that morally transformative consent transaction is a requirement of ethical research, then deceptive research without authorized deception *must* be regarded as nontransformative on LK/AA and therefore unethical. I would think that FT provides somewhat more room for morally transformative consent without prior authorization, although the extent to which that is so is far from clear.

Exploitation

It is often argued that avoiding exploitation is a core principle of research ethics.[95] I consider exploitation in considerable detail in Chapter 5. Here I want to briefly focus on one corner of the issue: can B give morally transformative consent to participate in research if A is exploiting B? I set aside those cases of harmful and patently nonconsensual exploitation in which A coerces or deceives B or in which B is suffering from a deficiency of information or competence. Rather, I focus on cases that are at least *arguably* consensual and mutually advantageous.

Consider *Rescue.*

> *Rescue.* B's car slides off a snow-covered road into a ditch late at
> night. A comes by and proposes to pull B out for $200 with his
> 4-wheel drive pick-up truck and a chain and says it will take
> 5 minutes. B believes that it would be hours before another
> person were to come by or before a tow service could help.
> Moreover, it is bitter cold. B agrees to pay.

In an earlier work, I describe this as a case of mutually advantageous and consensual exploitation.[96] The transaction is mutually advantageous because, *ex hypothesi*, it is better for B to be rescued for $200 than not to be rescued at all. It is arguably consensual because there is a consent token, because B understands that to which she is consenting, because it is rational for B to consent, and because A's proposal is not coercive, given that A does not propose to violate B's rights if she declines (assuming that A has no obligation to help).

Now despite appearances, it is not obvious that A is actually exploiting B in *Rescue*. If an entrepreneurial A roams the highway every night, his average pay may be less than $25 per hour if he charges $200 for a rescue and so A is not exploiting B. But if A is an opportunistic by passer in *Rescue,* then I believe that A is exploiting or taking unfair advantage of B. (I consider this issue in more detail in Chapter 5.)

Let us assume for the sake of argument that the terms of *Rescue* are exploitative. If so, does that exploitation render B's consent nontransformative? Interestingly, on LK/AA, the transformative quality of B's consent *cannot* turn on whether the terms of a transaction are exploitative. Suppose, on the one hand, that the best account of AA maintains that B's decision satisfies the mental state conditions for AA consent because B's plight is a "background circumstance" for which A bears no responsibility and that background conditions do not compromise autonomy. Then it would seem that B's consent in *Rescue* is morally transformative on AA, its exploitativeness notwithstanding. On the other hand, if the pressures of background circumstances—such as B's need to be rescued—do compromise AA, then the permissibility of A's action cannot turn on whether the terms of A's proposal are exploitative. For whether A proposes to rescue B for $5 or $200, B's background circumstances are such that B has no alternative but to pay. In either case, the exploitativeness of the transaction has no bearing on whether B's consent is morally transformative on LK/AA.

Things seem to be more complicated on FT. It might appear that what I have called mutually advantageous and consensual exploitation, such as in

Rescue, would be impossible on FT given that A has—by definition—not treated B fairly. But that would be too quick. For, as I have suggested, there is a distinction between procedural and substantive fairness and a case such as *Rescue* can involve at least two different types of moral transformation. Consider two questions: (1) does B's consent give A permission to tow B's car? (2) Does B's promise (consent) to pay A $200 obligate B to pay the full amount? I believe that the answer to (1) may be yes, because A has not coerced B and because B may be fully informed about the alternatives available to her and competent to choose among them. At the same time, the answer to (2) may be no. Why might this be so? We might say that there has been *procedural* fairness because A does not coerce or deceive B, but that there is *substantive unfairness* with respect to the terms of the agreement. It may turn out that procedural fairness is sufficient to render it permissible for A to proceed (tow the car) but that it is not sufficient to generate an obligation for B to pay A the full amount if A should go ahead and make the rescue or to remove B's grounds for complaint about the terms of the agreement. If the purpose of a consent transaction is to render A's action *permissible*, then fairness may be primarily procedural and so unfairness in the terms of the agreement does not render it impermissible for A to proceed. On the other hand, if the purpose of a consent transaction is to create an obligation for B to comply with unfair terms, then unfairness in the terms of the transaction may compromise that form of moral transformation. A more robust theory of *fairness* does have the resources to deal with the terms of a transaction *ex post*.

Is Consent to Research Special?

I have argued that bioethics has given uncritical endorsement to something like the autonomous authorization view and that the AA view of morally transformative consent has not been adopted in many non-bioethical contexts. When I say that the endorsement is uncritical, I do not mean that it is necessarily wrong (although I think it is wrong). Rather, I believe that bioethics has not sought to demonstrate why consent to participate in research (or treatment) should require a higher or different standard of morally transformative consent than is applied in other spheres such as contracts, sex, and gambling. One cannot simply assert that "medical research is different." Of course it is different. Sex is different from gambling. The question is whether there are characteristics of clinical research that justify different criteria of moral transformation.

At first glance, clinical research does not look all that different from a range of activities in which people take risks for which the law or widely held moral beliefs do not require anything *approaching* the traditional conception of informed consent, much less a version that requires comprehension of the sort that is thought incompatible with the therapeutic misconception. One can give consent to sexual relations that is *regarded* as morally transformative on the basis of virtually no information, even though it can carry significant emotional risk as well as the risk of pregnancy and disease. One can give consent to gamble that is regarded as morally transformative without being provided with any information as to the probability and magnitude of one's expected losses and while being plied with liquor by those to whom one is losing. One can give consent to work in risky occupations that is regarded as morally transformative without any information as to the level of the risk and, I might add, under the considerable pressure of the alternative of unemployment. Because participation in research often reflects altruistic motivations, it is important to note that one can make small and large charitable donations without any assessment of one's competence, without any information as to how the money will be spent, and while being subject to the personal pressure of direct solicitation or manipulative advertising. One can give legally valid consent to get a (relatively) permanent tattoo on a whim. One can give legally valid consent to marry another person on the basis of virtually no information about that person and without any assessment as to whether one understands the risks of such decisions.

It is possible, of course, that we should adopt something like the rigorous standards of informed consent to participate in research in most or all of these contexts. It is possible that we should relax the standards for informed consent in research and bring them closer to the standards that are applied in other contexts such as sex, gambling, donations, and marriage. But if we are right to adopt *different* standards in the various contexts, then we must ask why the criteria of moral transformation in research should be so different.

I suspect that the reigning conception of informed consent to participate in research along with its intense worries about comprehension and voluntariness cannot be justified by the special riskiness of participation in research because participation in much research is not, in fact, riskier in terms of physical or overall well-being than many activities where we operate with a much less demanding conception of morally transformative consent. And so that conception must be justified on other grounds. Without claiming exhaustiveness, here are a few possibilities. First, much of the apparatus of research ethics and subject protection may be understood as a "public relations" response to the legacy of historical abuses. I do not use this phrase derisively. It is crucial that society *trust* the research enterprise. Moreover, whatever the extent to which patient subjects are in the grips of a therapeutic misconception, such misconceptions are probably more common among the general public. Even if "insiders" understand the distinction between medical care and medical research, outsiders may not. We not only want them to trust the research enterprise, we do not want doubts about that enterprise to contaminate their general trust in the medical profession. An elaborate consent process may serve that goal.

Second, and as a general proposition, the criteria for morally transformative consent vary with the asymmetry of information, which is acute in the research context. The greater the asymmetry, the greater the obligation to ensure that the less knowledgeable party has the requisite information before her consent is treated as transformative or that there is a robust screening process in the background or both. Even if research is no more risky than many ordinary activities, it is more complex. Third, we may be particularly concerned about comprehension when people are likely to be confused. Research is similar to treatment in that it is often performed by the same sorts of people (physicians) or conducted in the same sorts of places (hospitals). Moreover, many participants are recruited for participation in research by their treating physicians and may therefore assume that what happens to them as a participant will be guided by their personal medical interests rather than the development of generalizable knowledge. Few people will confuse enrolling in the military with a cushy job, and so we do not worry (much) about the quality of the recruit's consent (perhaps we should!). Whereas people knowingly take risks in some contexts (gambling and jobs) because they receive what they regard as a benefit (entertainment and money), research subjects may be confused as to whether their participation is likely to be of benefit to them. Thus, while some have argued that researchers have a fiduciary relation with participants akin to the fiduciary relation between doctors and patients, it is more plausible to suppose that we need to be careful about the quality of a participant's consent precisely because researchers do *not* have a fiduciary duty to subjects of that kind. After all, to the extent that we think A has an obligation to advance B's interests, we need not worry so much about the quality of B's consent. We justifiably worry about consent in the research context precisely because there is considerable tension between the interests of researchers and subjects.

Fourth, I suspect that we view consent to research as special because it is, by comparison, a relatively *uncommon* experience. Most of us have consented to sex, commercial transactions, marriage, medical care, jobs, and the like. Many gamble and what appears to be an increasing number get tattoos. By comparison, relatively few of us consent to participate in clinical research that involves genuine risks. When consent contexts are more common, where the risks and benefits are better understood, and where we are likely to be on both sides of the consensual transaction, we may be less concerned with the quality of consent.

When all is said and done, are there good reasons to adopt a conception of consent to participation in research that is much more demanding than the conception we employ in other contexts? Perhaps, but probably less so than is often supposed. But this chapter is, as I said, only a "preface." My principal objective has been to advance the fair transaction model of consent. If I am on the right track, there is a range of issues that remain to be explored from the perspective that I have defended.

4 Should We Worry about Money?

Introduction

Financial payments to research participants have long been a fixture of medical research. In his famous experiments on yellow fever, Walter Reed paid subjects $100 to be exposed to the disease, an additional $100 if they became infected, and a payment to the family in case of death.[1] By demonstrating that yellow fever was transmitted by mosquitoes rather than by direct contact, Reed's research opened entire new fields of epidemiology and biomedicine. It also allowed the completion of work on the Panama Canal.

More recently, serious "adverse incidents" in a Phase I trial of an immunomodulatory compound—TGN1412—placed ethical questions about the use of financial incentives in the public eye. TGN1412 was developed by TeGenero AG, a German pharmaceutical corporation, for the treatment of lymphocytic leukemia and rheumatoid arthritis.[2] A Phase I trial of the compound was conducted in the United Kingdom by Parexel, an American contract research organization that assists the pharmaceutical industry "in bringing new products to market . . . with a focus on first-in-man clinical evaluation through to product commercialization."[3] In the first human clinical trials in March 2006, the compound caused catastrophic system failure in six subjects who received what was thought to be a sub-clinical dose that was 1/500th of the comparable dose found safe in animals. The subjects, all of whom were healthy volunteers, were to be paid £2,000 for their participation. Numerous questions have been raised about this study: Was the informed consent process adequate? Did the participants understand the risks of participation? Should the investigators have waited to observe the reaction in the first subject (or two) before proceeding to the next? Were the tragic results due to important breaches of the principles of ethical research or were they simply an unfortunate accident?[4]

The trial also (re)raised questions about the use of financial incentives in recruiting research subjects. The practice of paying subjects—both healthy volunteers and patients—to participate in research is now widespread. A website—rxgetpaid.com—advertises opportunities to participate in clinical research.[5] Another website—guineapigzero.com—describes itself as "an occupational jobzine for people who are used as medical or pharmaceutical research subjects."[6] Financial incentives are widely used in trials conducted by the private sector, but are also commonly used by academic institutions, particularly in trials without the prospect of direct medical benefit.

In this chapter, I focus on the ethics of providing financial payments to research *participants*. There are, of course, serious questions about the ethics of providing financial payment to *physicians* who refer patients to research. No one assumes that investigators will work without pay, but we have reason to worry about conflicts of interest when physicians are paid $12,000 for every patient whom they enroll.[7] These are serious matters, but they are beyond the scope of this chapter.

Some think that monetary payment is acceptable in Phase I trials with healthy volunteers for whom there is no prospect of a direct medical benefit. (Such payments are not typical in Phase I oncology trials with patients who have not responded to other treatments.) We understand that healthy volunteers would have no self-interested reason to participate in a test of toxicity and we do not think that altruism is sufficiently strong or widespread so as to generate enough participants. On the other hand, monetary payment is frowned upon in Phase II and Phase III trials which typically involve patient-subjects, even though it is used with some frequency there as well.[8] As Carl Elliott maintains, "Ethicists generally prefer that subjects take part in studies for altruistic reasons."[9] The general view seems to be that payments may be a necessary evil, but an evil nonetheless.

The general unease about the practice of payment is heightened when payment is regarded as an inducement rather than as compensation or gratitude for the burdens and inconveniences of participation. As John Harris puts it, "Most research ethics protocols and guidelines are antipathetic to inducements."[10] Australian policy states that "Volunteers may be paid for inconvenience and time spent, but such payment should not be so large as to be an inducement to participate."[11] Other guidelines imply that moderate inducements are acceptable, but it is crucial that they not be excessive or "undue." So whereas we are more likely to worry that ordinary workers are paid too little, the dominant worry in bioethics is that subjects may be paid too much.

It is not easy to assess the actual consequences of these worries on the research enterprise. We know that monetary payment is frequently made to research participants in all types of trials.[12] But that fact does *not* show that the worries make no difference to the frequency or magnitude of such payments any more than the fact that many people exceed the speed limit shows that speed limits make no difference to behavior. (I may drive 72 m.p.h. in a 65 m.p.h. zone, but I do not drive 85 m.p.h.) We know relatively little about the effects of these worries on the decision making of IRBs or, more importantly, on the researchers whose proposals to IRBs are (rightly or wrongly) also influenced by such worries or are predicated on their expectations as to how IRBs would respond. It is not that IRBs frequently disapprove protocols that involve what they consider to be inappropriate or excessive financial payments. The point is that we do not know what *would* occur in a counter-factual world in which there were fewer formal or informal constraints on the use of financial incentives. Do some potential protocols never see the light of day because the investigators know that it will be impossible to recruit participants given the constraints on financial incentives? Would researchers offer greater payments? Would the accrual rate of participants be much faster if researchers offered greater payments?

We must also consider how IRBs should understand financial payment in executing their specific responsibilities. The canons of research ethics require that the risks to subjects of participating in research must be reasonable in relation to the anticipated benefits to the subjects or to others. Although the "reasonable risk criterion" is uncontroversial when stated so broadly, it leaves entirely open what *counts as a benefit*. The (virtually?) universally held current view is that IRBs should *not* regard financial payment as a benefit to subjects in evaluating whether the expected benefits of a protocol are sufficient to justify the risks posed to participants. This view is rarely (if ever) defended, most likely because it is thought to be so obviously correct as not to require a defense. Here, too, we have no idea as to what would happen in a counterfactual world in which this view was rejected.

In one sense, the general antipathy to the use of financial incentives is surprising. If we widen the lens once again and place the practice of clinical research within a broader moral context, the default position would allow competent adults to offer or accept payment for participation in clinical research—so long as their conduct does not harm others. From that perspective, there is no reason to oppose what Robert Nozick slyly called "capitalist acts between consenting adults."[13]

A default position is not a final position. Even if we start from these liberal premises, there may be reasons to forbid or discourage or tightly constrain financial payment to research subjects. The principal purpose of this chapter is to consider what those reasons might be. In doing so, I mostly set aside reasons related to *scientific validity*. There may be good scientific reasons to limit or bar financial payment to participants if such payments motivated potential participants to conceal information that would compromise the quality of the results. There may also be scientific reasons to want research subjects to be drawn from all socio-economic categories, and that might be more difficult if financial payments are offered. But if we set such reasons aside, the question remains as to whether there are good reasons for regarding financial incentives with moral suspicion.

My plan is this. First, I begin with a general discussion of the assessment of risks and benefits of research and consider whether financial payment should be regarded as a benefit in that context. Second, I consider the alleged distinction between using financial payment as compensation and using it as an inducement or incentive. Third, I consider the principal argument for allowing research participants to receive financial payment, namely, that doing so respects their autonomy. Fourth, I consider four major lines of argument against the use of monetary incentives in clinical research (although each contains several subsidiary lines of argument): (1) compromised consent; (2) commodification; (3) equality or justice; (4) institutional integrity.

My main objective throughout is not to defend or promote the use of financial payments in clinical research, although my argument points in that direction. My main objective is to examine the major arguments against the use of financial payments. If my analysis is on the mark, it will be much harder to justify a constrained approach to the use of monetary payments than is commonly supposed.

I want to reemphasize that my task here is philosophical and not descriptive or programmatic. I do not mean to downplay the importance of the genuine horror stories of financial payment accompanied by fraud, unsafe and degrading conditions, inadequate review, and compromised consent.[14] My purpose here is to consider whether there are reasons to reject or severely constrain payments to research participants when these sorts of problems do not arise.

Risks and Benefits

As I noted in Chapter 2, the reigning regulatory and ethical frameworks for human research emphasize the *protection* of research subjects. Although informed consent was given pride of place in the wake of the Nazi experiments and other infamous examples of nonconsensual research, the current regulatory system emphasizes prospective risk-benefit assessment by independent ethics committees or IRBs as the principal means by which to protect subjects from undue risks of harm (see Chapter 2). An IRB must determine that a protocol satisfies several ethical criteria *before* the subject is given the opportunity to consent and these criteria cannot be overridden or ignored just because a subject would be willing to enroll in a study that does not meet them.

With respect to risks and benefits, IRBs have three major tasks: (1) to ensure that risks are minimized within the context of the study; (2) to ensure that benefits are enhanced when it is feasible to do so; (3) to ensure that the risks to subjects are reasonable in relation to anticipated benefits. With respect to the reasonableness of risk, "The Common Rule" says this:

> Risks to subjects are reasonable in relation to anticipated benefits,
> if any, *to subjects, and the importance of the knowledge that may
> reasonably be expected to result*[15] (emphasis added).

The Declaration of Helsinki includes similar wording.

> Every medical research project involving human subjects should be
> preceded by careful assessment of predictable risks and burdens
> in comparison with foreseeable benefits to *the subject or to
> others* . . . Medical research involving human subjects should only
> be conducted if the importance of the objective outweighs the
> inherent risks and burdens to the subject[16] (emphasis added)

As I argued in Chapter 2, the point of the *Reasonable Risk Criterion* (RRC) is to take certain options off the table in order to protect prospective subjects who might either imprudently expose themselves to risks, or place themselves at risk for the sake of a study that is unworthy of their sacrifice.[17] The present issue is how to interpret the principle that risks must be "reasonable in relation to anticipated benefits" or that research should be conducted only if "the importance of the objective outweighs the inherent risks and burdens to the subject" or what is somewhat misleadingly referred to as a favorable risk/benefit ratio. ("Ratio" is misleading because the question is not whether it is 2/1 or 3/1 or ½ or 1/3, but whether the net or sum total is positive or negative.)

At the most basic level we can distinguish between the *personal* and *social* benefits of research. Let us say that a protocol has a *personally favorable risk/benefit ratio* when the expected or *ex ante* benefits (whatever they are) to the subject exceed the expected or *ex ante* disadvantages, burdens, and risks to the subject. In assessing the risks and benefits of participation, we must do so from an *ex ante* rather than *ex post* perspective.

We can distinguish between three types of personal benefits to research participants: direct medical benefits, indirect medical benefits, and non-medical benefit. Research that is focused on the development of treatments or diagnosis may provide *the prospect of direct medical benefit* to the subjects when they receive the intervention or diagnostic technology under investigation.[18] Subjects may receive the prospect of direct medical benefit in a placebo controlled trial of an experimental treatment if they would otherwise not receive the standard treatment or did not respond positively to the standard treatment. On the other hand, subjects cannot expect to personally benefit in a placebo controlled trial of a new intervention if they would otherwise receive and benefit from the standard treatment, setting aside the possibility that the "placebo effect" may be more beneficial than the standard treatment.[19]

Participation in research may also provide *indirect* or *collateral medical* benefits. Subjects may receive general preventive medical care or diagnoses that they would otherwise not receive. Even if they would receive the standard care in a non-research setting, they may receive better care if they participate in a randomized controlled trial say because the level of care in a research hospital is superior or because they will be more closely monitored.

Subjects may also receive *non-medical* benefits. They may gain psychological satisfaction from altruistic participation in a study. They may enjoy interaction with investigators and other participants. As Lynn Jansen suggests, we can understand benefits so as to include anything that contributes to the advancement of a personal goal or project. On this view, a subject may "objectively" benefit from altruistic participation apart from any "warm glow" that they experience.[20] Participants may also benefit monetarily. There are disputes as to whether IRBs should count collateral medical benefits, psychic benefits, or monetary benefits in applying the reasonable risk criterion, but there is no reason to deny that they are regarded as benefits by the participants themselves.

Let us say that a protocol has positive *social* value when the expected benefits to present and future persons from the knowledge gained by the study exceeds its costs—*exclusive of the effects on the participants themselves*. Although I use the term "social value," the potential beneficiaries of clinical research certainly extend beyond the participant's own society and will ordinarily include present and future persons throughout the world. Calculating the expected social value of research is enormously difficult, but it is important to stress that a study may have considerable social value even if the drug, medical procedure, or diagnostic tool turns out to be inefficacious or no more efficacious than other alternatives. It was of great importance to determine that lumpectomies were no less effective than mastectomies in treating breast cancer, as it allowed women to undergo less disfiguring surgery without increased mortality.

Given the distinction between the personal and social value of research, we can say that a study has positive *total* or *overall* value when the *sum* of the expected *personal* and *social* value is positive, i.e. its risk/benefit ratio is favorable. Consider the following set of possibilities (Table 4.1), where + = a net expected benefit, ++ = a greater net expected benefit; - = a net expected loss; and 0 = no expected benefit or loss, and so forth.

Table 4.1

	Personal	Social	Total
1	+	+	++
2	0	+	+
3	-	++	+
4	--	+++	+
5	+	0	+

If we assume that a study must have positive *social* value, it would seem that (1) – (4) pass the test whereas (5) does not. Second, it seems that (1) – (4) are in principle compatible with a straightforward reading of the "reasonable risk" criterion. They have a positive risk/benefit ratio. It would seem, for example, that (3) and (4) are cases in which the "importance of the objective outweighs the inherent risks and burdens to the subject." If the relevant principle concerns the *overall* value of the research, then (2), (3), and (4) are actually on a par.

Case (5) raises an issue that is often ignored. Although (5) is unlikely to be an issue in academic research, it could easily arise in commercial research on "me, too" drugs that are structurally similar to currently available treatments and which offer no therapeutic advantages. Case (5) may provide direct medical benefit to the participants, but does not contribute much to generalizable knowledge. In my view, such research should not be barred on the grounds of *the protection of human subjects*. It might be thought that (5) violates the principle of non-exploitation, since we would be using people for no good purpose, but it is not clear that the subjects would have a complaint since *they* are better off being used and might well receive an eminently fair package of personal benefits. One might object to (5) on the grounds of allocation of social resources, but it's arguable that *society* cannot justifiably object to such research when conducted by private corporations.

Return to cases (3) and (4). Sven Ove Hansson says that "the received ethical approach to clinical trials . . . [does] not allow a person to sacrifice her own interests by taking part in a clinical trial that is beneficial to the wider community. . . ."[21] If we adopt the view of RRC reflected in Common Rule and the Declaration of Helsinki, it would seem that Hansson is wrong. Indeed, if Hansson is right, then there would be much less to worry about—for there would be no great tension between the interests of subjects and those of the wider community. But contrary to Hansson's claim, both documents adopt an *aggregative view* of reasonable risk. They place no *de jure* or principled limitation on the risks to which subjects may be exposed so long as the social value of the research is sufficient to outweigh them. None. On that view, (4), which exemplifies a "bad deal" or "bad choice" trial from the participant's perspective, is ethically permissible because the expected net harm to the participant is outweighed by the "importance of the objective."[22] On the aggregative view, the principles of subject protection are designed to protect subjects from risks that are not justified by a greater sum of benefits, but are not designed to protect them from even very high risks if the benefits to others outweigh those risks. People may, of course, refuse to enroll in trials such as (3) and (4), but that is a different matter.

Even though a literal reading of these documents supports the aggregative view, it appears that, *de facto*, IRBs are unlikely to approve high risk research such as (4) even if it also promises great social value—"IRBs tend to be very reluctant to allow even competent adults to be exposed to substantially more than minor net risks for the benefit of society."[23] According to Jerry Menikoff, IRBs tend to apply a "stricter test" of reasonable risk, one which asks whether the risks are reasonable to the *subject* and drops out the "benefits to society" factor.[24] Of course, IRBs might be legitimately concerned that that any consent obtained in a case such as (4) would be insufficiently competent or informed. But assuming that an adequate process for assuring the quality of informed consent is in place, there remains the question as to whether IRBs *should* allow high risk studies such as (4) to go forward. And there remains the question as to whether investigators should be allowed to use substantial financial incentives to overcome the reluctance of people to enroll in a study such as (4), just as employers pay extra to those who engage in risky labor.

Is Money a Benefit?

Ezekiel Emanuel has argued that "Excessively risky research ought not be permitted no matter what" and thus if IRBs are doing their job, we need not worry as to whether people might be induced by payment into participating in excessively risky research.[25] But to say that excessively risky research should not be permitted (period!) does not resolve the issue as to whether monetary payments might convert research that would *otherwise* be excessively risky into research that is not *excessively* risky, if the participants can *reasonably* regard such payments as compensating them for the risks.

On what I will call *the standard view* or *exclusion view*, IRBs should completely *ignore* the value of financial payments to participants in determining whether the risks of research are reasonable in relation to the anticipated benefits. If a protocol meets the reasonable risk criterion without counting the value of financial payment, then it is permissible for investigators to offer financial payments so long as they are not coercive or constitute an "undue inducement," but the value of those payments to the participants should have no bearing whatsoever on whether the protocol meets the reasonable risk criterion. By contrast, on what I shall call the *incorporation view*, IRBs should consider the value of financial payments as a benefit to participants in assessing whether the risks of research are reasonable in relation to the anticipated benefits.

The incorporation view receives support from what I will call *the linkage thesis*. Consider these two claims.

(1) An IRB should *respect* a person's *reasonable* judgment as to whether the benefits of financial payment outweigh the risks of participation if the protocol is *otherwise* approvable.

(2) An IRB should *incorporate* a person's *reasonable* judgment about the benefits of financial payment in determining whether the risks of research are reasonable in relation to the anticipated benefits.

The *linkage thesis* states that if one accepts (1), then one should accept (2). The standard view rejects the linkage thesis; it accepts (1), but rejects (2). Despite its widespread acceptance, I believe that the standard view is difficult to defend.

Although the canonical documents and laws do not directly address this issue, the standard view is (almost?) universally accepted. For example, the University of California at Irvine's policy states that "Payment to research participants for participation is not considered a benefit. Rather, it should be considered compensation for time and inconvenience or a recruitment incentive."[26] The Syracuse University Handbook for IRBs states that "Incentives for participation in research are not considered as benefits of the research and should not be reported as such on the IRB application."[27] Guidelines prepared by the Office of Human Subjects Research at the National Institutes of Health say this:

> The IRB should not view remuneration as a benefit to offset
> research risks in deciding whether a protocol should be approved.
> As in all cases, the IRB is charged with determining whether
> research risks are justified by the potential benefits of doing the
> research. Risks that are otherwise unacceptable cannot be made
> acceptable by offering increasing amounts of money to subjects.[28]

And whereas the FDA's 1989 guidelines reflected the incorporation view, it had changed its tune by 1995 when it emphatically stated that financial payments are *not* a benefit of participation.[29]

In rejecting the linkage thesis, the standard view implicitly distinguishes between the role of IRBs and investigators and the role of participants with respect to the benefit of financial payment. On that view, *IRBs* should *not* allow financial payment to be counted as a benefit in determining whether the risks of research are reasonable in relation to the benefits, but *participants* can *legitimately* regard payment as a benefit once the research is approved without respect to those benefits. In effect, the standard view uses a "*moderate altruist*" or *prudent subject* criterion. IRBs will ask whether the risks are such that moderate altruists could agree to participate *without* financial compensation. If it passes that test, the investigators could then offer financial incentives—*so long as the incentives do not compromise the subject's consent.*

The previous qualifying phrase is crucial. It might be thought that if a prudent person could reasonably choose to participate in a study, then we need not worry whether financial payments constitute an undue inducement. I disagree. For it does not follow that just because a moderate *altruist* would consent to accept a risk for the sake of others, that a *non*-altruist is acting reasonably in subjecting herself to the same risk. The transformative quality of consent is *motivation sensitive*.

Consider two kidney donors.

> *Altruistic Donor.* Larry David consents to donate a kidney to his friend, Richard Lewis. He does not expect that he or his family will receive any (non-psychic) benefit as a result.[30]
>
> *Egoistic Donor.* B consents to donate a kidney to a stranger because she falsely believes that she or her family will have preference in getting an organ should the need arise in the future.

Although Larry David gives valid consent, it is arguable that the Egoistic Donor does not give valid consent, given that her consent is rooted in a "donation misconception," and this is so even if it would have been perfectly reasonable for her to make such a donation if she had been altruistic.

A brief aside on altruism. Somewhat surprisingly, some bioethicists are uneasy with *more* than minimal or moderate altruism. Grant and Sugarman argue that "If the risks [from a study] are too high, it would be unethical to ask anyone to take them, regardless of whether they would be asked to volunteer or offered wages or incentives."[31] Why is this so? We might say that that risks are "too high" just in case it is unethical to ask anyone to take them, in which case the claim is simply a tautology. But precisely why is it unethical to *ask* people to consider taking high risks for the benefit of other people so long as they are free to say no? After all, we ask people to volunteer to serve in the military or to donate organs or join fire-fighting brigades.

In any case, the present question is not whether it is justifiable to ask people to participate in risky research on altruistic grounds, but how to apply the reasonable risk criterion if we assume that people are participating on (broadly) *self-interested* grounds. And IRBs cannot determine whether prospective subjects would be making competent and reasonable judgments without considering whether it would be *reasonable* for a participant to believe that the value of a financial benefit is sufficient to outweigh the risk.

I do not doubt that it will be difficult for IRBs to make such judgments. Here I make two points. First, evaluating whether it is reasonable to accept direct or collateral *medical* benefits in exchange for accepting medical risks is not vastly different than evaluating whether it is reasonable to accept collateral *financial* benefits in exchange for accepting medical risks. Second, IRBs *cannot* refuse to make such judgments if they are concerned to ensure that financial payments not constitute *undue inducements*. For to say that a financial payment constitutes an undue inducement is precisely to say that it would be unreasonable for the participant to accept the inducement in exchange for accepting a risk—given her motivations and aims.

Does it matter whether we adopt the standard view or the incorporation view? It depends. If IRBs should adopt an *aggregative* view of the reasonable risk criterion, then IRBs could approve high risk/higher social benefit research (as in (4) above) even if it does *not* count financial payment as a benefit. If research is permissible so long as the expected social benefits outweigh the risks to participants, the reasonable risk criterion would not exclude research that Emanuel and others might call "excessively risky." If, however, IRBs adopt a subject-oriented view of RRC that focuses on the *personal* risk/benefit ratio, then (4) would be rejected on the standard view but could be approved on the incorporation view if the financial benefits were sufficient to offset those risks.

If IRBs should reject the aggregative view such that we approve research only if it is not unreasonably risky to the participant *whatever* the social benefit, then it makes a significant difference as to whether they regard financial payments as a benefit to the participants. For by excluding financial payment from the risk/benefit assessment, IRBs may refuse to approve protocols that have considerable social value or, what is more likely, protocols may not even be proposed because it is anticipated that they will not be approved. If IRBs adopt the standard view on counting payment as a benefit and also adopt a subject-oriented rather than an aggregative view of *RRC*, they will inevitably fail to approve research that promises to be of value both to future patients and to the participants. If we do not come to grips with the potential upside to accepting the incorporation view, there is a substantial risk of perpetuating a sub-optimal state of affairs. Researchers want to go forward. Future patients would be better off. And prospective subjects would benefit from participation by their own reasonable lights. We should be very careful before we preclude a win-win-win solution.

To see why the choice between the standard view and the incorporation view is important, it will prove useful to ignore financial payment as compensation for time, inconvenience, and financial costs (such as travel) and focus solely on payment as a benefit that can offset risk. On the *off the books* or *monetary-exclusive* method adopted by the standard view, we do not count financial payments as a personal benefit of participation in research, although we do count the prospect of direct and, perhaps, indirect medical benefit. On the *on the books* or *monetary-inclusive* method adopted by the incorporation view, we include the expected value of financial payment as a benefit of participation in research.

If participation can reasonably be expected to be of *medical* benefit on the monetary-exclusive method and the research is socially beneficial, then it is unproblematic with respect to RRC. So, let us focus on cases in which the *personal* benefit from participation is *negative* on the *standard* view. In some cases, the net (overall) personal benefit is moderately negative (-); in other cases the net personal benefit is more negative (--) or (---). We can also estimate the monetary-inclusive personal benefit from research for cases in which investigators might be prepared to offer participants substantial monetary payment that will *reasonably* affect the participant's assessment of the overall personal benefit from participation. We also estimate the social value of the research. Given these estimates, we assess the overall or aggregative expected benefits of the research. In each set of cases (e.g., (6), (6a), (6b)), the *unmodified* number *excludes* financial benefits from the calculation as on the standard view (SV)) whereas the *modified* number *includes* the financial benefits of various magnitudes ((6a) and (6b)), as on the incorporation view (IV).

Now let us assume for the sake of argument that a protocol satisfies RRC only if it has positive overall value; that is, the social benefits are sufficient to

Table 4.2

	Overall Personal $$ exclusive	Financial	Overall Personal $$ inclusive	Social	Overall
6 (SV)	-	NC	-	++	+
6a (IV)	-	+	0	++	++
6b (IV)	-	++	+	++	++
7 (SV)	-	NC	-	+	0
7a (IV)	-	+	0	+	+
7b (IV)	-	++	+	+	++
8 (SV)	--	NC	--	+	-
8a (IV)	--	+	-	+	0
8b (IV)	--	++	0	+	+
9 (SV)	--	NC	--	++	0
9a (IV)	--	+	-	++	+
9b (IV)	--	++	0	++	++
9c (IV)	--	+++	+	++	+++

outweigh the risks to participants. If we focus on the standard view "unmodified" (SV) cases, then (6) is the only protocol in Table 4.2 that can be approved and to which prospective participants would even have the opportunity to consent. It is the only case of risky research that is "reasonable in relation to anticipated benefits" in light of "the importance of the knowledge that may reasonably be expected to result." Case (7) has a similar personal risk profile to (6), but less expected social value and thus does not produce net positive overall value, and therefore could not be approved. Note, however, that the modified or IV view versions of (7) *could* be approved as in (7a) and (7b). Indeed, if the payments are high, as in (7b), the protocol would not only be expected to be of moderate positive *social* value, but participation would be of positive *personal* value. Case (8) is a riskier cousin of (7). On the standard or exclusion view, (8) would certainly not be approved. Moreover, incorporation versions of (8) would not be approved if the payment were modest (8a), but could be approved if the payments were substantial (8b).

As an example of high risk/high social value research, (9) is the most interesting case. Assuming we reject the aggregative view and adopt a subject-oriented view of RRC, then (9) will not be approved on the standard view. On the incorporation view, however, IRBs might approve the protocol in (9a) and (9b). Moreover, if the payments are high enough, as in (9c), the research would not only be expected to be of substantial *social* value, it would also generate a positive *personal* benefit for the participants. The important point is that by refusing to regard financial incentives as a benefit to the subject, the standard view excludes protocols in which *both the society and the subjects* can expect to benefit from their respective points of view.

Now there may be moral reasons to adopt the standard or exclusion view that are unrelated to concerns about the protection of subjects. For example, refusing to count such benefits may contribute to general social trust in the research enterprise even if it works to the detriment of prospective subjects. But to the extent that we are concerned with the protection of the prospective participants themselves, there is a strong *prima facie* case for accepting the linkage thesis and adopting the incorporation view under which we would regard financial payment as a benefit to the participants that offsets the risk of participation. Put simply, *if it is reasonable for the subjects themselves to regard financial payment as a benefit that can offset risk, there is prima facie reason for IRBs to respect their judgment and to incorporate that judgment into their own assessment of the risk/benefit profile of the protocol.*

Once again, I say *reasonable*. The incorporation view assumes that participants are making reasonable judgments. I do not deny that participants may consent to participate because the offer of financial payments lures them to make unreasonable judgments about the risks and benefits of participation. And on the soft-paternalist model I have advocated in Chapter 2, IRBs have an obligation to determine—at a relatively broad level—whether it would be reasonable for subjects to participate on self-interested grounds. But IRBs *must* make that judgment on *both* the standard view and the incorporation view. And once they do make this judgment, it is difficult for them to say, in effect: "we have decided that it is reasonable for the subject to accept the risks of participation in light of the financial payment, but, for his own protection, we will not regard financial payments as a benefit to him."

Ruth Macklin would object to this entire line of argument. She argues that "to construe payment to subjects as a "benefit" of research is to distort the very meaning of the concept" and to do so would be inconsistent with the way in which that concept was "originally intended" to work. She notes that The Belmont Report states that "The term 'benefit' is used in the research context to refer to something of positive value related to health or welfare."[32] And she adds that it would "be stretching the meaning of the term 'welfare' to interpret it as including financial benefit to research subjects." Macklin may be right about the drafter's intention in The Belmont Report, but to construe payment as a "benefit" hardly distorts "the meaning of the concept" of a benefit, per se.

I have argued that insofar as we are concerned with the protection of subjects, we should prefer the incorporation view to the standard view. We should regard financial payment as a benefit to subjects that offsets risk. Nonetheless, let us assume for the sake of argument that the linkage thesis and the incorporation view should be rejected and that IRBs should continue *not* to regard financial payment as a benefit in determining whether a proto-col passes the reasonable risk criterion. If we adopt the standard view, then (6) is the only protocol in Table 4.2 that will be approved because it is the only (unmodified) case that has positive overall value. Still, even though (6) can be approved without regarding financial payment as a benefit, it may be difficult to recruit potential subjects into research such as (6) in the absence of financial payments. So setting aside worries about the application of RRC, we must ask whether there are reasons to eschew or constrain financial pay-ments to subjects.

Compensation, Incentives, and Risk

Australian policy states that "Volunteers may be paid for inconvenience and time spent, but such payment should not be so large as to be an inducement to participate."[33] Compensation is permissible, but incentives are not. Other canonical statements are silent on the permissibility of using financial pay-ment as an incentive. CIOMS says this:

> Subjects may be reimbursed for lost earnings, travel costs and other expenses incurred in taking part in a study; they may also receive free medical services. Subjects, particularly those who receive no direct benefit from research, may also be paid or otherwise compensated for inconvenience and time spent. The payments should not be so large, however, or the medical services so extensive as to induce prospective subjects to consent to participate in the research against their better judgment ("undue inducement").[34]

Note that while this statement says that "*undue* inducements" are not permis-sible, it does not say whether payments that are offered as inducements are permissible if they are not "undue."

I will consider the "undue inducement" argument below. The present question is whether there is a significant distinction between compensation and incentives. On one view, it is permissible to use financial payment to compensate subjects, but not to provide payment that would "more than compensate" for their burdens so as to provide an overall personal benefit. Moreover, the prevailing view is that it is permissible to compensate participants for the expense, time and inconvenience of participation, but not for the *risk of harm*. And so there are two distinctions at play here: (1) the distinction between compensation and incentives; (2) the distinction between compensating for burdens and inconvenience and compensating for risk.

Let us start with the second distinction between compensation for the burdens of participation and compensation for risk. It is certainly possible to draw a *conceptual* distinction between the (non-risk) *burdens* of participation as contrasted with *risks* to one's long-term well-being or health, although there is no agreement as to whether some procedures (such as lumbar punctures) fall into one category or the other. The burdens of participation include inconvenience, time, and pain or aversive experience, even when interventions such as blood draws do not pose a risk to one's long term health. I am not sure how to categorize some cases. More than 900 people have participated in malaria vaccine trials at Walter Reed Institute of Research. After receiving the study vaccine, they are exposed to malaria-infected mosquitoes. If they contract malaria, they are treated immediately and can be quickly cured. Although such studies have not resulted in any deaths or hospitalizations, participants typically experience flu-like symptoms for several days. A risk or a burden?[35] By contrast, participation in research can certainly entail genuine risk of serious illness or death, as in the TGN 1412 study or the gene therapy study that resulted in the death of Jesse Gelsinger.[36]

Although some think it is acceptable to compensate participants for burdens, but not for risks, there is certainly no *conceptual* bar to compensating people agreeing to accept the (*ex ante*) risk of harm. Now there are contexts in which we only compensate people for *actual* or *ex post* harm. If A's negligent driving increases the risk that B will be harmed, B does not have a claim against A for compensation if she is not palpably harmed. In other contexts, however, we regularly compensate people for assuming an increased risk of harm. High rise structural steel work may be no more burdensome than other construction work, but it may well be riskier, and it is arguable that pay should and will be responsive to that risk. To the extent that we regard participation in research as comparable to other risky endeavors or lines of work, it is difficult to see why we should treat risk as a noncompensable cost of participation.

With respect to the distinction between compensation and incentives, Grant and Sugarman suggest that it is relatively unproblematic to compensate or to seek to neutralize the burdens of participation. "Compensation means "rendering equal," a "recompense or equivalent," "payment for value received or service rendered," or something which "makes up for a loss." By contrast, they believe it is problematic for investigators to give people an incentive to do something that one would otherwise not have done or that would have (otherwise) been against their better judgment.[37]

Grant and Sugarman are right to distinguish what we might regard as "reimbursements" for burdens or costs incurred—and which are designed to take money "out of the picture"—and incentives that are designed to increase the probability that a person will enroll in a trial even though simply reimbursing people for burdens or costs incurred (e.g. travel expenses) will make it more likely that some people will participate. But some forms of compensation put pressure on this distinction. Investigators in a study of childhood malaria mortality in Malawi wanted to perform autopsies on children who had died from the disease. As an expression of gratitude, the investigators offered to provide a coffin and transportation of the body from the hospital to the parents' community to those parents who consented to the autopsy.[38] Interestingly, the investigators were reluctant to inform the parents that they would receive this compensation because they did *not* want to sway the parents' decision. Now there is an interesting question here as to whether this policy—however well intentioned—allowed the parents to make an appropriately informed judgment to *not consent* to the autopsy, given that they were denied information about the foregone benefits of their decision. The present point is that it was well understood that this form of compensation could also constitute a powerful incentive.

Sarah Edwards argues that monetary payment only qualifies as an inducement if it is "the *significant* factor" in one's decision-making.[39] I don't see why. The Seattle Biomedical Research Institute proposed a study of malaria vaccines in which healthy volunteers would be exposed to malaria infected mosquitoes. If a subject becomes infected, she will be immediately treated. The researchers plan to offer upwards of $2000 to participants. Dr. Patrick Duffy, head of the Institute, said: "I don't think most people would volunteer for this unless they felt like they were doing it for a larger purpose."[40] He may be right, but I assume that even those who have this larger purpose in mind are more likely to participate if they receive several thousand dollars. Given that the motivational structure of most people is complex, monetary payment is properly understood as an inducement so long as it makes it more likely that someone will do something—whether or not it actually motivates them to do so and whatever its relative weight in an individual's psychic economy.

It is logically possible, of course, that monetary payment might render some people *less* likely to participate in research. Richard Titmuss has famously argued that if we permit people to be paid for giving blood, some persons who would otherwise have donated will simply stay away (although, if true, it is possible that the increase in paid donors will exceed the decrease in unpaid donors).[41] They do not want to sell their blood, but they also do not want to donate what can be bought and sold. They want to make a gift of what is not available on the market. And the same *might* hold for research participation. If monetary payments to research participants discouraged participation, this would, of course, be a good reason to refrain from the practice. In any case, there is some evidence that Titmuss is wrong about blood donations and I have seen no evidence that the Titmuss hypothesis is true for research participation.[42] Moreover, there is at least some evidence that, for most people, multiple motivations co-exist rather peacefully. Financial motivations do not displace the desire to contribute to science, nor does the desire to contribute to science render financial motivations irrelevant.

Autonomy and Risks

The liberal default position is to allow competent adults to engage in voluntary transactions so long as they do not harm others. This would involve allowing investigators to offer financial payments to research participants and to respect the latter's decision to regard such payments as a benefit or compensation that offsets risk. As I argued in Chapter 3, there are both consequentialist and autonomy-based reasons for respecting voluntary transactions. Since parties typically expect to gain from voluntary such transactions, allowing them typically enhances the welfare of both parties as well as demonstrating respect for their autonomy. If we place participation in research in a wider context, it is obvious that we allow people to accept considerable risks for what they regard as beneficial or worthwhile. And while this should not need restating, I restate the obvious for I think its significance for research ethics has not been sufficiently appreciated. We allow people to take considerable risks engaging in activities which they enjoy, be it football, skiing, rafting, climbing Mt. Everest, or riding motorcycles (without helmets in many states). We allow people to put their family in a car and take a cross country trip or just a Sunday drive to see Grandma. We allow people to accept risks to their health or life in pursuit of relief from pain, injuries, chronic conditions, sexual dysfunctions, or aesthetic enhancements.

Because participation in research is more akin to (temporary) employment than to mountain climbing or the purchase of a car, we should bear in mind that we allow people to accept jobs that involve moderate or even very high risks of illness, accidents, and death. Some high risk jobs are located in the public sector—police, military, and fire fighters. But many private sector jobs are not without risk. Ordinary jobs such as delivering pizzas are not without risk, but some jobs are extremely risky. Timber cutters face a death rate nearly 30 times that of a typical workplace.[43] Lobster fishermen, structural metal workers, coal miners, and general aviation pilots also face great risks. In effect, the market provides a "risk premium" for many occupations. Timber cutters and lobster fisherman earn relatively high salaries for relatively low skilled jobs.

Or consider merchant sailors. Recruiters from shipping companies actively recruit Filipinos. A 2008 report indicated that more than 100 Filipinos were being held by the Somali pirates "who have made the Gulf of Aden a terrifying place to sail."

> [Marlon] Arguelles, 28, who was scanning the job notices, was looking for work as a ship's cook. Many of the recruiting agencies were offering $1,000 to $2,000 a month for the position. . . But he said he needed more than that to help care for his mother, who suffers from hypertension, and to pay for the education of his three younger siblings.
>
> So he perked up when he heard that one recruiter was looking for crewmen for an oil tanker that would pass through the Gulf of Aden . . . "I know it's dangerous, but the agency is offering twice the salary," Mr. Arguelles said. "Besides, think about it: the pirates haven't killed any crew members so far, so it could be harmless."[44]

We do not have anything like an occupational IRB that must approve the risk/benefit ratio of employment before we allow people to choose to be employed in a risky line of work. We rely mostly on consent. The Occupational Safety and Health Administration (OSHA) may seek to "minimize risk" within the framework of what may be inherently risky jobs, but we do not ban jobs that are inherently quite risky. As a manager of the Luneta Seafarer's Center in Manila put it, "It's up to the sailor whether to accept the offer," he said. "The important thing is he knows what he's getting into."[45]

Now it might be argued that we can and should distinguish between allowing people to accept risk in exchange for financial benefit in ordinary employment and allowing such trade-offs in medical research. As Macklin puts it: "[I]f we view health care, medical benefits, and the research that yields these goods and services as a special sort of social good, we can readily reject the idea that research involving human subjects should be treated no differently from other activities driven by market forces."[46] But it is not sufficient to say that "if" we view research as a "special sort of good" then we can reject the view that serving as a research subject in exchange for financial compensation is like cutting timber. For even if we grant that health care and medical research are "special" sorts of social goods, they might not be special in this way. It must be shown that there are good reasons for thinking that it is morally permissible to allow timber cutters to accept risks in exchange for higher pay than they would otherwise earn, but wrong to allow research subjects to accept risks in exchange for money that they would otherwise not receive. The claim that medical research is a "special sort of good" does not come remotely close to establishing this. Moreover, it is a mistake to think that the realm of the medical is of monumental moral significance, whereas cutting timber to provide for one's family is a morally unimportant activity because it is "driven by market forces." Mr. Arguelles took on a dangerous job so that he could care for his mother who suffers from hypertension and educate his siblings.

Is there a principled basis for claiming that people should be allowed to incur risks as a commercial sailor, timber cutter, or coal miner in exchange for money but that it is morally suspect when people incur risks participating in medical research in exchange for money? It might be thought that it is worse to compensate people for work in which one is a passive target or locus of risk as opposed to compensating people for risks incurred in the course of active work—cutting timber, delivering pizza, etc. One's pay may reflect the risks, but one is paid for what one does. By contrast, participants in medical research are often passive recipients of a risk producing intervention. One is being paid to be *used*.

The distinction between active and passive employment has some intuitive appeal, but it is difficult to say how much weight it will bear. Consider medical education. Medical students practice some procedures, such as the use of a stethoscope, on fellow students, but other procedures are considered too "personal" and so medical schools hire model patients on whom students can practice procedures such as a rectal exam for enlarged prostate. Carl Elliott finds this practice "oddly disturbing" and thinks that the work is "degrading."[47] Perhaps it is. At the same time, we should remember that many jobs involve unpleasant and dirty work—plucking chickens, shoveling manure, and cleaning toilets. Indeed, although Elliott finds the practice "disturbing," he does not claim that it should be stopped. Moreover, I assume that there would be few objections if a medical school offered *free* prostate exams, colonoscopies, or pelvic exams to uninsured persons so that students could learn how to do these procedures under supervision. I don't see an important distinction between being paid to do something and getting something for free for which one ordinarily has to pay.

Any case against paying people just to accept risks must decide what to do about Phase I research. Unlike other risky employment in which risk is an unintended but unavoidable consequence of employment, healthy volunteers in Phase I research (although not Phase II and Phase III research) are often employed precisely to put themselves at risk of harm and to incur other burdens of research. But few propose that Phase I research be by-passed or that that healthy volunteers not be paid. And so even if we can make a conceptual distinction between active work such as timber cutting and passive work such as being used as a subject in a Phase I trial, the distinction is of limited relevance to the legitimacy of financial payment.

Paul McNeill rejects the analogy between employment and research participation on different grounds. He argues that work is "not normally a risky practice," and that the risks are generally known in advance "and can be minimized by safe practices."[48] This is doubly wrong. First, the risks of *many* jobs are actually much greater than the risks of much clinical research. Second, while the actual effects of a particular study may not be knowable in advance, we can make reasonable estimates of the risks of certain types of research based on evidence from studies with animals, the results of Phase I trials (for later research), the chemistry of the drug, etc. We know, for example, that few participants in Phase I trials require hospitalization. There is simply no reason to think that the risks involved in research are of greater magnitude or predictability than the risks involved in timber cutting and coal mining.

McNeill also rejects the analogy between dangerous work and research participation on the grounds that participation in research is *less important* than dangerous work and so there is less reason to allow people to incur research-related risks. He argues that whereas some dangerous work is "necessary to society . . . the justification for research is always in terms of progress: some added benefit to society . . . ."[49] On this view, whereas fire fighting is necessary to preserve the society, research that would (merely?) cure diseases from which people suffer or die is not. McNeill approvingly refers to Hans Jonas's remark that "progress is an optional goal," that "there is no necessity about seeking new knowledge or finding 'new miracle cures."[50] Why is progress optional? Because, says Jonas, whereas a "slower progress in the conquest of disease would not threaten society . . . [it] would . . . be threatened by the erosion of those moral values . . . caused by too ruthless a pursuit of scientific progress . . ."[51]

It is difficult to respond to such lofty rhetoric, but the argument strikes me as silly and even pernicious. A few quick points. First, we do well to remember that yesterday's "miracle cure" which was the product of "nonnecessary" medical research is today's ordinary medical treatment. Second, it is not clear why the preservation of *society* is the right unit of analysis as contrasted, say, with the health of the discrete individuals who compose it. It is true, as Jonas writes, that "If cancer, heart disease, and other organic noncontiguous ills . . . continue to exact their toll at the normal rate of incidence (including the toll of private anguish and misery), society can go on flourishing in every way."[52] Society can go on flourishing amidst all sorts of misfortunes and immoralities, although Jonas seems to think that, in a "subtler sense," society "cannot 'afford' a single miscarriage of justice, a single inequity in the dispensation of its laws, the violation of the rights of even the tiniest minority, because these undermine the moral basis on which society's existence rests."[53] This I simply do not get. Third, even if there were reason to distinguish between factors that threaten to harm society as an ongoing enterprise and those that (merely) promise to benefit society, there is no reason to think that the latter are of little moral weight or of insufficient weight to justify allowing people to freely choose to offer their services to advance that goal in exchange for payment. We let people accepts employment risks to provide us with "frivolous" goods. We don't *need* lobsters. I see no reason to think there is more reason to respect a person's decision to accept the risks of lobster fishing than to respect her decision to accept the risks of participation in research.

Lynn Jansen thinks that not allowing people to participate in research—for any reason—*can't* disrespect their autonomy because people have no autonomy based right to participate in research.[54]

> *Unreasonable Optimism.* A is conducting a Phase I trial of a new treatment for colon cancer. Although A explains to B that there is no reason for her to think that she will be helped by this treatment, B says she is willing to participate. When A probes B's reasons, it becomes clear that despite what A has said, B is unreasonably optimistic that the treatment will work for *her*. Because A believes that B's consent is tainted by such optimism, A excludes B from the trial.

Jansen argues that for B to object to being excluded from the trial on this ground is for B to assume that she has "an autonomy-based claim to participate in clinical research" and that she is owed a "non-paternalistic justification for the exclusion." Jansen says that assumption should be rejected: "Exclusion from a clinical trial, whether for ethical or scientific reasons, does not set back the autonomy of anyone, since there is no general right to have the option to participate in clinical research."[55]

Jansen goes wrong and we can learn from her error. First, B is certainly not owed a *non*-paternalistic justification for being excluded if A has a sound (soft-)paternalistic justification for excluding her and unreasonable optimism may be one such reason. Second, if we assume that B is a competent decision maker, then B *can* reasonably claim that A fails to respect her autonomy. Jansen mistakenly conflates a right to be treated on the basis of certain *reasons* with a right to obtain some *opportunity* that one is pursuing. Consider racial discrimination. B may have a right not to be denied a job on the basis of her race even if she has no right to the job itself. Similarly, B may have a right not to be excluded from an opportunity for paternalistic reasons even if B has no general right to the opportunity.

If we confine ourselves to reasons grounded in the protection of subjects, respect for the autonomy of participants entails that IRBs cannot justify placing limits on the ability of prospective participants to receive financial payments as compensation for accepting risks if it is clear that the participants would be making an autonomous or reasonable judgment to do so. This does not mean that IRBs should approve research (such as (5) in Table 4-1) that exhibits a personally favorable risk/benefit ratio if it lacks sufficient social value. For the protection of subjects is not the only desideratum of ethical research. It does mean that *insofar as the IRB is concerned with the protection of research subjects* and *insofar as it seeks to respect the autonomy of prospective participants,* the default position should be not to constrain the ability of investigators to offer financial incentives to prospective participants.

This analysis may appear to have an unsettling implication. Respecting a prospective participant's autonomy or values requires that we evaluate the reasonableness of her participation in light of her own circumstances and values. Just as it might be reasonable for a person to accept the risks of a Phase I oncology trial if this represents her best chance for survival, it might be reasonable for an impoverished person to accept financial payment for unpleasant work or participation in a trial that involves non-trivial risks. We should avoid condescension. We don't ban commercial fishing on the grounds that the salaries may tempt poor people to risk their lives. We do not question the judgment of an unemployed single mother who accepts work as a custodian for $7.50 per hour. Similarly, IRBs should not conclude that just because it wouldn't be reasonable for middle class persons (them!) to accept a certain level of risk in exchange for a certain payment that it wouldn't be reasonable for poverty stricken persons to do so.

Objections to the Use of Financial Incentives: Autonomy and Compromised Consent

If the previous argument is on the right track, we should start from the assumption that respect for autonomy gives us reason not to bar or restrict the use of financial incentives. But we do not have to end there. This line of argument assumes that prospective subjects are making their decisions autonomously. That can be denied. The general thrust of autonomy-based objections to the use of financial payments is that such incentives can undermine the autonomy of the agent, and this is particularly so if the incentives are too great. As one who has spent too much of his life worrying about the concept of coercion, I have been struck by the pervasiveness of these worries, both in the literature of bioethics and in conversations with investigators and IRB members. I believe that most of these worries are misplaced. Incentives *can* compromise autonomy and can render consent non-transformative, but it is important to be clear about when and why this is so.

One oft-heard argument should be rejected out of hand. It is sometimes said that financial payments are worrisome when and because they motivate people to do something that they would otherwise not do. For example, an HHS document says that "The level of remuneration should not be so high as to cause a prospective subject to accept risks that he or she would not accept in the absence of the remuneration."[56] This is a complete non-starter. By itself, it is entirely unobjectionable to motivate someone to do something they would otherwise not do. If A persuades B to give blood or to give to charity by giving B reasons as to why she should do so, then A gets B to do something that B would otherwise not do. If A, a physician, tells B to take an antibiotic for her infection and B does so because B has confidence in A's judgment, then A gets B to do something that B would otherwise not do. If A induces B to mow his lawn by offering B a monetary payment, he gets B to do something B would otherwise not do. There is nothing problematic here.

There are two more plausible arguments to the effect that A's offer of incentives can compromise the autonomy of B's decision. Some claim that A's offer of financial incentives can effectively coerce subjects into enrolling. Second, A's offer of financial incentives may compromise the subject's capacity to rationally weigh the costs and benefits of her decision. This is the realm of "undue influence" or "undue incentives." Although coercion and undue influence are often conflated, they represent quite distinct worries. Coercion compromises the *voluntariness* but not (necessarily) the *rationality* of B's decision; "undue influence" compromises the *rationality* of B's decisions, although it need not compromise its *voluntariness*.

Coercion

It has been suggested that "attractive monetary incentives means participation in the study is no longer voluntary for some subjects, but rather a moneymaking enterprise . . . offering a large financial payment in exchange for volunteering may in itself be a form of coercion."[57] There are two claims here. First, it is suggested that if participation is a "moneymaking enterprise," then it is "no longer voluntary." This is false. Although we sometimes refer to volunteers as those who work without pay, it hardly follows that those who work for pay are not doing so voluntarily. A teenager may view shoveling neighbors' driveways as a moneymaking enterprise. He is not "volunteering," but it is perfectly voluntary. Second, the implication that larger payments are more coercive then smaller payments is also false. A large offer may be more efficacious in motivating B to shovel her driveway, but it is no more coercive.

So what is coercion? It is difficult (I think impossible) and unnecessary to provide a univocal account of the proper use of the *word* coercion. I have argued elsewhere that the "truth conditions" of a coercion claim—the claim that A coerces B to do X—vary with the purposes for which a coercion claim is made.[58] In some cases, we say that A coerces B whenever A threatens to make B worse off than B's *status quo* if B does not comply, even when such coercion is uncontroversially justifiable. So we may say that the state coerces its citizens to pay taxes without denying that such coercion is legitimate or even morally required. By contrast, there are contexts in which to say that A coerces B is to make a *normative* claim, for example, that B's consent is not transformative or that B is not responsible for what she has done or that agreements are not valid. The question here is clearly normative: Does A's offer of financial incentives render B's consent non-transformative? In the present context, no one says "It is true that incentives coerce, but it is legitimate to coerce citizens into participating in research by paying them."[59]

Putting aside some minor complications, I suggest that A coerces B to do X in a way that invalidates B's consent only if A proposes to violate B's rights or not fulfill an obligation to B if B chooses not do X. In other words, A's proposal is coercive only if A has no *right* to carry out his "declared unilateral plan," that is, what A proposes to do if his proposal is not accepted.[60] Call this the *rights violating view*.

It is commonly said that A coerces B to do X when A threatens to make B worse off than B's *status quo* if B does not do X. This is close to the truth, but it is not quite right. The "rights violating" approach is more accurate because it allows us to handle cases in which (1) A has a right to make B worse off than B's *status quo* or (2) A has an obligation to render B *better off* than B's *status quo*. To illustrate (1), a prosecutor does not coerce a defendant into pleading guilty to a crime in exchange for a relatively lenient sentence when he proposes to take her to trial if she does not plead guilty, even though both options—pleading guilty and going to trial—are worse than B's *status quo*. Why? Because the prosecutor has a *right* to take the defendant to trial and relative to what the prosecutor has a right to do, the prosecutor is actually making an offer of leniency and not a threat. We do not say that B is coerced if she settles a dispute with a plaintiff simply because the plaintiff has proposed to take her to court if she does not agree to a settlement. Otherwise, settlements would be impossible. To illustrate (2), if a physician has an obligation to provide a patient with free medical services, say because he is employed by the U.K. National Health Service, then he coerces a patient into paying him a fee if he proposes *not* to provide such services unless the patient pays. And this is so even though the physician does not propose to render B worse off than her *status quo* if B declines. Why? Because the physician's declared unilateral plan—not to provide B with free services—would violate B's right to free medical service.

Note that A's coercive threat does *not* necessarily nor even typically compromise the *rationality* of B's decision. Some threats do trigger a type of mental paralysis, but the standard cases of coercion are different.

> *Extortion.* A is a mobster. B owns a restaurant. A says to B: "You may find that the windows on your restaurant are broken unless you agree to hire my company to remove your garbage. Think it over. Talk to your friends. Talk to the police. Let me know if you want to hire my company next week."

B might make a perfectly rational decision to hire A's company. B may calmly weigh the costs and benefits of compliance. B may investigate the prospects of informing the police and decide that it is better to comply after learning that the mobster has the police in his pocket as well. B makes a business decision to comply with A's proposal, and yet A has coerced B to hire his company because his declared unilateral plan (to break the windows of B's restaurant) would violate B's rights.

If A coerces B to do X only if A proposes or threatens to violate B's rights if B does not do X, then A does not coerce B to do X if A proposes to give a benefit to B if B does X. Threats are coercive but genuine offers are not. Threats reduce the options available to the target, whereas offers expand them and one does not coerce another when one's proposal expands the options available to her. And this is true even if A makes what we might call an "unattractive offer." If B is earning $100,000 in her present job and A offers B a comparable job at $95,000, then A's offer expands the options available to B. It's just that the new option is less attractive than B's *status quo.*

If normal offers do not coerce, can *extremely* attractive offers coerce? Many seem to think so. Ruth Macklin has said that the question as to how large a payment constitutes a coercive offer is one for "which no clear answer is forthcoming."[61] I disagree. A clear answer is forthcoming: Genuine offers do not coerce. Period.

Joel Feinberg *appears* to disagree, and the italicized word is crucial. Consider one of Feinberg's famous cases (which I paraphrase).

The Lecherous Millionaire. B, who is poor, needs money to pay for expensive surgery that alone can save her child's life. A, a millionaire, indicates that he will pay for the surgery if B becomes his mistress for a period.[62]

Feinberg argues that A's proposal is a freedom-enhancing offer and not a threat because it adds to B's options. Nonetheless, Feinberg suggests that A's proposal is coercive because it rearranges B's options such that B has "no choice" but to accept."[63] I concede that Feinberg is on plausible *linguistic* grounds here. People often say that one is coerced or forced to do something when one has no reasonable alternative. But there is much less here than meets the eye. Feinberg writes that even though he is linguistically prepared to call A's proposal coercive, the important *moral* question is "what bearing . . . the coerciveness of an otherwise freedom-enhancing offer has on the consent which it produces." And from *that* perspective, Feinberg says that the "voluntariness of B's consent is *not* sufficiently reduced by A's coercive offer to be invalidated."[64] As Feinberg adds, A could "hardly be convicted of rape." So despite the apparent conceptual and linguistic disagreement, Feinberg and I agree on the substantive moral point, namely, that a freedom-enhancing offer does not coerce in a way that renders consent non-transformative.

Those who think that offers can coerce, sometimes appeal to the well known phrase from *The Godfather*—"My father made him an offer he couldn't refuse." But Don Corleone's proposal was coercive not because it was an exceptionally attractive offer, but because it was a paradigmatically coercive threat—"Either your signature or your brains will be on the contract." So this conceit does nothing to support the view that genuine offers can coerce in a way that renders consent non-transformative.

Now to say that offers do not coerce is not to deny that offers can be seriously immoral.

Bribe. A, a police officer, stops B for speeding. B offers to give A $100 if B does not write a ticket. A accepts.

It is immoral for B to offer a bribe to A and it is immoral for A to accept a bribe, but we do not think that B's offer of a financial incentive coerces A into accepting B's bribe in a way that negates or reduces A's responsibility for accepting it. Similarly, if A offers to pay B $10,000 to kill C, B could hardly claim that he committed the crime under duress. B could hardly say, "But I didn't do it voluntarily. A coerced me into killing C by offering a financial incentive." And we would not change our judgment if A offered to pay B $1,000,000.

Some think that A coerces B to do X when A's proposal leaves B with "no reasonable alternative" but to accept A's proposal. This is a natural but deeply mistaken view about coercion. It is a natural view because it is true that one generally has no reasonable alternative but to succumb to a coercive proposal. But it does not follow that one is coerced to accept A's proposal in a way that renders consent non-transformative *just in case* or *because* one has no reasonable alternative.

There are two ways in which we might interpret having "no reasonable alternative," and neither amount to coercion. On one view, one has no reasonable alternative when the utility *distance* between the alternatives is so great that it would be *irrational* to reject the better alternative, and (virtually) no one would do so. If A offers B $1,000 to mow his lawn (a one hour job), B may have no reasonable alternative but to accept, given the utility distance between the two options: (1) $1,000 + mowing A's lawn, and (2) 0 + not mowing A's lawn. Yet B is obviously not coerced.

A second and more plausible interpretation of "no reasonable alternative" focuses on the unacceptability of B's situation if she rejects A's proposal. On this view, A's offer is coercive if rejecting A's proposal would leave B in dire straits and this may be so even if A's offer is not that much better than B's *status quo*.

> *Volunteer Army.* B enlists in the Army because he lacks decent
>   civilian career opportunities.

Michael Sandel argues that "volunteer army" is a misnomer: "The difference between conscription and the volunteer army is not that one is compulsory, whereas the other is not; it is rather that each employs *a different form of compulsion*—the state in the first case, economic necessity in the second."[65] Sandel might be engaged in linguistic hyperbole to draw attention to the background facts that motivate some people to enlist in the military. Fair enough. But it is important to see that "necessity" as such does not constitute compulsion or coercion of the form that renders consent invalid. Consider:

> *Breast Surgery.* A biopsy has shown that B has a malignant tumor
>   in her breast. A, a breast oncologist, tells B that she must have

surgery or she will be unlikely to survive more than a year.
B consents.

B may have "no reasonable alternative" to accepting A's proposal, but A has surely not coerced B and, more importantly, we would *not* say that A has performed surgery on B's breast without B's voluntary and valid consent.

It is sometimes claimed that A's offer coerces B when A knowingly takes advantage of B's *vulnerability*. But this, too, can't be right. In principle, it is entirely unproblematic for A to take advantage of B's need for assistance or desire to strike an agreement. B would not agree to hire a plumber if her pipes were not frozen. Consider:

> *Desperation*. B is selling her house because she is taking a job in a
> different city. She listed the house for $300,000, but has
> lowered the price to $200,000 because the move is pending
> and she is desperate to sell. A agrees to pay $200,000.

Although A has taken advantage of B's vulnerable position, B can hardly claim that her agreement to sell has been coerced or that the contract is not valid. It is arguable that A should have offered to pay more, but if B signs the contract and then receives a better offer, she cannot claim that the contract is not binding because she signed out of desperation. So, those who claim that offers of payment to prospective research subjects who are in vulnerable positions render them incapable of giving voluntary consent must explain why there is no coercion of the vulnerable in *Desperation* but there is coercion of the vulnerable to participate in research. I doubt they can do so.

It might be argued that there is a moral distinction between desperate situations that arise from misfortune (as in *Breast Surgery* and *Desperation*) and desperate situations that arise from injustice. This may be true. *Ceteris paribus* (all things being equal), we have a stronger duty to remedy or rectify desperate conditions that are due to injustice than those due to misfortune. But the difference between misfortune and injustice has little bearing on the voluntariness of transactions that occur within the framework of those conditions when the alleged coercer did not create or has no duty to rectify those conditions. Consider:

> *Domestic*. A advertises for a house cleaner and offers to pay
> minimum wage. B, who has been unjustly fired from her
> previous job, accepts because she needs to support her family.

Even though B is driven by "economic compulsion" to accept A's offer and even though B's poor background condition is clearly due to injustice, A has not coerced B into accepting her job. B has claims of rectification against her former employer, but has no claim against A. Similarly, if B accepts an offer to participate in research because her dire background conditions arise from injustice, it does not follow that her decision is involuntary or coerced.

The issue here is not just conceptual. To regard B's decision as coerced in *Desperation* or *Domestic* would have unfortunate consequences for both A and B. Recall the fair transaction model of consent transactions. It would be unfair to A to void the agreement when A has no responsibility for creating or rectifying B's background conditions. As Robert Goodin has observed, if any wrong in the past could upset an agreement or invalidate consent, then no one could be secure in acting.[66] More importantly, it would be unfair to B. For if B's decision were regarded as coerced or non-transformative, then A will avoid transacting with B—much to B's regret. So when IRBs bar research or constrain the level of financial incentives on the grounds that the financial incentives are coercive, they are denying prospective subjects an opportunity they might welcome.

It might be objected that my argument has a conservative bias, that it somehow "accepts" the status as defining a person's entitlements.[67] Not so. The argument only claims that we must distinguish between moral objections to a person's background circumstances and moral objections to transactions that occur within those circumstances. David Rothman writes that "abject poverty is harsh enough without people having to bear the additional burdens of serving as research subjects."[68] But if research participants are *benefiting* from participating in research all things considered, we might just as well say that abject poverty is harsh enough without denying people the opportunity to make their lives somewhat less miserable by participating in biomedical research and receiving financial payments that they would not otherwise receive. We can grant that people "do not have enough options and that society has been unjust to them in not extending more options, while nonetheless respecting and honoring the choices they actually make in reduced circumstances."[69] Wars can be fought on multiple fronts simultaneously, although I have chosen to fight only one of those wars in this project. This is not, however, the end of the story about compromised consent.

Undue Inducements and Irrationality

Offers of financial payments can render consent non-transformative if the prospective subject cannot make a competent and rational decision response. This is the realm of undue influence—not coercion. As Bishop Butler put it, "Everything is what it is and not another thing."[70] I have previously referred to such proposals as "seductive offers."[71] Seductive offers are genuine *offers*, because A does not propose to violate B's rights if B should reject the proposal. Seductive offers are *seductive* when B's decision-making in response to the offer is flawed or compromised. The phrase—seductive offer—is somewhat misleading because "seductiveness" is a feature of B's *decision-making* in *response* to an offer and not a feature of the offer itself. A given proposal may be a non-seductive offer to an agent who can rationally weigh its advantages and disadvantages while constituting a seductive offer to an agent whose decision-making is flawed. Similarly, an inducement is "undue" in virtue of the target's inability to respond to that inducement in a rational manner. It is *not* a function of the magnitude of the inducement.

The phrase "undue inducement" or "undue influence" appears in some of the canonical statements of research ethics, in regulatory documents, and in the work of bioethicists. The Common Rule states that "An investigator shall seek such consent only under circumstances that provide the prospective subject or the representative sufficient opportunity to consider whether or not to participate and that minimize the possibility of coercion or undue influence."[72] An HHS document that elaborates on the Common Rule states that while paying research subjects is a "common and, in general, acceptable practice. . . IRBs must be sensitive to whether any aspect of the proposed remuneration will be an undue influence."[73] The Syracuse University IRB handbook states that "Incentives or payments must not be of such an amount as to result in undue influence on an individual's decision to participate, especially in the case of persons who are poor."[74]

The key word is *undue*. I believe that an inducement should be regarded as undue only when it triggers irrational decision-making given the agent's own settled (and reasonable) values and aims. As *The Official IRB guidebook* (33) puts it, an offer is troublesome if it is so "attractive that [it can] *blind* prospective subjects to potential risks or impair their ability to exercise *proper judgment* about the risks of participation" (emphasis added). An inducement is *not* morally problematic if it is *genuinely* too good to refuse. It is problematic if it *seems* to be too good to be refused and would be refused if the agent's judgment were not blinded or clouded or impaired. Distortion of judgment is the key.

An agent's decision-making may be distorted by the offer of inducements in at least two ways. An agent experiences *tunnel vision* when the lure of the payment causes the patient to ignore or give inadequate consideration to other relevant interests—including the interests of others. An agent experiences *decisional myopia* when she is aware of her other interests, but the lure of the inducement causes her to overweight the short-term benefits and underestimate or underweight the long-term costs of accepting the proposal. Just as drug addicts display what George Ainslie calls "hyperbolic discounting" of the future costs of their behavior, prospective participants may excessively discount the future costs of their participation.[75] Moreover, even if B recognizes—on a cognitive level—that she should not accept A's proposal, she may experience weakness of will. Just as people may accept the offer of an alcoholic beverage or a piece of pie even though they recognize that it is not in their interest to do so, someone might accept the offer of financial payment for participation in research even though she recognizes that doing so does not advance her long term interests.

Some commentators do not adequately attend to the distinction between distorted and non-distorted responses to inducements. Consider once again the study of malaria mortality in Malawi in which investigators were prepared to pay for burial expenses for the deceased children whose parents agreed to an autopsy. Lemmons and Nwabueze say this:

> . . . economic pressure and the need to offset expenses related to a decent burial could conceivably become an incentive for many poor families to participate when they might otherwise prefer not to. The voluntariness of the consent could be undermined as much in this case as when, for example, $10,000 is paid to university students in developed countries for participating in a study that offers no benefits.[76]

They are wrong in both cases. I see no reason to think that university students are acting involuntarily in accepting $10,000 to participate in a study, if their judgment that the payment is adequate compensation for the risk is not distorted. Similarly, if poor Malawian parents were to authorize autopsies for their deceased children "when they might otherwise prefer not to" precisely to be able to provide a decent burial for their children, there is no reason to think that their reasoning is distorted, although it is possible that they are overweighting their present desire and underestimating the anguish they will come to experience.[77]

Another oft-encountered interpretation of undue inducements should also be rejected. The Council for the International Organization of Medical Sciences worries that the offer of monetary payments may "induce prospective subjects to consent to participate in the research *against their better judgment*"[78] (emphasis added). Similarly, Grant and Sugarman state that "A destitute person may be induced to do something *against his or her better judgment*, and even almost against his or her will, by the offer of a large amount of money."[79] But what does that mean? The phrase "against one's better judgment" sometimes conveys that we do something reluctantly or that one's choice violates an important value. For example, a professor might say to a student, "It's against my better judgment but I'll grant your request for an extension on your paper." The professor does not think that he acts involuntarily or that he is not responsible for his decision or that granting the extension is against his better judgment, *all things considered*. A's offer of money (or medical benefits) may motivate B to do something that *would* have been against her better judgment in the absence of the offer, but that does not show that acceptance of the offer is against her better judgment *given* the value of the offer to her.

It is important to distinguish between two claims:

(1) an inducement distorts the subject's judgment such that the subject consents to participate when doing so does not advance his interests;

(2) given the subject's objective circumstances, an inducement actually renders it rational for the subject to participate.

In (1), the offer constitutes an undue inducement because the subject's judgment is distorted. In (2), the inducements are large enough to render participation *compatible* with the participant's better judgment. She is making a reasonable judgment that she is better off accepting the proposal.

In commenting on the TGN 1412 trial, Benjamin Hale writes that some of the participants were members of an "economically vulnerable population; members who, presumably, would have made a different decision had they been in a position in which their personal valuations of the incentive were not *clouded* by their economic standing."[80] The key word here is "clouded." The question is not whether economically vulnerable people would make a different decision than they would make if they were not economically vulnerable. I would not hire a plumber if my pipes were not frozen. The issue is whether the decision-making of economically vulnerable people is "clouded" or distorted by their economic standing.

It is sometimes argued that an offer constitutes an undue inducement or compromises voluntariness if it is "so large or in excess that it is irresistible in this context."[81] Once again, we must be careful. We cannot say that an offer is irresistible just because one finds it hard to reject it, for that is true of all choices for which we have strong desires. We might say that a proposal is irresistible just in case no reasonable person (in that person's situation) would reject the proposal, as when a person of modest means is offered $1,000 to mow a lawn. But that would rob the concept of any moral punch.

If "irresistibility" is to do any moral work, it must involve distortion of judgment. An offer might be so tempting—irresistible—that the target accepts it even though the target realizes or should realize that it is in her long-term interest to decline. In a famous study of the capacity for delayed gratification, 4-year-olds were left in a room with a bell and a marshmallow.[82] If they rang the bell, the investigator would come back and they could eat the marshmallow. If they didn't ring the bell and waited for the investigator to return on his own, they could then have two marshmallows. Many found the offer of an immediate marshmallow to be "irresistible." Even though some understood that they would be better off if they waited, many seemed not to be able to defer gratification. It would be problematic for investigators to prey upon this sort of irresistibility, but there is no reason to think that this often occurs.

Here we encounter what Macklin regards as the "paradoxical case of payment."

> The paradox can be stated as follows: the higher the monetary payment, the greater is the benefit; the greater the benefit, the more acceptable is the research. However, the greater the monetary payment, the more potential subjects are unduly influenced to participate . . . the more coercive the recruitment, the more unacceptable is the research.[83]

Now, given that Macklin does not think that payment should not count as a benefit at all, it is not clear that the first part of the paradox gets going on her terms. But if we set aside the conflation of coercion and undue inducement and if we assume that payment is a benefit (at least from the subject's point of view) and that increasing such benefits renders research more acceptable, the paradox can be unraveled once we see that the relationship between the magnitude of the financial payment and the rationality of the potential subject's decision may not be linear.

Suppose that we can evaluate protocols in terms of the utility effects on participants across four dimensions: (1) the burdens and risks of participation as assessed by a rational decision-maker; (2) the value of financial payment as assessed by a rational decision-maker; (3) the "objective" risk/benefit ratio (the sum of (1) and (2)); and (4) the "perceived" risk/benefit ratio by a given decision-maker. The *perceived* risk/benefit ratio (4) may be more favorable than the *actual* risk/benefit ratio (3) if the lure of a financial payment causes the agent to underestimate or excessively discount the long-term risks of participation (1) or overestimate the value of financial payment (2). (The perceived risk/benefit ratio may be less favorable than the actual risk/benefit ratio, but, interestingly, we do not worry about cases in which a person makes an irrational decision not to participate.)

Consider three possible protocols: (a) – (c).

Table 4.3

	(1) Actual Risk	(2) Actual Financial Benefit	(3) Actual R/B Ratio	(4) Perceived R/B ratio
(a)	-50	25	-25	-20
(b)	-50	40	-10	10
(c)	-50	60	10	30

An egoistic or prudent subject would refuse to participate in (a) because she believes (it so happens correctly) that the risk/benefit ratio is unfavorable. By contrast, the subject might agree to participate in (b) and (c) because she believes that the risk/benefit ratio is favorable. We might say that (b) constitutes a case of *undue* inducement because the subject's decision-making is distorted by the offer of financial payment. A rational decision-maker would believe that the payment does not actually compensate her for the risks and burdens, although she believes that it does. On the other hand, (c) is *not* a case of undue inducement. Even though she overestimates the extent to which she benefits from participation, a rational decision-maker would correctly believes that she can expect to benefit from participation. When we compare (a) and (b), the larger payment (b) constitutes an *undue* inducement because it motivates the subject to make an *irrational* decision. But when we compare (b) and (c) the larger payment does *not* make the inducement "more undue" as it were. To the contrary. It actually renders participation compatible with the subject's interests.

Now it might be argued that IRBs are not in a position to make the assessments reflected in Table 4.3. How are they to evaluate the actual and perceived value of the financial benefits to participants? Although they clearly cannot and should not attempt to do this on an individual basis, the question is whether they can make an overall judgment about the class of prospective participants or some sub-groups. In any case, and as I argued above, IRBs cannot *avoid* making such assessments *if* they are to consider whether a protocol is offering undue inducements. *The logic of the concept of undue inducement requires it.* An IRB cannot claim that a financial payment of some magnitude will motivate many or most prospective participants to make an irrational decision unless they have a basis for assessing its irrationality.

Grant and Sugarman introduce a different and interesting angle on undue inducement. They argue that while incentives are always designed to motivate "someone to do what they otherwise might not," there is something ethically suspect about using an incentive to get "someone to do something to which they are *averse* . . . And the ethical problem is multiplied where the aversion is a principled one or a matter of moral scruple."[84]

Start with simple—non-moral—aversion. I'm not sure I understand the distinction between: (1) getting someone to do something they would otherwise not do in the absence of an incentive and (2) getting someone to do something to which they are averse. If I would not work unless I were paid for doing so, does it not mean that I am averse to working without being paid? Grant and Sugarman might say that I'm not averse to teaching college students but I might be averse, say, to teaching middle school students or mowing lawns. I don't think this reply will work. For whatever sum of money that would be sufficient to motivate me to teach college students (to which I would be averse in the absence of being paid that sum), there is a greater sum that would be sufficient to motivate me to teach middle school or mow lawns. Here we are reminded of the (apocryphal?) story in which George Bernard Shaw asked a woman if she would sleep with him for a million pounds. When she said that she would, he asked if she would do so for one pound and sixpence. "Certainly not?" the woman huffed, "what do you think

I am?" Shaw responded, "We've already established that. Now we're merely haggling about the price." Now it is true that some people genuinely enjoy their work. Indeed, some people work for free—think retired people who do volunteer work in hospitals. Still, most people who enjoy their work would be averse to working without pay. So, as a general matter there is no important distinction between giving people an incentive to do that which they would otherwise not do and giving people an incentive to do that to which they are otherwise averse.

In response, Grant and Sugarman might claim that things are different if the aversion is "a principled one or a matter of moral scruple," as for example, if one tried "to induce religious people to work on the Sabbath by offering large incentives," or if Shaw's prospect had a moral objection to non-marital or commercial sex.[85] This is tricky. I share the intuition that inducing someone to violate what they take to be an important principle (observing the Sabbath) is different from inducing one to do something they find unpleasant (mowing lawns) but not immoral, and this is so even if one's moral principles are of doubtful validity. It does seem perverse to offer Mormons a large cash incentive to participate in a study of the effects of caffeine on the brain (the research may require people who have never consumed caffeine), even if there is nothing intrinsically wrong with the consumption of caffeine. But I am not sure to what extent this intuition is defensible.

First, people do not all place the same weight on their moral commitments as contrasted with their non-moral interests. Second, and more importantly, even if an offer may motivate B to violate *one* of her moral values, people have multiple values and commitments. Consider this case.

> *Family.* A wants to hire B. The job would require that B spend much
> of her time traveling. B tells A that she is reluctant to accept
> because she thinks she has an obligation to her spouse and
> children to work close to home. A raises the offer. B accepts.

Grant and Sugarman might argue that A is acting wrongly in making the offer to B because he is seeking to get B to do something to which she was averse on moral grounds (her obligation to her family). I disagree. First, there is some moral reason to endorse a "moral division of labor" as between employers and prospective employees, such that employers should be encouraged to advance the interests of their organizations and leave it to prospective employees to protect their own interests and commitments. Second, it might be objectionably paternalistic for A to not offer B a payment on this ground.

Unless A has reason to think that his offer will distort B's judgment, A shows respect for B's autonomy by allowing B to make her own decisions in the light of her own value structure and by not preemptively short-circuiting B's decision process. Third, and as I noted above, people have *multiple* aims, projects, and obligations. B may believe that she has an obligation to spend time with her family, but she may also believe that she has a greater obligation to provide for them financially. Hale says that the jury is "still out" on whether a desire to make one's family more secure is a "permissible reason" to accept a financial incentive.[86] But what would a jury need to know? *Ceteris paribus,* I would think that such a desire is among the most praiseworthy reasons for action.

To further exemplify the previous point, recall the grisly example in which malaria investigators considered offering Malawi parents a coffin and burial expenses if they allowed an autopsy to be performed on their deceased child. Although the parents might have had moral objections to autopsies, it was also of moral importance to them to provide a decent burial for their children. Given that financial incentives might actually enhance the recipient's capacity to fulfill some of one's moral obligations, it is difficult to see why there should be any general reason to avoid using financial incentives to motivate people to do things to which they are *otherwise* averse on moral grounds.

In sum, an offer of financial payment to a prospective subject constitutes a morally problematic undue inducement only if a subject's response to the offer is irrational or her reasoning is distorted. Absent a showing that participants are making irrational judgments in response to offers of financial payment, there is no reason to reject them on this ground.

The Right to Withdraw and Completion Bonuses

Just as bioethics has worried about the relation between financial payment and the decision to *enroll* in research, it has also worried about the relation between financial payment and the decision to *withdraw* from research.

It is accepted wisdom that one has a right to withdraw from research, by which it is meant that there should be no penalties for withdrawal. As with many other principles of research ethics, this principle is thought to be so uncontroversial as not to require much explication or defense. I think it needs both.

The standard view is that to have a right to withdraw from a trial means that one should be able to withdraw "without penalty or loss of benefits to which the subject is otherwise entitled."[87] Note, however, that to say that subjects have a *right* to withdraw does not mean or entail that it is always morally legitimate for them to do so, although I think some would endorse this stronger claim. For one can have a moral right to do what is otherwise wrong. For example, one may have a right to engage in offensive speech, but it may be wrong to do so nonetheless. I simply see no reason to think that it is always morally acceptable to withdraw from a research protocol without good reason, and this is particularly so when investigators have made considerable investments in each subject and when withdrawal will seriously compromise the data. There might be good reason not to penalize people for withdrawing or even not to demand such reasons, but I see no reason to think that participants should always have a free moral pass to stay or leave.

The accepted view is not only that that research subjects have a right to withdraw at any time, but, in addition, that the right is *inalienable*. It is a right that that cannot be waived or traded by one's own voluntary actions. It is not clear why this is so. After all, most of our rights—including many of our most cherished rights—are eminently alienable. Indeed, our rights are valuable, in part, precisely because we can waive them in exchange for something of greater value. I can't be forced to work against my will, but I can certainly agree to work in exchange for wages. I may have the right to wear whatever color shirt I prefer, but I can waive that right if I want to work at a restaurant that requires its staff to wear black. One may have a right to freedom of speech, but one can sign a confidentiality (or non-disclosure) agreement as a condition of being hired.

Of greater relevance to the present topic, there are numerous ordinary contexts in which people can and should be able to make commitments that involve substantial penalties for non-fulfillment. As a general proposition, whenever the parties to an agreement must perform non-simultaneously (as when A hires B to fix a leaky faucet), then the party that first incurs the cost (A pays or B performs the service) may want to be assured that the other party will perform. If B wants to borrow money from A at Time-1, B had better be able to bind herself to pay A at Time-2, or A will not loan her the money. Given this, the default moral position is that research subjects should be able to make a similar commitment to investigators.

Having said this, we are sometimes justified in treating a right as inalienable. In effect, minimum wage laws give people a right not to work for less than a specified wage that is not waivable and could not be waivable if it were to serve its intended purpose. In most states, one cannot make a legally binding commitment not to divorce one's spouse. In effect, the right to divorce is inalienable. Some jurisdictions give people an inalienable right to rent (or give landlords an inalienable duty to provide) a "habitable" dwelling that meets certain minimal standards of safety and comfort. One cannot agree to rent an uninhabitable apartment even if one wanted to do so in exchange for lower rent. Setting aside special contexts such as boxing matches or surgery, one has an inalienable right not to be victimized by battery. As a general rule, one cannot consent to be beaten. And until such time as voluntary euthanasia is permitted, one has an inalienable legal right not to be killed. B may *forfeit* her right not to be killed, as when A kills B in self-defense, but B cannot simply waive her right not to be killed, thereby rendering it permissible for A to kill B.

What justifies treating a right as inalienable? In some cases, we treat a right as inalienable because it is difficult to determine whether a waiver is based on morally transformative consent. If A is fighting with B outside a bar, how can we tell whether B agreed to fight? It is better to assume that B did not agree and treat the right not to be beaten as inalienable. In other cases we may treat a right as inalienable because we think it is essential to living an autonomous life. Mill famously argued that one should not be free to sell oneself into slavery—"The principle of freedom cannot require that he should be free not to be free. It is not freedom, to be allowed to alienate his freedom."[88] For similar reasons, we may treat the right to divorce as inalienable because we think it crucial that people preserve freedom of choice in areas of life that are of the most profound consequence to their well-being. Somewhat less famously, Mill noted that treating some rights as inalienable helps to solve collective action problems.[89] Although it might be in the interest of an individual to agree to work for less than a certain wage rather than remain unemployed, it may be better for the *class* of unskilled workers (including many of those individuals) that they *not* be able to agree to work for less than a minimum wage.

All these exceptions to the contrary notwithstanding, the moral default position is that a right is alienable at the discretion of the right-holder. So if we assume that one starts with a right to withdraw from a research protocol at any time, it simply does not follow that one should be barred from waiving that right in exchange for opportunities or benefits that one would not otherwise receive and which one has no pre-existing right to receive. Given that investigators may need to make considerable investments in research subjects, it is possible that it would be better for investigators and subjects if subjects were able to make a binding commitment to remain in the protocol.

To illustrate the previous point, suppose that A were to allow B to choose among these three options in a research protocol in which there is no prospect of a direct medical benefit to B, but which requires a large investment by A for each participant.

(1) B receives no financial payment and may withdraw at any time without penalty.

(2) B receives $5000 for enrolling in the protocol but also agrees to repay the $5,000 + a penalty of $1,000 if she withdraws from the protocol. Both parties put their funds (or collateral) in an escrow account to be administered by an impartial third-party.

(3) B receives $5000 for enrolling in the protocol and agrees not to withdraw from the protocol on pain of being held in contempt of court for breach of contract.

Let us assume that (3) is off the table as it involves what contract law calls "specific performance" and that (1) is perfectly acceptable. The present question is whether (2) might be acceptable. I assume that if B chooses (2), she has effectively waived her right to withdraw without penalty. Note, however, that it might be perfectly rational for both A and B to prefer (2) to (1) even if, *ex ante*, B knows that there are risks and burdens to remaining in the protocol that could be avoided by choosing option (1). If we say, however, that B has an *inalienable* right to withdraw from a protocol without penalty, then we effectively preclude B from choosing the option (2) that she and A would both prefer. It may be justifiable to preclude B from choosing (2), but it is not clear why.

Let us assume for the sake of argument that subjects do have an inalienable right to withdraw from a research protocol at any time, except, perhaps, when abrupt withdrawal might endanger their health or the health or safety of others (We may not allow psychiatric patient/subjects to leave the hospital during a washout period from medication). The present question is this: Is the right to withdraw from research compromised by a payment schedule that contains a substantial completion bonus or, as in the TGN1412 trial, where the receipt of the entire payment is conditional upon completion?

Many seem to think so. Some institutions appear to ban completion bonuses entirely. The Syracuse University IRB Handbook says this:

> Incentives must not be provided on a schedule that results in coercion or undue influence on an individual's decision to continue participation. That is, incentives must not be withheld as a condition of an individual completing the research. If an individual withdraws early, payments or incentives must be prorated to reflect the time and inconvenience of the individual's participation up until that point.[90]

Other institutions place restrictions on the *proportion* of the financial payment that can be made as a completion bonus. The University of California at Irvine's regulations state that "Participants who withdraw before completion of the study should receive accrued compensation in a timely manner" and that while the "entire payment" should not be contingent upon completion, "payment of a small proportion as an incentive for completion is acceptable, providing that such incentive is not coercive."[91] The University of Vermont's policy states that "bonuses contingent on performance are allowed beyond the base, as long as they do not constitute more than half of the total amount that a subject may be compensated."[92]

Are completion bonuses problematic? A payment schedule cannot constitute a problematic *undue* inducement simply because it induces participants to remain when they "would otherwise have withdrawn," for that is the whole point of an inducement. After all, even a *pro rata* payment scheme affects a participant's willingness to withdraw. If one receives half the payment for completing half the protocol, one must remain in the protocol if one wants to receive the rest. So we must say that a completion bonus is an *undue* inducement only if it induces subjects to remain in a study when it gets them to make an irrational judgment to remain in the protocol.

The Common Rule states that "the subject may discontinue participation at any time without penalty or loss of benefits *to which the subject is otherwise entitled*" (emphasis added). Consider the TGN1412 study in this light. The first page of the consent document says participants can leave the trial at "any time without giving a reason and my rights will not be affected." But the document also states: "If you leave the study and exercise your right not to give a reason or are required to leave the study for non-compliance, no payment need be made to you."[93] Greg Koski, a physician and former head of the U.S. Office for Human Research Protection, said that this was "very coercive language . . . It's a bait and switch."[94]

Koski wrongfully equates a coercion argument and a "bait and switch" argument. Bait and switch is a manipulative strategy by which A lures B to do X and then gets B to switch to Y, as when A advertises a mattress for $100 and, once B is in the store, says, "Actually, that mattress isn't very good. Let me suggest that you buy this other mattress for $500." People often succumb to bait and switch techniques because they have incurred the cost of responding to a solicitation and want to get something for their efforts. Given that prospective subjects are often lured by the prospect of a financial payment and then informed about the risk and schedule of payments, there is some plausibility to the "bait and switch" complaint if they would have declined to participate if they had received (and adequately processed) the information up front.

Let us consider the argument from coercion. The Common Rule puts its finger on the crux of the issue because everything turns on the phrase: "to which the subject is otherwise entitled." I have argued that A coerces B to do X only if A's declared unilateral plan (in this case – not to pay) would constitute a violation of B's rights. On the strictest view, a subject is not "otherwise entitled" to *any* of the benefits of participation in research unless we assume that the investigators would have an obligation to provide those benefits even if the subject chose not to enter the protocol. On a less strict interpretation, we could say that participants are entitled to a fair share of the financial payment (if any), and thus a proposal to withhold benefits to which the subject was entitled as a matter of fairness if she withdrew would qualify as coercive. But that bootstrapping argument assumes what has to be shown, namely, that completion bonuses or a completion-only payment schedule are unfair.

There are many contexts in which it is perfectly fair to pay someone only if the job is completed, for example, an indexer for a book or a portrait painter. So barring some argument that explains why participation in research is fundamentally different, we can't bootstrap an argument from fairness into an argument from coercion.

If completion bonuses are not coercive, they could still constitute an undue inducement.

> . . . if the research is painful, debilitating, or distressing . . . a completion bonus can be seen as undue influence, not because it is the same as coercion, but because it can be used as a seductive pressure to overcome the subject's reasonable resistance to what he or she is being asked to suffer.[95]

We have to be careful here. The important question is not whether it is reasonable for a subject to resist and to want out of the study at the time of the suffering (Time-2). The question is whether the subject can reasonably agree, at Time-1, to a payment scheme that exerts pressure on her to overcome what she may anticipate is reasonable resistance to suffering at Time-2. Just as it was reasonable for Ulysses to asked to be tied to the mast because he knew—in advance—that he would find it difficult to resist the call of the sirens, it may be reasonable for a subject to agree to be paid (mostly) upon completion precisely because she realizes that—at a later point—she may want to withdraw.

Suppose that A's research requires 12 people to complete a trial that requires blood draws at 2, 4, and 6 month intervals after the last intervention. The data from non-completers is useless. A has $36,000 available for payment to subjects. If A offers pro-rata compensation, A expects 1/3 of the subjects to withdraw. So A has a choice between two payment schedules. On (PS1) A will enroll 18 people at $200 per session for 12 sessions. If 1/3 drop out, A will end up spending about $2000 a person, since some will receive less than $2,000 because they drop out quickly. Those who complete the study will receive $2,400. On (PS2) A enrolls 12 persons at $3,000 a person ($250 per session), payable only on completion. A is indifferent as between (1) and (2). A gets 12 completers for $36,000 either way. Some participants may well prefer (2) to (1). They would rather have more money and would be prepared to accept the risk that they would be paid nothing if they drop out. Would it be unfair for the investigators and subjects to agree to (PS2)? I can't see why. Just as I pay less for collision insurance premiums by agreeing to a large deductible and absorbing a greater risk of financial loss, we might think that subjects should be able to receive more money by absorbing the risk that they will want to withdraw.

Is a *"pro rata"* approach superior on grounds of fairness? Two points. First, if we are to evaluate a payment schedule in terms of fairness, we must consider it from the perspective of both A and B. Fairness is bi-lateral. A *pro rata* payment schedule *could* be unfair to A given that B's participation in a study may be of little or no value to A if B does not complete the protocol. Second, it is possible that the burdens or risks of participation in a protocol increase over time, and that a completion bonus more accurately reflects that fact. Suppose that some of the burdens on participants are similar to doing pushups. The first ten are easy; it's the second ten that are hard. If paying $100 for 20 pushups is a fair deal, a pro rata approach ($50 for the first 10;

$50 for the second 10) might be unfair, as it would fail to match the compensation to the actual burden. A similar principle might apply to research, as when a Phase I toxicity trial increases the dosage over time.

It is not my purpose to argue for a general practice of offering large completion bonuses. I have argued, however, that completion bonuses are generally compatible with a subject's right to withdraw from research and that specific limitations on completion bonuses are difficult to justify.

Objections to the Use of Financial Payments: Commodification

Aristotle remarked that usury was the most "hated sort" of exchange, not because it involved (as we now define it) excessive rates of interest, but because it is a "most unnatural" mode of gaining wealth.[96] Usury seeks to make "a gain out of money itself." Many contemporary commentators have adopted a similar view about the sale of one's body or bodily services, whether it take the form of selling sex or procreational labor or bodily organs or participation in clinical research. In his Tanner Lecture, "What Money Can't Buy: The Moral Limits of Markets," Michael Sandel considers "the degrading effect of market valuation and exchange on certain goods and practices."[97] Call this *the commodification argument*. It maintains that monetary incentives are improper when they wrongly commodify a human activity even if the decision to engage in that activity is uncontroversially voluntary, informed, competent, and so forth. Along these lines, Elizabeth Anderson objects to commercial surrogacy on the grounds that it commodifies procreational labor and degrades the women who serve as surrogates.[98] In discussing a proposal to allow the sale of kidneys, Leon Kass puts it this way: "Selling our bodies, we come perilously close to selling out our souls. . . . if we come to think ourselves like pork bellies, pork bellies we will become."[99]

The commodification argument has figured prominently in discussions of financial incentives in research. According to Ruth Macklin, "Payment to patients to serve as research subjects is an ethically unacceptable commodification of research practice."[100] Carl Elliott writes "Perhaps there is something inherently disconcerting about the idea of turning drug testing into a job."[101]

It is not clear just what force such arguments are meant to have. We can distinguish between three claims about the commodification of research: (1) commodification is a wrong-making feature of the practice of paying research subjects; (2) paying research subjects is generally wrong, all things considered; (3) society should seek to *regulate* or *prohibit* the practice. Even if we accept (1), and it is not clear that we should, note that (1) does not entail (2) and (2) does not entail (3). Claim (1) does not entail (2) because (2) requires us to evaluate all the values at stake and which may outweigh the (assumed) wrong-making feature of commodification. In addition, (2) does not entail (3) because a moral regime that values autonomy and liberty may well favor allowing people the right to engage in behavior that it judges to be wrong, particularly if it does not involve harm to others. But this is to concede too much too soon. We must first determine whether we should accept (1).

I suspect that much of the appeal of commodification arguments turns on linguistic aesthetics or question-begging rhetoric. Who could support something as ugly as the commodification of clinical research? Who wants to treat participation in research as comensurable with money? Who could want to defend participation in research as a "purely commercial activity"? But derisive language aside, what are the *arguments* for thinking that there is something inherently morally suspect about buying and selling participation in research?

When one looks more closely, one finds several related but distinct claims. Grant and Sugarman argue that "a regime of payments for objectified uses of the body might erode the collective respect for personal dignity in the culture."[102] Call this *the degradation argument*. Michael Sandel argues that market exchanges assume that "all goods can be translated without loss into a single measure or unit of value."[103] Call this the *incommensurability argument*. Alex John London argues that support for financial incentives is rooted in "a purely economic view of individual interests"[104] Call this the *economic view of individual interests* argument.

Degradation

Consider commercial surrogacy, which typically involves an agreement between a couple that is unable to conceive or bear a child and a woman (the surrogate mother) whereby the surrogate is paid to become pregnant via artificial insemination with the male's sperm (or, in some cases, have a fertilized ovum implanted) and waive parental rights to the child when born. According to Sandel,

Treating children as commodities degrades them by using them as instruments of profit rather than cherishing them as persons worthy of love and care. Contract pregnancy also degrades women by treating their bodies as factories and by paying them not to bond with the children they bear.[105]

Setting aside the plausibility of this view in the surrogacy context (is the child degraded if the adoptive parents treat the child as an object of love?), is a practice of paying research participants degrading to the overall practice of medical research or to the participants themselves?

Should we accept the degradation argument? Ruth Sample argues that degradation involves "treating someone or something as having less value than that person or thing actually has."[106] But if the wrong of degradation lies in the way A *treats* B, it does not follow that B actually comes to have less value as a result of A's treatment. Suppose A has contempt for homeless people and spits on B, who appears to be a homeless man lying on the sidewalk, but who is actually an undercover police officer. A may *treat* B as having little value, but I can't see that B now has less value in his own eyes or, for that matter, in any objective sense.

The previous point suggests that we should distinguish among a psychological, a social, and an objective or moral account of degradation. Let us say that a person is psychologically degraded if she *feels* less worthy if she does X (or if X is done to her). So a police officer may not feel psychologically degraded in the previous case, but a homeless person might feel differently. Let us say that there is social degradation when others *regard* a person as less worthy if she does X (of if X is done to her). And let us say that a person is objectively degraded when she *is* less worthy or ought to be regarded as less worthy if she does X (or X is done to her). A professional who has been laid off from his job might feel degraded by working at Wal-Mart, but there is nothing objectively degrading about such work. A woman may or may not feel degraded by working as a stripper, although others may think she has degraded herself (and this independent of whether she is objectively degraded). Feminists have sometimes argued that being a housewife is objectively degrading to women because it fails to value her or her potential in an appropriate way, and that this is so even if—indeed especially if—she and others are so fully socialized into accepting this role that she does not feel degraded.

To say that we can distinguish between these forms of degradation is not to deny that there are important connections among them. Our self-conceptions are related to the way others respond to us. If people treat B as less than fully human (social degradation), B may come to feel less than fully human (psychological degradation). But applying this taxonomy to participation in clinical research, I know of no systematic evidence that those who participate in research in response to financial incentives regard themselves as degraded by their participation. In suggesting that "a regime of payments for objectified uses of the body might erode the collective respect for personal dignity in the culture," Grant and Sugarman appeal to what I have called "social degradation."[107] I agree that it "might." But whether such a regime of payments actually has such an effect is, of course, an empirical claim and I know of no evidence that it has such effects.

Finally, it might be argued that the commodification of participation in research is objectively degrading to the participants even if they do not feel degraded or are regarded as degraded by the society. But why? It might be thought that paying participants treats them merely as means rather than as ends in themselves. As a general rule, however, we do not treat others merely as a means when we require and seek their consent as a condition of any interaction. Still, it might be argued that consent is insufficient to block this charge if the person is prepared to treat herself or her body "merely as a means" to an unworthy end. In my view, this Kantian charge does not work if it assumes an unjustifiably narrow perfectionist view as to what constitutes legitimate ends of human activities. Rather than pursue that issue here, I will simply say that if A seeks B's consent before transacting with B and if B is making a reasonable judgment about the relationship between payment and ends that are deserving of our respect, then this objective degradation/treating merely as a means argument gets no or little traction.[108]

Commensurability

The argument from (in)commensurability claims that monetary payment for a service implies that "all goods are commensurable, that all goods can be translated without loss into a single measure or unit of value."[109] So if a subject participates in research in exchange for money she supposedly assumes that her participation is commensurable with the marginal amount that would have been necessary to secure her participation. And, the argument goes, this sort of equation is conceptually mistaken and morally objectionable.

I find this argument entirely unpersuasive. First, the conceptual claim that two goods are incommensurable is often asserted without argument. Assuming that the claim "X and Y are incommensurable" is not true by definition, then we need to know what must be shown before such a claim is accepted. And I do not know what that is. How do we know that X and Y cannot be translated into a single measure or that they cannot be exchanged without (much) loss? Second, it is not at all clear that those who exchange goods or services for money assume that those goods are services actually *are* commensurable with money. I might trade lessons in bioethics for lessons in bridge, but I can't see how this commits me to commensurability between bioethics and bridge. And I don't see why things should change if I were to trade my lessons for money. Consider the buying and selling of a kidney—a favorite example of the incommensurability camp. It is preposterous to think that the buyer equates the money that he spends with the value of his own life and no reason to think that the seller equates the value of his kidney with the money he receives. Those who advance the incommensurability claim seem to believe that because money is fungible and has no intrinsic value, it is therefore of lesser value than many of the goods or services for which it is exchanged and which do have intrinsic value. But precisely because money is fungible, it can be used to purchase goods or services that do have intrinsic value. It may seem crass if B sells a kidney for $25,000. It seems less crass if B uses that $25,000 to educate her children or to get medical care for them. Somewhat ironically, it is the critics of commensurability that reify the value of money.

Third, even if two goods cannot be translated "without loss" into a single measure, it is not clear whether any such loss is of moral consequence. One can't translate Shakespeare into French or Cervantes into English "without loss," but, it hardly follows that it is wrong to try. Indeed, given the value created by such translations, it would be wrong not to try. Although a broken arm or the loss of an eye or the loss of one's spouse cannot be translated into monetary terms "without loss," courts and juries must still attempt to put a reasonable dollar figure on such injuries. The entire practice of compensation for injuries or damages would be impossible without assuming *some* form of commensurability. Here, too, it would be wrong not to try to commensurate what some regard as incommensurable.

And this raises a fourth difficulty for the worry about commensurability. We are constantly required to make choices among various alternatives. Suppose that Jane must decide whether to take a job that she would find more intellectually challenging but that also involves considerable travel and time away from her husband. Jane might say "But the values—my job and time with my husband—are incommensurable; I can't weigh them against each other." Then what? Jane still has to decide. And suppose that Jane makes a conceptual mistake in coming to her decision. She wrongly assumes that her deliberative process presupposes that the values at stake are commensurable, say in units of utility. It hardly follows that she is acting *immorally* in making her decision.

And this brings us to the crucial issue. Those who wave the flag of incommensurability do not seek to make a mere conceptual point. They mean to argue that we are doing something wrong when we treat goods that have a "higher value" as exchangeable with goods that have "lower value;" that we are not recognizing the unique meaning or significance of the different goods and the special claims that are associated with them. I find the specification of this wrong to be rather elusive although I do not deny the intuitive appeal of this sentiment. The general idea seems to be that participation in research should be an act of altruism or commitment and that paying people for participation detracts from its social meaning, just as giving cash to one's spouse as an anniversary present is not a way to convey one's love (although it also seems perfectly fine for parents to give their children large gifts of money as a wedding present).

How much moral weight can this bear? Despite references to the moral loss associated with commensurating the incommensurable, few argue that this loss is sufficient to render such exchanges wrongful all things considered, when the things to be considered include the ends that people can achieve precisely because of such commodification and the respect for their autonomy that allowing such choices involves. And with a few possible exceptions, such as laws against prostitution, it is rarely argued that this disvalue is sufficient to prohibit people from entering into such transactions and so the policy consequences of this line of argument appear to be very weak indeed beyond suggesting that we squirm a bit as we allow such transactions.

The Economic View of Individual Interests

Closely related to the argument from commodification, it may be thought that it is of moral importance why people do what they do. We may prefer that soldiers fight for love of country rather than for love of gore or for love of money. We may prefer that athletes play for the love of the sport rather than for fame or filthy lucre. We may prefer that professors prepare inspiring lectures because they want their students to learn rather than for the adoration of their students or as a way to secure tenure. We may prefer that people donate organs or eggs or sperm out of a desire to help others rather than for cash. And we may prefer that people participate in research because they think the research is valuable rather than in response to financial incentives. Are motivations important? If so, why?

Motivations may be of considerable contingent importance insofar as they affect performance. It is, however, an empirical question as to whether the preferred motivations do lead to better outcomes. Do football-loving football players play harder than money-loving football players? Do avaricious restaurateurs serve inferior food? Are patriotic soldiers more effective than mercenary soldiers? If so, that is a reason to prefer the selection of patriotic soldiers, other things being equal. If research participants are more likely to comply with the protocol if they are motivated to contribute to generalizable knowledge, then that is a reason to prefer such participants, other things being equal.

Of course, other things are not always equal. In particular, we may have an insufficient supply of persons who have the appropriate motivations. We may prefer having enough soldiers to having an insufficient number of country-loving soldiers. We may prefer a money-seeking egg donor to no donor at all. And we may prefer an adequate number of partially compliant research participants to an inadequate number of fully compliant participants.

The present question is whether there are other intrinsic or non-consequentialist reasons to worry about motivations. I have argued that a person might reasonably regard the value of financial payment as greater than the disvalue of the burdens and risks of participation. In an insightful commentary, Alex John London contends that this line of thought reflects a morally problematic "purely economic view of individual interests."[110]

The notion of an economic view of individual interests is ambiguous. It could be understood as claiming that a person's interests are fundamentally financial. Neither London nor I nor any self-respecting economist thinks that. More plausibly, the economic view claims that a person's interests are defined in terms of their preferences or well-being (or something along those lines) or utility and that one can maximize one's interests by making trade-offs among various goods and values. On this view, a prospective participant asks whether the package deal of participation is better than not participating. On that view, although B would not choose some humiliating action for free, she might choose the package deal that includes humiliation and a sufficient amount of money. All that matters is that the option is "worthy of choice" in the sense that she reasonably chooses it in light of all her values.[111] Think Shaw's apocryphal bed-mate.

On the economic view of individual interests, a prostitute may regard the option of accepting money for sex as "worthy of choice." London finds this problematic. But why? If prostitution is wrong, it's not necessarily wrong because it's contrary to the interests of the prostitute, all things considered, although it may well be contrary to *some* of her interests. We may think that prostitution is intrinsically wrong or that it is wrong because it has undesirable effects on social attitudes towards sexual relations, the family, or women.[112] But neither argument requires or implies that prostitution is wrong because it is contrary to the interests of the prostitute.

London might reply that it is bad for people to think about their interests as a utility or preference maximizer rather than as an integrated person seeking to live a moral life. On the economic view, it is in one's interests to be moral if but only if one cares about being moral. By contrast, there is a long philosophical tradition that holds that one has an objective interest in "doing the right thing" whether or not one cares about it. On this view, it is bad *for* a person to do what *is* bad. As Robert George puts it, "Every immoral choice . . . corrupts the chooser; every such choice integrates moral evil into the chooser's will, thus unreasonably damaging that aspect of the chooser's own well-being which consists in establishing and maintaining an upright moral character."[113] So, if it were morally objectionable to participate in research for pecuniary reasons, then receiving money for participation would be contrary to the objective moral interests of those who are paid.

Two points. First, note that George argues that immoral choice is damaging only to "that aspect" of well-being that consists in upright moral character. So unless the moral aspect of well-being always trumps its nonmoral aspects, the ways in which an immoral choice advances the chooser's well-being may outweigh the moral aspect in which it does not. Second, a choice is damaging to one's moral character only if the choice is objectively wrong. George thinks that engaging in homosexual conduct is harmful to one's moral character because he believes that homosexuality is objectively wrong. But if engaging in homosexual relations is not wrong, then it can't be harmful to one's character on that account. It follows that if serving as a research subject in exchange for money is *not* wrong, then doing so can't be contrary to the moral component of one's interests in the first place.

London's final argument against the use of financial incentives claims that there is "moral danger" in paying research subjects who do not share the goals of the research because it is morally important that "research subjects be motivated to advance the common good rather than their own individual good."[114] Here London reprises Jonas's view that subjects should identify with the goals of research.

I have two replies. First, if there is moral danger in participation in research that is motivated by financial gain rather than altruism, there would seem to be comparable moral danger if people participate in research because there is a prospect of direct or collateral *medical* benefit. In neither case are people motivated to "advance the common good rather than their own individual good."[115]

Second, it is not clear why it is of moral importance that research subjects "share the mission" of the research enterprise apart from the consequentialist reasons discussed above. Although it might be important that a person's actions tend to "advance the common good, "it is not clear why it is important that a person's actions are *motivated* to do so. Firefighters, police officers, sanitation workers, teachers, road repair crews, and soldiers all work to directly advance the common good. Their motivations are no doubt complex, and some are at least partially motivated by the desire to serve. But all such workers are paid and would not otherwise serve. In other cases, people can advance the overall good (if not the "common good") of the society when they produce or provide services or products that people want (or come to want), be they iPods, organic foods, computers, software, video games, books, or Viagra. Here, once again, people's motives are complex, but few would engage in these enterprises if they were not paid. As Adam Smith famously noted, "It is not from the benevolence of the butcher, the brewer, or the baker that we expect our dinner, but from their regard to their self-love."[116] And that does not make the baker's bread inferior. I don't see why the same can't be true of a research participant.

To press this line a bit further, note that John Rawls's conception of a just society does *not* require that individuals are motivated in their everyday life by the pursuit of justice.

Ideally the rules [of a just society] should be set up so that men are led by their predominant interests to act in ways which further socially desirable ends. The conduct of individuals guided by their rational plans should be coordinated as far as possible to achieve results which although not intended or perhaps even foreseen by them are nevertheless the best ones from the standpoint of social justice.[117]

Rawls prefers to use institutions and government coercion to promote desirable ends rather than to rely on a radical change in individual motivation or what Jerry Cohen calls an "extravagant degree of socialization."[118] If a good set of social rules motivates people to be led by their "predominant interests" to promote social justice, I do not understand what constitutes the "moral danger" in allowing a practice in which research subjects to be motivated by their conception of their own good when doing so leads them to serve the interests of medical science and future patients.

I am prepared to grant that we should think more highly of the *persons* who participate in research for altruistic reasons, although I wouldn't want to press that too far. And so from an aretaic or "virtue ethics" perspective, motivations surely matter. But even if we were to grant that it is morally preferable that people be motivated to participate in research for altruistic reasons, I do not see that this view has important implications for the formulation of policy with respect to payment to research subjects. One would have to say a *lot* more to show that the motivations of participants are of sufficient importance to bar or severely constrict payment to research subjects if doing so would significantly impair the research enterprise.

Soft Externalities[119]

It is sometimes argued that even if a transaction between the parties does not have palpable harmful effects on other identifiable individuals (hard externalities), the legitimation of such activities may give rise to unwanted and untoward social and psychological effects (soft externalities). So it is said that if we treat sexuality or procreational labor or bodily organs or our immune system as tradable commodities, we will come to have a diminished sense of ourselves and each other. This argument need not claim that the relevant practice is "intrinsically" degrading. Rather, it claims that by some unspecified causal mechanisms the practice affects the way we *regard* human beings. And if regarding organs or sexuality or children as alienable property can have such consequences, treating the human body as alienable property for the purpose of medical research can also have such consequences.

But will it? It is impossible to say with any confidence. There is no reason to assume that the legitimation of market transactions will reduce our concern for the object or practice. The market in pets does not cause people not to respect the value of their pets. That adoptive parents are willing to pay a surrogate to bear a child for them does not mean that they or others will regard the child as anything other than an object of love. Of course, the absence of evidence does not mean that the claim is necessarily false. We cannot entirely dismiss the worry. Any change in social practices can have unintended and undesirable consequences and this includes liberal favorites such as the acceptance of same sex marriages. Still, the mere possibility that acceptance of such practices might upset the social-psychological ecosystem is hardly sufficient reason to condemn or bar changes that are otherwise defensible.

It is important to see that the "soft externalities" argument is fundamentally consequentialist. It maintains that a decision to allow or prohibit transactions between consenting adults must take account of their effects on others. Fair enough. But from this perspective, one can't count just the negative externalities of the practice. They would have to be weighed against the positive consequences. So even if a more robust legitimation of the practice of offering financial payments to research participants would have some negative soft externalities, those effects might be exceeded by its positive effects on the scope and pace of clinical research and so is unlikely to support an overall negative evaluation of the practice.

Objections to Financial Payments: Equality, Justice and Exploitation

In this section, I want to consider objections to the use of financial payments that are rooted in concerns about justice and equality. In principle, the worries could go both ways. On the one hand, it is sometimes argued that a commitment to justice precludes or constrains financial incentives to participants. On the other hand, it can also be argued that a commitment to justice requires payment as an expression of reciprocity or gratitude or compensation. Whereas those who worry about the validity of consent seem to be concerned that financial payments not be too high, those that worry about the exploitation of research participants might argue that financial payments are often too low.

Equality

Setting aside issues of financial incentives for the moment, there is a more basic question as to the moral perspective that should underlie the assessment of risks and benefits. In Chapter 2, I argued that because prospective subjects are not capable of evaluating research protocols, IRBs effectively attempt to make the judgments that prospective participants would hypothetically make if they were rational consenters. Alex John London has argued that this soft paternalistic perspective on risk/benefit assessment is wrong or incomplete. Instead, IRBs should adopt a "social perspective" that is rooted in a commitment to moral equality. The fundamental challenge is to see that the risks of research "are consistent with an equal regard for the basic interests of study participants and the members of the larger community whose interests that research is intended to serve."[120]

But what does that mean? London argues that we can gain some traction by distinguishing between a person's *basic interests* and *personal interests*. We all have a basic interest in our health, but some of us have personal interest in music or athletics or our pets, and others do not. We need not get precise about that distinction here. The central point, says London, is that the practice of medical research should be committed to an equal regard for everyone's *basic* interests. Such a commitment would permit individuals to sacrifice some of their *personal* interests in order to advance the *basic* interests of others, but research "must not pose risks to the basic interests of participants that are inconsistent with the same degree of concern that is shown for the basic interests of other community members."[121] London notes that we all incur some risk to our basic interests in pursuit of our personal interests (travel, wealth, etc.) in the course of daily life. The challenge, says London, is to "establish when incremental risks to an individual's basic interests violate the underlying commitment to moral equality."[122]

T.M. Scanlon has developed a similar distinction in a way that could justify restrictions on financial payment to research subjects. He argues that even if a person were to value a personal interest or "preference" more than a basic interest, society has no obligation to support the preference even if it does have an obligation to support the basic interest.[123] Although an individual might prefer a new television to health care, society can legitimately use its resources to purchase health care for her but refuse to buy her a television. It might seem, then, that IRBs could refuse to allow participants to risk their health for the sake of non-basic interests. The subject may be entitled to make this trade-off but others need not help her do so.

Even if the equality perspective were the deep moral truth about risk assessment, it is unlikely to be helpful to IRBs. First, the principle of equal concern is notoriously indeterminate. After all, some argue that utilitarianism is the *only* view that instantiates equal concern for all. As Bentham put it, "each person should count for one and no one for more than one." Thus a standard worry about utilitarianism is that its commitment to equal regard for everyone's interests is so strong that it would require people to sacrifice or be sacrificed in order to advance the interests of others. So, far from justifying special priority for the interests of *subjects*, a commitment to equality might require prospective participants to take risks to their basic interests in order to show equal concern for "the basic interests of *other community members*" who stand to gain from the research. This understanding of equality can, of course, be challenged. As is well known, Rawls argues that utilitarianism does not take seriously the distinction between persons and that when properly understood, a commitment to equal concern and respect requires a commitment to basic rights or liberties, equal opportunity, and priority to the worst off.[124] Needless to say, we will not resolve these issues here. The present point is that the principle of equality is unlikely to be of great help to those engaged in risk/benefit assessment.

Let us suppose, however, that we accept London's basic framework. London argues that from this perspective, it "is permissible to ask individual community members to alter, risk, or even to sacrifice some of their *personal interests* as part of an effort to advance or secure the *basic interests* of others."[125] It is permissible to ask them to adopt—as a personal project—participation in research that uses time and energy that might have been devoted to other personal projects and to "endure experiences" that are unpleasant or painful. At the same time, says London, it is *not* permissible to ask or invite people to accept risks to their basic interests that "are inconsistent with the same degree of concern that is shown for the basic interests of other community members."[126]

It is not clear whether this view says much about the legitimacy of financial payment to research participants. After all, people have *multiple* basic interests. It is one thing to provide B with a new television in exchange for accepting the risks of research. But allowing B to receive financial payment in exchange for incurring incremental risks to one basic interest (her health) may well permit B to provide for another basic interest such as food or shelter. It is also important to distinguish between what a commitment to moral equality requires, in particular, of medical researchers as opposed to what it requires of the broader society. London says that we must ensure that "when individuals whose basic interests are threatened or restricted by sickness or disease participate in research they receive a level of care that is consistent with an equal regard for the basic interests of participants and non-participants alike."[127] And so it might be thought that if society does not provide prospective subjects with an appropriate standard of care, then it would be wrong to enroll them in a randomized controlled trial that does not guarantee that level of care to all participants. But that moves too quickly. If it is *society's* responsibility to provide such care, it does not follow that *investigators* should be saddled with those obligations. It may turn out that the best theory of the responsibilities of investigators does impose such obligations on investigators, but that must be established independently.

Finally, and perhaps most importantly, a commitment to moral equality can be understood as requiring equal respect for people as autonomous agents. From this perspective, we should not use risk-benefit assessments to preclude subjects from assuming risks to their basic interests for what they reasonably regard as compensating financial benefits.

Exploitation

I consider exploitation in clinical research in less developed countries in the next chapter. Here, I briefly explore the claim that financial payment in developed societies can also be exploitative. Worries about exploitation can go two ways. It may be thought that if participants are offered too *little,* they will be exploited because they will not be adequately compensated for their participation. On the other hand, it may be thought that if investigators offer too *much* financial compensation, then subjects may be exploited because they are induced into participating in research that does not serve their long-term interests in order to serve the interests of the affluent.

> The key is to strike a balance between a rate of payment high enough that it does not exploit subjects by underpayment and low enough that it does not create an irresistible inducement. There is no *a priori* way to set this level, but the general rule should be that the sponsor pay a fair wage for the labor and not increase the wage in order to entice subjects to unwelcome research with a higher level of risk.[128]

Beauchamp identifies a voluntariness (or consent) worry and a justice worry. We have already considered the first worry. Recall the discussion of Table 4.3. If (as in (b)), a given level of financial payment will motivate most (or too many) prospective subjects to make an irrational assessment of the risks and benefits of participation, then such incentives should be rejected. But there is no reason to reject financial payments on voluntariness grounds if, as in (c) the subjects are making a reasonable—nondistorted—judgment.

Even if we assume that subjects give morally transformative consent to participate in research in exchange for financial payment, it may be argued that payment can be so low as to be disrespectful, unfair, or exploitative. Joan McGregor rightly claims that an exchange is not "sanitized" from a moral point of view just because it is mutually advantageous and consensual. She is, however, wrong to maintain that "Taking advantage of people's desperation, misfortune, or illness constitutes clear cases of unfair advantage taking."[129] McGregor ignores the distinction (as do many) between A's taking advantage of an unfairness or misfortune to B and A's taking unfair advantage of B. A fair and honest tow truck operator takes advantage of misfortune, but he does not take *unfair* advantage of misfortune.

So when does someone take *unfair* advantage of another? As I indicate in Chapter 5, a consensual and mutually advantageous transaction is exploitative when B receives too little or pays too much for rendering a service or receiving some good.

> *Umbrella.* A, a store owner, normally charges $10 for an umbrella. B, who is wearing an expensive suede jacket, wants to buy an umbrella from A. A sees that it is pouring and tells B that the umbrella will cost $50.

This transaction is consensual because there is no coercion (A is not threatening to violate B's rights if she refuses to pay) and because B's judgment is not distorted. The transaction is mutually advantageous because both A and B gain from the transaction. Nonetheless, A is arguably exploiting B because A is taking unfair advantage of B's circumstances.

Although I think that *Umbrella* is a case of unfair advantage taking, it is not easy to explain why this is so. Although some say that a transaction is exploitative when the exploiter gains much more than the exploitee, the exploited person usually gains *more* utility from a transaction than the exploiter. The utility gain to B (who preserves an expensive jacket) is probably much greater than the utility gain to A (who gets, say, $40 more than usual). Indeed, it is precisely because the exploiter stands to gain relatively little that he can threaten to walk away from the transaction and has more bargaining power.

Umbrellas are hard enough, but it is particularly difficult to specify a fair level of financial payment for labor or services, particularly when they are not obviously driven by market forces. It is easy to endorse the principle that "equals should be treated equally," but that formal principle of equality says nothing about the appropriate basis on which people should be treated equally.[130] Consider payment for serving on juries. We might treat jurors equally by giving everyone the same nominal amount or by giving everyone a similar proportion of their foregone wages. On the latter view, we treat a radiologist and a truck driver equally only if a radiologist receives a larger payment than a truck driver because serving on a jury requires the radiologist to sacrifice more income than the truck driver. Shamoo and Resnik argue that this approach would be "patently unfair because two different subjects could receive different payments for the same type of work."[131] But this is not obviously unfair if we are compensating people for their time rather than their work. Although many would recoil at the proposal to adjust the financial payment to the participant's opportunity cost, many of those same persons would not object to my former university's policy under which the fee for parking is adjusted to one's salary even though all were receiving the same good. Consider income taxes. If it is fair for those who *earn* more to *pay* more in taxes on the principle that the degree of sacrifice should be sensitive to income, it is hard to see why it is unfair to adjust what one *is paid* as reflecting a principle of equal sacrifice.

I have argued elsewhere that we could understand a fair price (or wage) as the price that hypothetically would be reached by a highly competitive market under conditions of full information.[132] Fifty dollars is an unfair price for an umbrella because A is taking advantage of his monopoly power (the only place B can purchase an umbrella without first ruining her jacket) where the hypothetical market price is, say, $10. On the other hand, a fair price for a house in La Jolla is greater than a fair price for an equivalent house in Indianapolis because a similar house will be purchased for a higher price in La Jolla than in Indianapolis when everyone is fully informed and when sellers have multiple possible buyers and vice versa.

Just as a "fair market price" for a house is the price that would be reached in a competitive market, the fair price for labor is the wage that would be paid under suitable background conditions. In a highly competitive market, employers cannot afford to pay less than the market wage because they would be unable to hire if they did and they cannot afford to pay more than the market wage because they would incur an erosion in their profits.

Grady and Dickert prefer a "wage payment" model that would specify a standard payment for all participants at something like the wage for unskilled labor. They reject a "market" model that would put no constraints on the level of payment and a "reimbursement model" that would compensate subjects for their opportunity costs and thus pay more to high income subjects than to low income subjects.[133] (I suspect that the "market model" and the "reimbursement model" are close to extensionally equivalent). But, as I have argued, one cannot reject the reimbursement (or market) model simply by appeal to the principle that "equals should be treated equally."

In addition to arguing for the wage payment model on grounds of fairness, Grady and Dickert argue that it will help "to contain the cost of research" and avoid a situation in which well funded research or research on potentially lucrative drugs drives out less well funded research and research on disease mechanisms and rarer diseases.[134] There may be social utility in limiting payment, but if Burger King and McDonald's were to agree to set a common wage, we would loudly complain that their anti-competitive behavior was depriving workers of a fair wage. It is possible that some such concerns should apply here as well and that fairness requires much greater compensation and better conditions than are often offered, even though this might raise the cost of each study, thereby leading to higher taxes or reduced expenditures for other objectives or fewer studies or higher prices. If we have to pay more for wine in order to adequately compensate the grape pickers, so be it. Much the same may be true for medical research.

Fair Subject Selection

The final justice related worry about the use of financial incentives concerns the principle of fair subject selection. The Common Rule says that the selection of subjects must be "equitable."

> In making this assessment the IRB should take into account the purposes of the research and the setting in which the research will be conducted and should be particularly cognizant of the special problems of research involving vulnerable populations, such as children, prisoners, pregnant women, mentally disabled persons, or economically or educationally disadvantaged persons.[135]

This statement actually focuses on consent rather than equity. The core idea seems to be that we should not take unfair advantage of a person's vulnerabilities to get them to agree to participate in research when doing so does not advance their interests or when they would not do so if they were able to rationally assess the risks and benefits of participation.

By contrast, most discussions of the principle of fair subject selection focus on the distribution of benefits and burdens of research among various groups or classes. In the present context, it may be thought that the use of financial incentives to recruit participants will result in the disproportionate representation of the poor or minorities. Call this the problem of *demographic disproportionality*. Suppose that a research protocol involves some inconvenience and risk and that investigators are prepared to offer $1,000 to participants. It may well be that many low-income persons would find an offer of $1,000 sufficient to entice them to participate but that few suitable subjects with annual incomes over $75,000 would be willing to participate for that amount. Under such conditions, the subject pool will be disproportionately drawn from those with lower incomes. Ezekiel Emanuel argues that if we want to reduce demographic disproportionality, then "the solution would seem to be to raise the incentives to make the rich deem it worthwhile to participate too."[136] This will not solve the problem. Any feasible level of financial payment will attract the poor disproportionately. Would this be a cause for concern?

There might be scientific reasons to worry about demographic disproportionality. It might be important that a study control for confounding factors such as income, educational level, etc. The present question is whether such a study would violate the principle of fair subject selection? The Belmont Report says that "Injustice may appear in the selection of subjects, even if individual subjects are selected fairly by investigators and treated fairly in the course of research."[137] Belmont seems to be claiming that subject selection can be unjust when it exhibits demographic disproportionality even though no individual has been treated unjustly. Along those lines, CIOMS states that "Equity requires that no *group* or *class* of persons should bear more than its fair share of the *burdens* of participation in research"[138] (emphasis added). This statement raises two distinct questions: (1) are groups or classes of persons the sorts of entities that can bear burdens or receive benefits?; (2) if so, are groups or individuals actually bearing the *burdens* of research?

Although we sometimes speak as if groups can bear burdens or receive benefits, I believe that researchers cannot treat *groups* fairly or unfairly because they don't interact with groups at all in a relevant way. One can treat an individual unfairly *because* one is prejudiced against members of a group. One may believe "most X's are lazy" and thus refuse to hire an X who is not lazy. Moreover, treating an individual unfairly because she is a member of a group can have effects on other members of that group, as when individuals "identify" with people who share a certain trait. But one would still not be treating the *group* unfairly. And *if*—and this is a big *if*—all individuals are treated fairly and respectfully, it is hard to see why we should care if those individuals come disproportionally from some demographic groups.

Demographic disproportionality is sometimes an important *signal* or evidence that individuals may have been or even probably have been treated unjustly. When a disproportionate number of those accepted or rejected for some good or opportunity come from one group or another, we may have reason to examine the selection process with special care. When we do so, we will find that demographic disproportionality sometimes signals unjust treatment and sometimes does not. It is unlikely that the disproportionate representation of African Americans in the National Basketball Association is due to unfairness to whites. It is unlikely that the greater longevity of women is due to unfairness to men in the distribution of health care. It is, by contrast, more likely that the underrepresentation of African Americans among coaches in the National Football League is due to unfairness to blacks. It is unlikely that the overrepresentation of males in prisons is due to discrimination against men, but the overrepresentation of African Americans in prisons may well reflect discrimination in the legal process against blacks or a higher rate of criminality among African Americans that is itself the result of a history and pattern of social injustice in the background. Still, demographic disproportionality is not a moral problem in its own right.

Recall that CIOMS states that "Equity requires that no group or class of persons should bear more than its fair share of the *burdens* of participation in research."[139] Even if we assume that a principle of equity can apply to groups, the word—burdens—is ambiguous as between two senses. In an expansive sense, we can say that participants bear the burdens of research because participation frequently involves at least some inconvenience or element of risk or aversive experience. In a narrower or more restrictive sense, we could say that participants bear the *burdens* of research if and only if they can expect to be worse off *all things considered*. In the latter sense, participants are not bearing the *burdens* of research if they can reasonably expect to *benefit* from participating in research, all things considered, anymore than teachers bear the burdens of teaching. And if monetary payment could render participation that is *otherwise* burdensome into participation that is beneficial all things considered, then there would be no issue as to the equitable distribution of the *burdens* of participation with respect to that class of research.

What about active recruitment? CIOMS says that "It is unjust to selectively recruit impoverished people to serve as research subjects simply because they can be more easily induced to participate in exchange for small payments. In most cases, these people would be called upon to bear the burdens of research so that others who are better off could enjoy the benefits."[140] This is puzzling. First, if the impoverished subjects are actually bearing *burdens,* all things considered, then it's unlikely that they are giving morally transformative consent unless they are particularly altruistic. We would then have a consent problem, not a justice problem.

Let us assume that "impoverished people" actually benefit from participating in research, all things considered and that they are capable of giving and do give morally transformative consent. If demographic disproportionately results from a process of announcing and advertising the opportunity to participate in research then the researchers have not "selectively recruited" impoverished people. It just so happens that the impoverished are more likely to volunteer. I cannot see why this would be wrong. Suppose, for example, that the XYZ waste removal company provides waste removal for a wealthy and mostly white suburb in a large metropolitan area. XYZ advertises for employees to drive garbage trucks and empty the garbage into the trucks. It turns out that while the metropolitan area is 20% African American, virtually all of the applicants are African Americans who are unemployed or who find the prospect of working for XYZ more attractive than their present job. Although African Americans are disproportionately bearing the "burden" of waste removal, there is no reason to think that XYZ has acted wrongly in recruiting and employing African Americans and this is true even though the employees are providing a service for affluent whites. If the overrepresentation of a racial group among sanitation workers is morally unproblematic, it is not clear why the overrepresentation of the impoverished among research participants is also morally unproblematic, if they benefit from their participation and give morally transformative consent.

Now demographic disproportionality could have indirect negative social consequences or soft-externalities even when it is intrinsically morally benign. People might assume that demographic disproportionality results from wrongful discrimination even if it does not. If African Americans themselves come to believe blacks are overrepresented in research and that participation in research is exploitative, burdensome, and inadequately consensual, they may come to distrust the research enterprise and the profession of medicine—even if those beliefs are false. I have seen no evidence that demographic disproportionality in research has such effects, but if it does, these are factors that must be weighed. That said, demographic disproportionality is not a problem in and of itself.

The Argument from Professional and Institutional Integrity

I have argued that insofar as we are concerned with the interests and autonomy of research subjects, there is little reason to discourage the use of financial incentives or to set limits on the amount of payments so long as prospective subjects are capable of making a reasonable decision in response to such offers. I have also argued that there are no general moral objections to the use of financial incentives in research on grounds of commodification or on grounds of justice, exploitation, or fair subject selection.

There is, however, an entirely different perspective from which one might raise ethical objections to the use of financial incentives. On this view, financial incentives do not wrong subjects, but they are inconsistent with the values and aims of the practice of medicine and medical research. These concerns are easiest to see if we focus on what I have called the linkage thesis and the incorporation view. For if this line of argument cannot be sustained as a critique of the incorporation view, it is unlikely to be successful as a critique of the use of financial payments as an incentive.

To refresh the reader's memory, the linkage thesis concerns the relation between the following two claims:

(1) An IRB should respect a person's reasonable judgment as to whether the benefits of financial payment outweigh the risks of participation if the protocol is otherwise approvable.

(2) An IRB should incorporate a person's reasonable judgment about the benefits of financial payment in determining whether the risks of research are reasonable in relation to the anticipated benefits and therefore approvable.

The linkage thesis states that if we accept (1), then we should also accept (2). I argued above that it is very difficult to resist the force of the linkage thesis *insofar as we are concerned with the interests and autonomy of research participants.* Still, it can be argued that the linkage thesis is incompatible with the integrity of the medical and research enterprise. On this view, it may be reasonable to regard financial payment as offsetting risk from the *subject's* perspective, but it does not follow that it is reasonable to regard payment as offsetting risk from an institutional perspective.

Along these lines, Mark Kuczewski has argued that "opposition to the use of financial incentives . . . is probably best conceived as a concern for the integrity of the medical profession, not as a concern about coercion or compromised autonomy. It is a concern that once the general public sees biomedical researchers as mercenary in the pursuit of their agenda, the trust of the medical professions will similarly erode."[141] This is partly right, but mostly wrong or irrelevant to the present concern. Kuczewski is right that the aversion to the use of financial incentives is not best conceived as a concern about coercion or compromised autonomy. On the other hand, the concern that biomedical *researchers* will be perceived as mercenary has little bearing on the legitimacy of financial payments to *research subjects.* Moreover, it is not clear why the public's response to the agenda of biomedical researchers should affect the public's trust in the *medical profession.* Finally, and of more theoretical importance, it is a mistake to conflate a worry about the public's *perception* of the research enterprise or the medical profession with a concern for the *integrity* of researchers or the medical profession itself.

There are, however, two related lines of argument that deserve a careful hearing. Both arguments refer to the special mission or aims of medicine and academic research. To put this argument in a broader context, there are often good reasons to endorse some sort of moral division of labor. A parent is legitimately more concerned with the interests of her child than the interests of other children. A lawyer is legitimately concerned with the interests of her client to the exclusion of the interests of her adversary. A breast cancer lobbyist is legitimately concerned with securing funding for research on breast cancer even if this means that fewer and perhaps insufficient resources will be devoted to other diseases such as prostate cancer. Similarly, the medical profession is concerned with the promotion of health and should not engage in practices inconsistent with this aim. It may be argued, for example, that a physician would not be justified in tattooing a patient although it would be perfectly legitimate for the patient to get a tattoo from a tattoo artist (could the physician do this after hours?).

This perspective affects our present topic in two ways. First, consider the role of (treating) physicians in referring or encouraging patients to participate in research for which they will receive financial payment. Ruth Macklin says this:

> Although many people in our society place themselves at considerable risk of physical, psychological, social or legal harm for the sake of obtaining money, it is wrong for *physicians* to put their *patients* in that position. Because they are rendered more vulnerable by their illness, patients might be more readily influenced by the lure of money[142] (emphasis added).

Macklin's point sets the stage for an argument from the institutional integrity of medical research, but she does not actually advance such an argument here. She provides no evidence that patients are especially prone to be influenced by money as opposed to treatment of their illness. Moreover, in suggesting that patients are more "readily influenced by the lure of money" because they are ill, she is actually pointing to a problem with their consent, not with the integrity of the physician's practices.

Macklin's point can be reframed in terms that raise a legitimate concern about institutional integrity. From that perspective, the relationship between physicians and patients is not compromised in Phase I research with healthy volunteers who are not patients, but it may be compromised when a physician refers or encourages a patient to participate in Phase II or Phase III research if participation is unlikely to best serve the patient's medical needs.

Consider the incorporation view in this light. Suppose that a physician believes that participation in a trial is not optimal for his patient from a *medical* perspective, but knows that the patient needs money and that the payment adequately compensates the patient for non-optimal medical treatment. It could be argued that even if participation is entirely reasonable from the *patient's* perspective given the "trade-off" between the value of financial payment and the disvalue of non-optimal medical treatment, this is not a choice that a *physician* should encourage a patient to make. The physician's role is to advance the patient's *medical* interests, and not her interests, writ large. It is less clear whether a physician could legitimately encourage a patient to participate in research for the sake of contributing to *medical science* when doing so involves some medical risk to the patient. On the one hand, recommending participation is inconsistent with the physician's obligation to advance the health of her particular *patient* to whom she has a fiduciary responsibility. On the other hand, it is arguable that physicians have multiple commitments and inviting altruistic participation in research is to ask the patient to share the physician's interest in advancing *health* and that seems entirely unobjectionable so long as the patient gives morally transformative consent.

A full assessment of this line of argument is beyond the scope of this project. Here I want to make an empirical point and a theoretical point. The empirical point is that the conception of a physician's role sketched above is incompatible with a wide variety of practices in which physicians actually engage. Physicians remove kidneys from live donors, and while such procedures may promote the recipient's health, they do not promote the health of the donor. Physicians perform cosmetic surgery, although some argue that this practice is based on a "consumerist" model of medical practice that is at odds with the legitimate goals of the medical profession.[143] Physicians assist the civil justice and criminal justice system. They testify as experts in civil trials. They testify as forensic psychiatrists with respect to the sanity of defendants, sometimes for the prosecution, sometimes for the defense. Physicians assist athletic teams where their job is complicated because they work for the team and not the patient and because the athletes may be prepared to sacrifice their health in order to perform. Now it is possible that physicians should not engage in some or all of these practices noted above, although I am inclined not to object to any of them on the grounds of role morality or integrity. The present point is that there would be a significant price to adopting an exclusively "health-promoting" view of medical practice.

The theoretical point concerns the source of appeals to role morality. Roughly speaking, there are two approaches to justifying the special aims and restrictions on professionals. On a "bottom-up" view, such roles are justified because they advance the interests of patients or clients or society as a whole. On a "top-down" or "essentialist" view, such roles are justified because they are intrinsic to the character of the relevant profession. So if one asks why doctors should not assist in executions, some will say that this is something that *doctors* should not do even if capital punishment is otherwise justifiable. Why? Because it's inconsistent with a certain understanding of the practice of medicine.

I shall assert but not defend the proposition that the first—bottom-up— view is a more compelling strategy for defending the obligations and constraints of various professions. From that perspective, lawyers have an obligation of zealous advocacy or confidentiality because assigning such obligations ultimately (not always proximately) serves the interests of clients or society and not because such obligations are somehow intrinsic to lawyering. Similarly, on a bottoms-up approach, "Treatment is the end of medicine, not by fiat, but because most individuals who consult a physician desire it. The ethical obligations of that office are not inherent in the role or defined independently of the desires of the parties to the relationship. They are chosen in view of the ends that this knowledge serves."[144] On this view, even though cosmetic surgery does not advance the *health* of the patient, it is compatible with ethical medical practice if patients reasonably want such interventions and physicians are well trained to provide it. After all, what is derisively referred to as a "consumerist" model of medical practice in which physicians cater to the sundry demands and desires of patients can also be described more sympathetically as an "autonomy facilitating" model in which physicians enable persons to achieve the aims that they autonomously choose and which physicians are in a position to facilitate. On this view, if it is legitimate for the cosmetic surgeon to regard the patient's psychic well-being as a benefit that she can help promote, then it is arguably legitimate for a physician to regard the patient's financial well-being as a benefit that she can help promote.

Finally, let us consider the argument from *institutional* integrity in the context of academic medical research. The appeal to institutional integrity challenges the claim that the value of financial payment to the subject can be considered in applying the reasonable risk criterion. On this view, the proper aim of such institutions is the advancement of health and the diagnosis, treatment, and cure of disease. An IRB can approve a protocol if it is determined that the risks to subjects "are reasonable" in relation to anticipated *medical* benefits, while leaving it to prospective participants to consider the benefit of financial payment in deciding whether to participate. At the same time, such institutions should not make their decisions on the basis of considerations that are beyond their special values and aims. It may be legitimate for such institutions to allow prospective subjects to altruistically accept risk to their health in order to advance the health of *others*. For promoting the health of *others* is the whole point of medical research. But, on this view, an academic research institution should not regard financial payment as a benefit that can offset the risks of participation.

It is important to see that the institutional integrity argument is rooted in a concern for the values of the institution and *not* (at least not proximately) in a concern for the interests of research subjects. I am skeptical that this argument will be more successful than appeals to the role of physician for the reasons I developed above. I suspect that those who are worried about the ethics of financial payment have simply assumed that they could justify their views within a subject protection framework and have therefore not seen the need to develop an alternative line of argument.

Although I am skeptical that the appeal to institutional integrity will justify not regarding financial payment as a benefit, it is difficult to assess its force because I know of no sustained argument in its defense. I suspect that those who are worried about the ethics of financial payment have simply assumed that they could justify their views within a subject protection framework and have therefore not seen the need to develop an alternative line of argument to support their conclusion.

Consider an interesting off-hand comment by Ruth Macklin. Macklin describes her experience on an IRB which considered a protocol "that involved paying psychiatric outpatients for participation in a study in which they were briefly hospitalized, discharged, and required to return in a few days for a second test."[145] Because many patients did not return for the second test, the study could not be completed, and so the investigators proposed to pay the patients at the end of the protocol. Macklin revealingly and uncritically notes that a subcommittee charged to examine the use of financial payments "did not even *consider* the possibility that payment to subjects could be a benefit, which would then produce a more favorable benefit-risk ratio."[146] If one doesn't *consider* the possibility that payment is a benefit to subjects, one is unlikely to develop arguments that would justify rejecting that view.

Conclusion

I have made two principal claims in this chapter. First, I argued that we should seriously reconsider the standard view that financial payment should not be regarded as a benefit for the purpose of risk/benefit assessment. Second, I argued that even if financial payment should not be regarded as a benefit, it does not follow that there should be any general ethical objection to financial payment to participants in protocols in which the anticipated risks of participation are clearly reasonable in relation to the anticipated benefits. If I am right, we should stop worrying quite so much about money.

Even if some of my arguments are wrong—they can't *all* be wrong (can they?)—my argument may serve an important Millian function for those who believe that financial payment to subjects is deeply problematic. As Mill famously argued, "He who knows only his own side of the case, knows little of that."[147] Mill went on to say that to appreciate the force of arguments against one's own view, it is important not to hear them as arguments one invents for the purpose of refuting them, but to "hear them from persons who actually believe them; who defend them in earnest." I do believe them and have tried to defend them in earnest.

5 Exploitation in Clinical Research

Introduction

The concept of exploitation is not explicitly included in the four canonical principles of bioethics—autonomy (or respect for persons), non-maleficence, beneficence, and justice.[1] Nonetheless, bioethicists have appealed to the language of exploitation in a variety of contexts. It is frequently claimed that the sale of kidneys for transplants exploits the sellers. It is said that charging high prices for anti-retroviral therapies exploits those with AIDS. It is said that psychotherapists who have sexual relations with their patients are engaged in exploitation. It is said that commercial surrogacy exploits the surrogate mothers. It has been argued that stem cell research treats "nascent human life as raw material to be exploited as a mere natural resource."[2]

The concept of exploitation has also come to play an especially important role in discourse about the ethics of clinical research. Indeed, some bioethicists have argued that the principle of non-exploitation is a rationale—even *the* underlying rationale—for many of the oft-mentioned principles of ethical research such as social value, scientific validity, informed consent, fair participant selection, and favorable risk-benefit ratio.[3] On this view, "the fundamental ethical challenge of all research with humans is to avoid exploitation."[4] It may be said that research that has no social value or is not scientifically valid exploits research participants because they are being "used" for no good end. To use people for research without their informed consent is to exploit or take unfair advantage of them. To subject subjects to unreasonable risks is to exploit them, and so on.

Accusations of wrongful exploitation in research are most frequently invoked with respect to research with vulnerable populations such as prisoners, other institutionalized persons, low-income persons, and the desperately ill. The charge seems particularly poignant in the international context when poor citizens in less developed countries (LDCs) are used as subjects in research that is primarily designed to benefit those in developed countries—"the specter of exploitation is the most serious ethical issue in multinational clinical research."[5] Accusations of exploitation are sometimes directed at research conducted by academic or non-profit organizations, but are especially applied to the growing practice in which pharmaceutical corporations "outsource" medical research to contract research organizations that, in turn, conduct many of their studies in LDCs—"A huge population with a diversity of diseases that are untreated—yes, that is the 'India Advantage'" (Igate Clinical Research, Inc.).[6]

Such accusations reached fever pitch when investigators conducted placebo controlled trials in LDCs when proven effective treatment was available in developed countries. It was argued that whereas it may be legitimate to recruit subjects into a placebo controlled trial under clinical equipoise, when medical science has no reason to think that the intervention is superior to no treatment (all things considered), it is grossly unethical to recruit subjects into a placebo controlled trial of an intervention when an available intervention is clearly superior to no treatment. To set the stage for the discussion, consider two examples.

The Short-Course ART Trial (SCAT)

Placebo-controlled trials had unequivocally established the efficacy of a "long course" (ACTG 076) use of the antiretroviral drug zidovudine for reducing maternal-fetal transmission of HIV.[7] The protocol involved administering the drug orally to HIV positive women during pregnancy, administering the drug intravenously during labor, and subsequently administering the drug to the newborn infant. When studied in developed countries, the regimen promised to save the lives of one in seven infants born to HIV positive mothers. Unfortunately, the efficacy and use of the 076 regime could not be confidently extrapolated to LDCs. First, the drug might not be as efficacious in LDCs due to differences in immune status and breastfeeding practices. Second, even if the 076 regime proved to be efficacious in LDCs, many thought that its use was not administratively or economically feasible. It would prove too expensive, compliance with the regime would prove virtually impossible for many women, and many LDCs lacked the medical infrastructure to support its administration. Given these facts on the ground, investigators wanted to determine whether a cheaper and simpler "short course" use of zidovudine would be at least reasonably effective in reducing maternal-fetal transmission of HIV even if it would not be *as* effective as the 076 regimen.

To test the short course regimen against the long course regimen in a *superiority study* or *active controlled trial* (ACT) would not answer the scientific question. If the 076 regimen were found to be better than short-course anti-retroviral treatment (ART), it would be unclear if and to what extent it was better than no treatment, and that was what the researchers wanted to know. It would have been impossible to conduct *a placebo controlled trial* (PCT) of the short course regimen in a developed nation where the local standard of care would have included the 076 regimen. It would not be approved by an IRB and even if it were approved, women would not consent to participate if the long course were available. By contrast, it was feasible to recruit subjects to a PCT of the short course treatment in a LDC where the local standard of care was to receive no treatment at all. Half a loaf is better than none. The placebo controlled trials were conducted but were widely condemned as unethical and exploitative because the investigators deliberately withheld a proven effective intervention from those in the control group.

The Surfaxin Trial[8]

Respiratory distress syndrome (RDS) is a common and potentially fatal disease in premature infants, caused by insufficient surfactant in the lungs. Surfactant is a protein fluid that reduces alveolar surface tension, enabling proper lung inflation and aeration. Several replacement surfactants such as *Exosurf* had been approved by the U.S. Food and Drug Administration (FDA). The use of surfactant replacement therapy is the standard treatment for RDS in the developed world. It is not a viable option in many LDCs because of its high cost (over $1,000 per child).

In 2000, a private U.S. drug company, Discovery Labs (DL), planned a study to demonstrate the efficacy of a new synthetic surfactant, Surfaxin, which was thought to be easier and cheaper to manufacture and which might have fewer side effects than surfactants derived from animal tissue. The principal target market for Surfaxin was the United States and Europe, as it would prove unaffordable in LDCs. The FDA does not require that a product be shown to be superior to other interventions. It requires only that it is safe and effective. For several reasons, which need not concern us here, DL proposed to conduct a multi-centered, double-blinded, randomized, two-arm *placebo* controlled trial involving 650 premature infants with RDS in Bolivia and other sites in South America. In the original proposal, DL agreed to provide endotracheal tubs, ventilators, and antibiotics for all study participants. Parents of infants with RDS would be asked to give consent for their babies to participate. After intubation with an endotracheal tube, half the infants would receive air suffused with Surfaxin and half the infants would receive ("sham") air without any drug, although they would *not* be denied a treatment to which they would otherwise have had access. Indeed, the ventilator support with sham air was known to improve survival and was superior to the treatment generally available to Bolivian infants with RDS.

Although the short-course HIV trial received more extensive discussion, the *Surfaxin Trial* (ST) was criticized on similar grounds. Both protocols involved withholding effective therapy from participants in the control group. Moreover, unlike SCAT, which was designed to test an intervention for use in LDCs, ST would be using infants in a poor nation to test the efficacy of a drug that would be primarily used in wealthy nations. In the face of intense criticism, DL withdrew its proposal to conduct a PCT in Bolivia and, instead, conducted a multi-centered ACT at sites where ventilation and surfactant therapy were ordinarily available.

Because my purpose is to use these cases as examples of alleged exploitation, references to ST in this chapter will refer to the *original* study design for a PCT in Bolivia (and other LDCs) and not the actual ACT that was eventually conducted.

The Exploitation Complaint

As I indicated above, many bioethicists have claimed that much clinical research (such as SCAT and ST) in underdeveloped societies exemplifies wrongful exploitation. Although these charges have considerable rhetorical force and their intuitive appeal is difficult to deny, they are not based on a careful examination as to what constitutes exploitation or its moral force.

Here are some typical statements, accompanied in italics by some questions that they raise.

1. "Unless the interventions being tested will actually be made available to the impoverished populations that are being used as research subjects, developed countries are simply exploiting them in order to quickly use the knowledge gained from the clinical trials for the developed countries' own benefit."[9] *Questions: would there be no exploitation of the research subjects if the intervention were made available to impoverished population? Who are the victims of exploitation? The subjects? The countries?*

2. ". . . the placebo-controlled trials are exploitative of poor people, who are being manipulated into serving the interests of those who live in wealthy nations. . ."[10] *Questions: what is manipulation? Would such trials be exploitative if the subjects gave competent, uncoerced, and rational consent?*

3. ". . . there is always the nagging possibility that the assurances of such benefits may offer inordinate inducements to poor and impoverished populations and thus represent another form of exploitation."[11] *Questions: what makes an inducement "inordinate"? Would people be less exploited if there were no inducements? Are such inducements inordinate only if they compromise consent? Is it less exploitative to provide a small inducement than a large inducement? Is the possibility of receiving life-saving treatment an undue inducement?*

4. "If the knowledge gained from the research in such a country is used primarily for the benefit of populations that can afford the tested product, the research may rightly be characterized as exploitative and therefore, unethical."[12] *Questions: Are subjects exploited just because the tested product is used for wealthy nations? Are workers in developing societies who produce athletic shoes exploited just because the product is typically unaffordable in their own society?*

5. "If the results of a clinical trial are not made reasonably available in a timely manner to study participants and other inhabitants of a host country, the researchers might be justly accused of exploiting poor, undereducated subjects for the

benefit of more affluent populations of the sponsoring countries.[13] *Questions: What if the trial is unsuccessful? If the results are not available in any society, does it mean that no one is exploited? Why do "other inhabitants" of a host country have a claim to be benefit from the efforts of participants?*

6. "Residents of impoverished, postcolonial countries, the majority of whom are people of color, must be protected from potential exploitation in research. Otherwise, the abominable state of health care in these countries can be used to justify studies that could never pass ethical muster in the sponsoring country."[14] *Questions: do the principles of ethical research require that if a study design were unethical in one society (given its conditions) that the study must be unethical in another society (given its conditions)? If $10 per hour is a fair wage in the United States for a manufacturing job, is it unethical to pay people less in a country where the average wage is $1 per hour?*

7. ". . . it is a fundamental ethical principle that those involved in research in developing countries . . . should not take advantage of the vulnerabilities created by poverty or a lack of infrastructure and resources."[15] *Questions: does one exploit another just because one takes advantage of their vulnerabilities? Do roofers exploit home owners when they take advantage of the vulnerabilities created by leaky roofs? Does it matter whether the vulnerable person benefits from or consents to participation?*

As these statements suggest—and one can find numerous additional similar statements in the literature—many commentators seem to accept what I call *The Exploitation Argument.* Reduced to its essentials, that argument maintains something like this:

(1) If a practice *is* exploitative, it should not be permitted.
(2) Placebo *controlled* trials (PCTs) that withhold proven effective therapy (such as ST) are exploitative.
(3) Therefore, such PCTs (or other exploitative practices) should not be permitted.

As it stands, this argument moves much too quickly. First, despite the ease with which accusations of exploitation are advanced, it is not clear when a practice or transaction is properly described as exploitative (2).

Indeed, it is not clear who are thought to be the victims of exploitation—the research subjects, the community, the nation? Until we have a better grip on the concept of exploitation, we cannot say with confidence that (2) is true. Second, it is not clear whether we should accept (1). There is an important and neglected distinction between the *ethics of interaction* between researchers and subjects and *the ethics of intervention* with the interaction between researchers and subjects. I shall argue that whereas it is wrong for researchers to exploit subjects, it simply does not follow that we should seek to prevent such exploitation.

My Plan

The major purpose of this chapter is to attempt to shed some philosophical light on a topic that has generated too much rhetorical heat and too many question-begging arguments. Here, once again, we need to widen the lens. To properly assess these claims about the exploitative character of much clinical research, we must step back and examine the concept of exploitation with care. The claim that clinical research is exploitative is sometimes true. But it is important to determine just when it is true and to get clear about the moral force of that truth. Drawing on some earlier work, I first develop some analytical distinctions about the concept of exploitation and about the forms it can take. In particular, I will distinguish between *harmful and nonconsensual exploitation* and *mutually advantageous and consensual exploitation*. I also seek to identify the essential elements of exploitation.[16] Second, I explore the *moral force* of exploitation and, in particular, the arguments for *prohibiting* mutually advantageous consensual exploitation. After all, the question for research ethics is not only whether a practice is properly *described* as exploitative, but what we should *do,* given its wrongfulness. Third, I try to bring those analyses to bear on the ethical issues that arise with respect to use of placebo-controlled trials in cases such as SCAT and ST. Although my analysis of exploitation also applies to other issues, such as the provision of post-trial treatment to subjects, I will mention them only briefly in this chapter because I consider such issues in more detail in Chapter 6. In considering the alleged exploitativeness of PCTs, I focus on ST rather than SCAT because it presents a greater challenge to my argument. Although both trials withhold proven effective treatment from the control group, the aim of SCAT was to develop an intervention that would benefit people in LDCs. If it was exploiting the poor, it was exploiting the poor for the benefit of the poor. If, as I shall argue, it is actually quite hard to justify interference with such trials when they benefit people in wealthy nations, there is certainly less reason to interfere when they would benefit people in LDCs.

A caveat. I will mostly set aside questions as to whether allegedly exploitative practices are compatible with the principles articulated in any of the canonical codes of research ethics such as the Declaration of Helsinki, the CIOMS Ethical Guidelines for Biomedical Research Involving Human Subjects, The Belmont Report, or The Common Rule. For example, the Declaration of Helsinki states that: "The benefits, risks, burdens and effectiveness of a new method should be tested against those of the best current prophylactic, diagnostic, and therapeutic methods."[17] If researchers were to comply with this passage, it would seem that they could not conduct PCTs such as SCAT or ST. I will, however, not be concerned as to whether ST can be rendered compatible with this or any other similar provision, say by claiming that "best current . . .method" could be understood in local terms, where the "best current . . . method" might be no treatment at all. The question here is whether a PCT such as ST is wrongfully exploitative and whether it should be prohibited for that reason. If the best answers to those questions are incompatible with the provisions of any particular document, so be it.

The Concept of Exploitation

The word "exploitation" can be used in a non-moral or non-derisive sense, where it means simply to "use" or "take advantage of." So we might say, "The basketball player exploited his great jumping ability." We are interested in *wrongful* exploitation. Although one finds multiple and quite different accounts of wrongful exploitation in philosophical literature, most—although not all—are compatible with the claim that *A exploits B when A takes unfair advantage of B*.[18] One problem with such a broad account is that there will "be as many competing conceptions of exploitation as theories of what persons owe to each other by way of fair treatment."[19] Consider a few examples which might be thought to involve exploitation.

> *Student Athletes.* A, a major university, provides B with a scholarship to play on its football team. A gains considerable revenue, but, like most athletes, B gets little education, does not graduate, and does not go on to play professional football.[20]

Kidneys. A, who is affluent, offers to pay B $25,000 for one of his
kidneys for purposes of transplantation. B, who is poor, agrees
in order to better provide for her family.[21]

Nazi Trials. A, a Nazi medical scientist, wishes to discover how long
a person can live in freezing water. He places B, who has been
placed in a death camp, in freezing water. B dies within an hour.

Surrogacy. A pays B $10,000 to become impregnated with A's
sperm (through artificial insemination) and to waive her rights
to the child after birth.[22]

Psychotherapy. A, a psychotherapist, proposes to B, his patient,
that they have sexual relations. B, who is infatuated with her
therapist, agrees.[23]

Lumber. There has been a hurricane in Florida. A, a lumber
retailer, triples his price for lumber. B, who needs lumber to
rebuild, pays A's price.

Lecherous Millionaire. B's child will die unless she receives
expensive surgery for which the state will not pay. A, a
millionaire, proposes to pay for the surgery if B will agree to
become his mistress. B agrees.

Rescue. B's car is stuck in a snow drift late at night on a rural road.
A comes along in his pick-up truck and offers to pull B out for
$200. It will take A two minutes to complete the job. B agrees.

Let us refer to a statement that A's interaction with B is wrongfully
exploitative as an *exploitation claim*. The first task of a theory of exploitation
is to provide the truth conditions for an exploitation claim. We want to know
whether it is *true* that A exploits B in *Lumber* or *Rescue*. Yet the truth of an
exploitation claim settles less than is often thought. For even if A wrongly
exploits B in *Lumber* or *Rescue*, it does not follow as a matter of moral logic
that we should prohibit or regulate the transaction between A and B. After
all, in *Rescue,* B might say, "I know that he is exploiting me, but I'd rather be
exploited than left here." And so the second task of a theory of exploitation
is to provide an account of its *moral force*. In particular, we must determine
when and why we are justified in prohibiting or regulating or interfering with
exploitative transaction.

Let us first attend to the first question. What are the truth conditions of an
exploitation claim? When is a transaction exploitative? Consider the following
proposed accounts of exploitation.

1. "[T]o exploit a person involves the *harmful, merely instrumental utilization* of him or his capacities, for one's own advantage or for the sake of one's own ends."[24]

2. "It is the fact that the [capitalist's] income is derived through *forced, unpaid, surplus [wage] labor, the product of which the workers do not control,* which makes [wage labor] exploitive."[25]

3. "Exploitation necessarily involves benefits or gains of some kind to someone. . . Exploitation resembles a zero-sum game, viz what the exploiter gains, the exploitee loses; or, minimally, for the exploiter to gain, the exploitee must lose."[26]

4. "Exploitation [in exchange] demands . . . that there is no reasonably eligible alternative [for the exploitee] and that the consideration or advantage received is incommensurate with the price paid. One is not exploited if one is offered what one desperately needs at a fair and reasonable price."[27]

5. "Common to all exploitation of one person (B) by another (A) . . . is that A makes a profit or gain by turning some characteristic of B to his own advantage . . . exploitation . . . can occur in morally unsavory forms without harming the exploitee's interests and . . . despite the exploitee's fully voluntary consent to the exploitative behavior. ."[28]

6. "Persons are exploited if (1) others secure a benefit by (2) using them as a tool or resource so as (3) to cause them serious harm."[29]

7. "An exploitative exchange is. . . an exchange in which the exploited party gets less than the exploiting party, who does better at the exploited party's expense. . . [T]he exchange must result from social relations of unequal power . . . exploitation can be entered into voluntarily; and can even, in some sense, be advantageous to the exploited party."[30]

8. "[E]xploitation is a psychological, rather than a social or an economic concept. For an offer to be exploitative, it must serve to create or to take advantage of some recognized psychological vulnerability which, in turn, disturbs the offeree's ability to reason effectively."[31]

9. "Exploitation, at its heart, is not just about unfair shares or garden-variety degradation; it is about wrongfully exacting benefit from another's actual vulnerability."[32]

All these accounts are compatible with the general claim that "A wrongfully exploits B when A takes unfair advantage of B," but there are some important differences among them. Some accounts are technical definitions of exploitation specific to a Marxist approach (1). Some accounts invoke the Kantian notion that one wrongfully exploits when one treats another instrumentally or merely as a means (1, 6, 9). On some accounts, someone is exploited only if she is harmed (1, 2, 3, 6), whereas others allow that the exploited party may gain from the relationship (4, 5, 7). On some accounts, the exploited party must be coerced (2, 4) or exhibit a defect in the quality or validity of the consent (8), whereas other accounts maintain that exploitation can be fully voluntary or consensual (5, 7).

I think it best not to put rigid constraints on what counts as exploitation. While some exploitative transactions are harmful to the exploitee, as is obvious in *Nazi Trial* and is likely in *Psychotherapy,* we often describe as exploitative cases in which both parties gain, as might be true in *Student Athletes, Surrogacy, Kidneys, Lumber, Lecherous Millionaire,* and *Rescue.* It will, therefore, be useful to make two sets of distinctions. First, we can distinguish between *harmful exploitation* and *mutually advantageous exploitation.* By harmful exploitation, I refer to those cases in which the exploiter gains by harming the exploitee. By mutually advantageous exploitation, I refer to those cases in which both parties—including the exploitee—reasonably expect to gain from the transaction as contrasted with the pre-transaction *status quo* or more accurately, as contrasted with their pre-transaction rights or entitlements. In any case, it is the *advantageousness* that is mutual, not the exploitation.

We can similarly distinguish between *nonconsensual exploitation* and *consensual exploitation.* By nonconsensual exploitation, I refer to cases in which the exploitee does not token consent or does not give morally transformative consent. Setting aside the possibility that exploitation itself may render consent non-transformative in certain ways (see Chapter 3), consensual exploitation refers to cases where the exploited party has given consent that would *otherwise* be regarded as morally transformative; that is, the consent is voluntary, competent, informed, and so forth.

The two distinctions overlap but are not equivalent. There can be cases of mutually advantageous but nonconsensual exploitation. If, in a version of

Rescue, A threatened to hurt B if B did not agree to pay A $200, B has not given morally transformative consent because he was coerced, but the transaction might still be mutually advantageous. There can also be cases of harmful but consensual exploitation, as when a self-loathing B allows A to benefit by harming her. Nonetheless, because these distinctions tend to converge, and because it will simplify matters, I shall rely on the distinction between harmful non-consensual exploitation (HNE) and mutually advantageous and consensual exploitation (MACE).

HNE is typically morally worse than MACE, but it is of less theoretical interest. It is not difficult to explain why it is wrong to harm another or to act without another's consent and it is relatively easy to justify prohibiting such actions. By contrast, it is more difficult to explain why and when MACE can be wrong and whether and why we might be justified in prohibiting or refusing to enforce such transactions. And so it is on those latter cases on which we will focus.

The elements of exploitation

Let us start with the claim that A exploits B when A takes unfair advantage of B. Taking unfair advantage could be understood in two ways. First, it may refer to some dimension of the *outcome* of the exploitative act or transaction, that is, the transaction is substantively unfair. And this, it seems, has two elements: (1) the benefit to A, and (2) the effect on B. We may say that the benefit to A is unfair because it is wrong for A to benefit by harming B in a case of HNE (in addition to the wrong of the harm itself) or because A's benefit is excessive relative to B's benefit in a case of MACE. Second, to say that A takes unfair advantage of B may imply that there is some sort of defect in the *process* by which the unfair outcome comes about; for example, that A coerces B into giving (apparent) consent or that A deceives B or fails to provide B with relevant information or manipulates B. If mutually advantageous and consensual transactions can be exploitative, then a defect in consent is not a necessary condition of exploitation. Rather, a moral defect in the *outcome* is both *necessary and sufficient* to constitute exploitation.

The Outcome of a Transaction

In assessing the exploitativeness of a transaction, we must consider two dimensions: its effect on A and its effect on B.

Benefit to A

A cannot take *unfair* advantage of B unless A gets some *advantage* from the transaction with B. Recall *Student Athletes*. If a university expects to *lose* money on its athletic programs, we cannot say that it *exploits* its athletes, although it may mistreat them if it does not provide them with appropriate educational opportunities. It is not accidental that all of the discussions of the exploitation of student athletes refer to those programs that generate income. The athletes can hardly claim that the university is making a profit at their expense when the university is not making a profit.

We can see the relevance of the "benefit to A" by contrasting exploitation with other forms of wrongdoing, such as discrimination, oppression, and neglect. A does not exploit B if A refuses to hire B on racial grounds, for A does not gain from the wrong to B. Let us say that A oppresses B when A deprives B of freedoms or opportunities to which B is entitled. If A gains from the oppressive relationship, as when A enslaves B, then A may both oppress and exploit B. But if A does not gain from the oppression, the oppression is wrong but not exploitative. Perhaps most important for present purposes, exploitation is a *transactional* or *interactional* norm. A does *not* exploit B when A *neglects* or *ignores* B as in *Non-Rescue*, where A sees B's plight but doesn't stop.

Although A exploits B only when A gains from the transaction with B, we can be relatively open ended as to what *counts* as a benefit to A. With respect to type of benefit, A may gain money or sexual pleasure or status or even scientific knowledge. A researcher could exploit his subjects while trying to advance perfectly benevolent ends as might have been true in SCAT. A university may exploit some athletes in order to build a better library or support scholarships for academically talented students or to support athletic programs that lose money.

The previous examples suggest that we can distinguish between *direct* and *indirect* exploitation. In direct exploitation, the exploiter is the primary beneficiary of the transaction. In indirect exploitation, the "exploiter" may generate benefits for others who are not parties to the transaction. The beneficiaries of the transaction may not be morally culpable, but it is only because the transaction serves to benefit them that we can say that others were exploited to benefit them.

On my view, A can exploit B if A can expect (*ex ante*) to benefit even if he does not benefit *ex post*. Suppose that A hires B and C to dig oil wells.

B and C are illegal immigrants and A pays them a sub-minimum wage. Each is required to dig a well by himself. A expects to find oil 50% of the time, a rate that is sufficient to generate a hefty profit. B's well turns up dry. C's well generates oil. If we adopt an actual benefit or *ex post* approach, then A exploits C, from whose efforts he makes a profit, but does not exploit B. I prefer to say that A exploits *both* B and C, because A has a positive *expected value* from the efforts of both B and C.

The effect on B

A's transaction or interaction with B may affect B in three ways. It may have no effect on B. It may be harmful to B. It may be advantageous to B. Let us consider each.

No Effect

There are cases in which B is not directly affected by A's utilization of B, what Feinberg refers to as *harmless parasitism*, as when A follows B's tail-lights in a dense fog. A uses B to his own advantage, but his use of B has no effect on B's welfare (assume that B is not bothered by A's headlights in B's mirror). There are also cases in which A's utilization of B has no palpable effect on B, but where it might violate B's privacy or autonomy or control. If A uses B's medical history as data without consulting B, it is arguable that B has not been harmed, but that B has been exploited. But if we define harm so as to include a violation of B's rights, and if B's rights are violated in such cases, then we could say that B has been harmed.[33]

B is Harmed

For present purposes we do not need an elaborate account of harm. In the standard case, A harms B by rendering B worse off. But worse off than what? In most cases, A harms B when A renders B worse off than B's prior *status quo*. In other cases, we might refer to B's trajectory or B's rights.

> *Cancer.* B has incurable cancer. If untreated, B's condition will decline rapidly and B will die in 6 months. A proposes a treatment that will slow the worsening of B's condition.

We would not say that A's treatment has harmed B in *Cancer* even though B is worse off after A's intervention, because A's intervention promises to render B *less* worse off than she would otherwise have been.

> *Inheritance.* C's will leaves $1,000,000 to B. A, the attorney for the
> estate, bills the estate an excessive amount, leaving B with
> $900,000 rather than $950,000.

In my view, A has harmed B even though A's actions leave B better off than
her pre-transaction *status quo*, because A's actions leave B less well off than
she has a right to be. Consider this case.

> *Tissue.* A uses tissue taken from B in the course of a standard
> medical procedure to develop a therapy that generates a profit
> for A. A makes no payment to B.[34]

If B has a right to a portion of A's profit—and I need take no position on that
here—then B is harmed in *Tissue* because A's action leaves B worse off than
she has a right to be.

B Gains

In cases of mutually advantageous exploitation, the transaction is beneficial
to B by reference to the "rights based" baseline just discussed. By that standard, B may gain in *Student Athletes, Lumber, Surrogacy, Kidneys, Lecherous
Millionaire, and Rescue.* True, A's transaction with B may leave B worse off
than the position to which B has a "general" right. For example, B may have
a right to have the state pay for her child's medical care in *Lecherous Millionaire.* Even so, B certainly has no right that *A* pay for her child's care, and so
the transaction between A and B should be understood as beneficial to B.

   In assessing the effect of a transaction on B, it is important to keep the
following considerations in mind. First, in asking how A's action affects B's
interests, we must be careful to adopt an *all things considered* point of view.
There are, after all, negative or harmful *elements* in virtually all uncontroversially beneficial transactions. If B pays money for a good that is clearly worth
the price, the payment is a negative element in the transaction, but the transaction is still advantageous to B all things considered. Similarly, although the
sale of a kidney has significant negative elements, a seller might reasonably
think that the value of the money exceeds the value of the costs or risks.

   Second, and as with assessing benefits to A, we should adopt an *ex ante*
point of view. Suppose that A enters into a business transaction with B,
where B expects (*ex ante*) to gain eighty per cent of the time and lose twenty
per cent of the time, as when A sells B land on which B hopes to find oil. We
could *say* that the transaction is harmful to B in those cases where B fails to

find oil, but it is not harmful in a way that has any moral significance if B's *ex ante* utility is clearly positive.

Third, we should resist the temptation to say that a transaction is harmful to B because A violates B's more abstract (Kantian) right not to be treated merely as a means but always as an end in herself. Along these lines, Allen Buchanan argues that exploitation occurs "whenever persons are harmfully utilized as mere instruments for private gain," and adds that this could apply to business transactions between two affluent bankers—"Each harmfully utilizes the other as a mere means to his own advantage."[35]

It is not clear what to make of this view. First, on one plausible reading of the Kantian maxim, one treats another *merely* as a means only when one treats "him in a way to which he could not possibly consent," as in cases of coercion and fraud because doing so undermines B's capacity as an autonomous decision-maker.[36] On this view, the bankers are *not* treating each other *merely* as a means to their own ends if each banker's treatment of the other banker requires the other's consent. Second, even if treating another as a means is a *way* of harming her, we would still want to distinguish between those cases in which A imposes a palpable harm on B from those in which B is not harmed apart from the harm that derives from being treated as a means. So the Kantian view does not deny the distinction between harmful exploitation and mutually advantageous exploitation.

When Are Mutually Advantageous Transactions Unfair? If clinical trials such as ST can be beneficial to the participants, then we need an account of a fair transaction if we are to make good on the claim that those trials are exploitative. And while many commentators write as if it were obvious when and why a transaction is unfair, I know of no non-problematic accounts of fair transactions, including one I have defended elsewhere.[37]

Some people adopt what Rawls calls a "pure procedural" view of transactional fairness.[38] They are inclined to argue that if a transaction is mutually advantageous and genuinely consensual then it simply cannot be unfair and (wrongfully) exploitative. Others, like me, have the intuition that transactions such as *Lumber* and *Rescue* can be unfair and exploitative, even if it is difficult to explain why.

We might say that a transaction is unfair when the goods exchanged are "incommensurable," as might be thought of the exchange of a bodily organ for money—"You can't put a price on a kidney." There are two problems here. First, it is not clear whether and when goods are ultimately incommensurable. (See Chapter 4) Second, if goods are incommensurable and we cannot *compare* what the parties receive, it is difficult to claim that the alleged exploitee receives too little and that the exchange is therefore unfair.

It might be argued that a mutually advantageous transaction is unfair or exploitative when A takes advantage of B's vulnerabilities or desperate situation to strike a deal. Joan McGregor writes that "Taking advantage of people's desperation, misfortune, or illness constitutes clear cases of unfair advantage taking."[39] This is surely wrong. The claim (1) "A is *taking advantage of unfairness* to B" does not entail (2) "A is *taking unfair advantage* of B." Consider the following examples.

> *Generic.* A proposes to sell B the generic version of a life-saving
> drug for a fair price. B accepts.
> *Surgery.* A proposes to amputate B's leg for a fair fee. Because
> B will die unless she agrees to the amputation, B authorizes
> A to perform the surgery.

A takes advantage of B's vulnerability in the sense that A makes a profit. Nonetheless, A does not exploit B in either case because a transaction is exploitative only if the distribution of the benefits is *unfair.* And here it is not.

Some philosophers, such as Allen Wood, have argued that it is degrading to have others take advantage of one's vulnerabilities and that such degradation—not unfairness—is the central wrong of exploitation.

> Proper respect for others is violated when we treat their
> vulnerabilities as opportunities to advance our own interests or
> projects. It is degrading to have your weaknesses taken advantage
> of and dishonorable to use the weaknesses of others for your ends,
> even if the exploitative arrangement is voluntary on both sides and
> no matter what the resulting distribution of benefits and harms.[40]

These claims have a pleasant ring, but it's not clear precisely what Wood is claiming or whether we should accept these claims. If taking advantages of "weaknesses" refers to the target's personal characteristics and decision-making infirmities, then the arrangement may not be fully voluntary. If the "weaknesses" or "vulnerabilities" are circumstantial, then it's not clear that there's anything wrong, per se, with using them for one's own ends. We do well to remember that the whole point of many legitimate occupations—plumbing, roofing, automobile repair, medicine—is to (non-pejoratively) take advantage of people's vulnerabilities. Although the providers of such services act wrongly when they take *unfair* advantage of those vulnerabilities, they do *not* act wrongly simply because they regard those vulnerabilities as an opportunity to advance their own interests.

Moreover, even if B's present situation is unjust and not merely unfortunate, it does not follow that the transaction *between A and B* is unfair or exploitative.

> *Unjust Firing*. B has been unjustly fired from a law firm where she
> was making $150,000 per year. A community college offers her
> a position to teach law courses for $40,000 per year, the
> maximum salary that it can offer.

A is taking advantage of the unfair situation in which B finds herself, but A is not taking unfair advantage of B. B's complaint is with the law firm, not the community college.

The dominant and superficially attractive view is that a mutually advantageous transaction is unfair when "the exploiter's gain is disproportionate when compared to the exploited person's gain."[41] On examination, this, too, can't be right. First, history matters. Certainly the fairness of the distribution of the results of a transaction is sometimes a function of the parties' contributions to or investments in the transaction. If A contributes $4,000 and B contributes $1,000 to a joint enterprise that yields a profit of $5,000, it does not seem unfair if A gets the lion's share of the profit.

Second, it is paradoxical but true that if we measure the parties' gains by the marginal utility they receive from a transaction as compared with the baseline in which there is no transaction at all, then the alleged exploitee typically gains *more* from an exploitative transaction than the exploiter.

> *Unfair Surgery*. A, a surgeon, knows that all the other surgeons
> in the area are on vacation. B will die without surgery.
> A proposes to perform the surgery for three times his
> normal fee. B accepts.

We would *not* say that B exploits A in *Unfair Surgery* because B receives a disproportionate gain from the transaction. After all, although A receives an excessive payment, B gets her *life*. Rather, we would say that A exploits B even though B gets *much* more value from the transaction than A. It is true that there is an immense inequality of bargaining power in this case. A has B "over a barrel." But on closer inspection, the exploiter's power over the exploitee typically stems precisely from the fact that the exploiter does *not* stand to gain too much and can walk away from the transaction more easily than the exploitee.

This suggests that we cannot evaluate the fairness of a transaction by comparing how much utility the parties can expect to receive from the transaction. Rather, we must measure the fairness of their gains against a *normative standard* as to how much the parties *ought* to gain. Unfortunately, that standard is not easy to specify.

I have elsewhere suggested that we might use a "hypothetical market" criterion of a fair transaction, where the terms are fair if they were the terms that would be agreed to by rational informed bargainers in a competitive market environment or what we sometimes call "fair market value."[42] For example, if I want to sell my house to a friend for a *fair* price, then I will try to discover what would (hypothetically) be paid for the house in an actual competitive market. The question is *not* how much I paid for the house (my profit) or what the buyer can afford. Fairness is market dependent. If the *actual* market in which A and B operate is highly competitive, A does not exploit B if A pays B the market price.

> *Burger King.* Burger King pays its workers $8.00 per hour,
>   similar to what McDonald's and Wendy's pays its
>   workers. Burger King's employees claim that they
>   are exploited.

I suggest that Burger King does *not* exploit its workers if, as seems likely, they could not afford to pay more, given that it operates in a highly competitive environment. It may be unjust that B has a low income, but we should not condemn Burger King, which is constrained by the market. Here, as elsewhere, ought implies can. Exploitation is tied to the set of feasible options available to A. After all, if Burger King paid more, then it would have to raise its price (losing customers and then profits) or maintain the same price but reduce its profit margin (losing shareholders). By contrast, A can arguably afford to sell at the normal price in *Lumber*, and that is why raising its price might be exploitative.[43]

Robert Mayer disagrees. Mayer argues that A engages in "structural exploitation" whenever A gains from a transaction that does not raise B's baseline to an acceptable level *regardless* of what A could feasibly provide to B. On his view, Burger King may exploit its workers if it fails to provide, say, a livable wage even if Burger King's profits are relatively low.

The low wages they receive are not adequate compensation for the work despite the fact that they represent the 'fair market value' of this labor in a competitive economy. Anyone who makes a profit by paying such low wages is an exploiter, even if competitive pressure makes it infeasible to pay more.[44]

I don't get it. Mayer may be right to claim that B would earn more in a more just better world, but if the point of claiming that A *exploits* B is that A is acting *wrongly*, I do not think anything is gained by saying that A exploits B in cases of structural exploitation. .

We appear to be stuck. Although I cannot produce a non-problematic theory of fair transactions, I remain convinced that some mutually advantageous transactions are unfair and exploitative. At the same time, I am reluctant to endorse the spirit of Justice Potter Stewart's view of pornography ("I shall not attempt to further define pornography, but I know it when I see it") because our intuitions about the fairness of transactions are often erroneous.[45] For example, we may think it unfair for a lender to charge a high rate of interest to a penurious borrower, but such rates may be necessary to compensate the lender for the high risk that the loan will not be repaid. Here is a test: do those who loan money to penurious borrowers earn supra-competitive returns? Suppose that A_1 loans money to poor people at 25% per annum whereas A_2 loans to rich people at 8% per annum and that A_1's net profit from such loans is no greater than A_2's profit given the high rate of default. I see no reason to think that A_1 is a (wrongful) exploiter but that A_2 is not. As Shaher Lifshitz has argued, it is the net gain to the *provider* that determines whether an agreement is exploitative and not the needs of or gains to the recipient.

> *Professional Rescue.* B's car is stuck in a snow drift late at night on a rural road. A is a self-employed professional rescuer. He roams the roads during snow storms, offering to tow people for $200. His net income is $20 per hour. A offers to pull B out for $200. It will take A two minutes. B agrees.

I believe that A has *not* exploited B in *Professional Rescue* because A does not earn an unreasonable amount on a per hour basis.

Although I am painfully aware that I have not presented a non-problematic principle of fair transactions, I am disinclined to abandon our strong intuition that mutually advantageous and consensual transactions can be substantively unfair. For present purposes, I will simply assume for the sake of argument that some mutually advantageous transactions are unfair by reference to an appropriate normative standard.

When Is A Transaction Consensual?

Although I have argued that one can consent to be exploited, the claim that A exploits B is often associated with the claim that B does not give morally transformative consent to the transaction. At first glance, it seems plausible to argue that A does not exploit if B voluntarily agrees to what might otherwise be an unequal or unfair distribution of advantages and burdens. Motive is important. I do not think that a hospital exploits its volunteer workers even if others are paid for comparable work if the volunteers prefer to work altruistically for no pay than not to work. Intentional altruism aside, although a transaction can be exploitative even if B's decision is voluntary, well informed, and rational as in *Lumber* and *Rescue,* the *moral force* of exploitation may turn on whether the exploitation is consensual. In particular, there may be good reason to prohibit nonconsensual exploitation, but to *permit* consensual exploitation. We have at least *prima facie* reason *not* to interfere with a person's autonomous choice to allow herself to be exploited.

Because I considered consent in some detail in Chapters 3 and 4, I will make only a few brief remarks here.

Voluntariness

We generally say that consent is voluntary when it is not coerced. I have argued that A coerces B to do X *in a way that renders B's consent non-transformative* only if A proposes (threatens) to violate B's rights if B chooses not do X. On this view, A does *not* coerce B in cases such as *Lumber, Lecherous Millionaire, Surgery, Kidneys,* or *Surrogacy.* For A does not propose to violate B's rights if B rejects A's proposal in any of these cases. Whatever we think about A's proposal in *Lecherous Millionaire,* A has made an offer not a threat, and offers do not coerce. The mere fact that B may have no reasonable alternative to accepting A's proposal does *not* entail that B's decision is coerced. We would not say that A commits a battery in *Surgery* on the grounds that B has no reasonable alternative but to agree to surgery. Moreover, even if B's background situation is unjust, it does not follow that A's proposal is coercive. Even if a just society would provide for B's daughter's surgery in *Lecherous Millionaire,* B has no right that *A* pay for her surgery. And so whatever else we think about A, his proposal does not coerce B into having sexual relations with him.

Information

B's token of consent may not be morally transformative if there are defects in B's information such that B's decision is not likely to advance B's interests considered from an *ex ante* and *all things considered* point of view. In some cases, B's informational deficiencies may be due to fraud, as when A deliberately sets back the odometer in a car that he is selling. In other cases, A may withhold or fail to disclose information that A has an obligation to provide. And so B's agreement to purchase a home from A is not binding if A fails to tell B that the roof leaks. And in the paradigmatic medical context, B's consent to surgery is not valid if A fails to inform B of the risks that are involved.

Competence

Even if A provides B with all the relevant information, B may not have the competence to process that information. We often assume that minors and those with mental impairments do not have the cognitive or emotional capacities to give morally transformative consent. Those who lack adequate education may be unable to make reasonable evaluations of the alternatives. Moreover, even if B is an otherwise competent person, her competence can be temporarily disturbed as in *Psychotherapy*, where B may be in the grips of transference. Furthermore, B's judgment can also be distorted when A makes what I call a *seductive offer*, where the lure of short term benefits causes B to excessively discount the long-term costs and to make a decision that does not serve her long-term interests, as *may* be true of cases such as *Kidneys* and *Surrogacy*.

Consensual Exploitation

All that said, there are numerous cases of alleged exploitation where B would not have agreed to A's proposal under better or perhaps more just background conditions, but where A has no special obligation to repair those conditions or to transact with B, and where B is fully informed as to the consequences of various choices and fully capable of making such choices. Without prejudging whether these transactions are actually exploitative or unfair, I suggest that such conditions *may* obtain in *Kidneys, Surrogacy, Lecherous Millionaire, Lumber,* and *Rescue.* Precisely because B's objective situation is what it is, it may be reasonable for B to agree to proposals to which those who are better situated would not agree.

Once again, I do *not* deny that A's transaction with B may be wrongfully exploitative even if B gives morally transformative consent. Moreover, I do not preclude the possibility that a transaction should be prohibited even if it is mutually advantageous and consensual. The present point is that we should *not* treat B's consent as non-transformative on grounds of coercion, information, competence, or rationality, just because the transaction is exploitative.

What Is the Moral Force of Exploitation?

The moral force of harmful and nonconsensual exploitation is relatively unproblematic. If a transaction is a case HNE, there is at least a *prima facie* case for prohibiting it. But what could justify not allowing the parties to enter into a mutually advantageous consensual transaction or refusing to enforce its terms given that such refusal is effectively equivalent to prohibiting the transaction? Consider a version of *Rescue.*

> *Cash-Poor.* B is prepared to pay A $200 to tow his car, but has
> only $50 in cash. He has no checks. He is prepared to sign an
> IOU for $150.

If it is known that the state will not enforce such agreements on the grounds that it constitutes an "unconscionable contract," A may be unwilling to rescue B. Can such a policy be justified? Perhaps.

Let us assume that the following (Table 5.1) represents the utility gains of A and B in *Rescue* as contrasted with the baseline in which A does not rescue B.

I intentionally stipulate that B gains more *utility* than A in the *unfair* transaction (2) to emphasize the earlier point that the exploitee often gains more utility in an exploitative transaction than the exploiter. It is entirely possible, for example, that B would have paid $500 to be rescued under the circumstances, but that we would still regard $200 as an excessive and unfair price.

Table 5.1

		A's payoff	B's Payoff
(1) No Transaction		0	0
(2) Unfair Transaction	($200)	4	6
(3) Fair Transaction	($50)	2	8

Rescue raises an interesting question about "comparative wrongness." Is A's behavior in (2) morally worse than in (1)? One might think that the wrongness of A's behavior must track the outcome for B, such that A's behavior in (1) must be worse than A's behavior in (2) because B is worse off in (1) than in (2). I consider this issue in more detail in Chapter 6.

In any case, the present question is not whether A's behavior in (2) could be wrong given that A's behavior in (1) is permissible, but whether it is possible to justify interfering in exploitative transactions such as (2) given that we do not require A to aid B in (1). After all, those who claim that a practice is exploitative typically claim or assume that exploitation provides a reason for intervention. Those who argue that commercial surrogacy exploits the birth mothers also maintain that surrogacy contracts should be unenforceable or entirely prohibited.[46] Those who argue that a market in kidneys exploits the poor typically argue that such sales should be banned. Those who argue that studies such as SCAT or ST are exploitative believe that such studies should not be allowed. Those who support intervention may assume or argue that the practices are nonconsensual or harmful, but we need to ask whether intervention can be justified if the transactions are consensual and mutually advantageous.

That line of argument is more difficult to sustain. As a starting point, it seems reasonable to assume a moral default position in which we should not interfere with or prohibit transactions which are beneficial to both parties and to which both parties consent. Consider, once again, the payoff structure of *Rescue* as described in Table 5.1. Suppose A proposes (2) (where B pays $200). B counters that they should agree on (3) (where B pays $50). A rejects (3) and tells B that it is either (1) (no transaction) or (2). Given these options, B is prepared to accept (2). At first glance it seems that society is not justified in preventing B from accepting (2), its unfairness notwithstanding and that it should also be prepared to enforce its terms, as in *Cash-Poor*, if doing so is necessary to facilitate such transactions.

Reasons for Intervention

In this section I consider seven arguments for intervention with mutually advantageous consensual exploitation. Although I do *not* think that most of these arguments are successful, at least one argument is quite plausible.

Paternalism

As we saw in Chapter 2, we may be justified in interfering with transactions on paternalistic grounds in order to protect B from making a decision that does not advance her own interests. But a paternalistic argument for interference simply does not apply in the present context if the exploitative transaction is *advantageous* to the exploitee. We can hardly forbid B from agreeing to pay the exorbitant price in *Rescue* on paternalistic grounds if A would otherwise leave her stranded. Similarly, we could not justify preventing parents from allowing their infants to participate in ST on paternalistic grounds given that the infants can expect to be better off if they do participate. So we can set paternalism aside as a justification for interfering with MACE.

Externalities

We might interfere with mutually advantageous and consensual transactions because they impose harm or negative externalities on others or because interference provides benefits or positive externalities to *others*. For example, even if commercial surrogacy is beneficial to the participants directly involved, it might have negative effects on the way in which society perceives and treats women or children.[47] And even if *Lecherous Millionaire* were beneficial to B, a system which allows A to take advantage of society's failure to provide health care may postpone the day in which society fulfills its obligation.

    Three points about this line of argument. First, if a transaction between A and B has negative effects on others, there is a *prima facie* case for intervention, although there are some contexts in which we do and probably should ignore such harms. If A offers B a job for which C has applied, the transaction between A and B has a negative effect on C. But this hardly constitutes a reason to interfere with the transaction because C has no right to be protected from competitors. Second, it is an empirical question—and often an extraordinarily complex empirical question—as to whether interfering with a practice would actually reduce negative externalities or promote positive externalities. The assertion that commercial surrogacy has harmful effects on the way in which society regards children and women does not show that commercial surrogacy actually has those effects.[48] Third, even if the externalities argument provides a rationale for intervention, it has nothing to do with the interests of the exploitee or exploitation as such, and so we can set it aside.

Strategic Intervention

What I call "strategic intervention" is the most plausible justification for interfering with MACE. It is, in essence, a collective action argument. The core idea is best explained by an example. Thomas Schelling once argued that professional hockey players preferred to wear helmets for safety but that few players would do so voluntarily because they believed that wearing helmets compromised performance, putting them at a competitive disadvantage, and also detracted from their "macho" reputation.[49] Schelling argued that virtually all players would prefer that the NHL *require* them to wear helmets, in which case they can gain the safety benefits of helmets without bearing the competitive or reputational costs. Wearing hockey helmets constituted a collective action problem among the players that could be solved by *strategic intervention*. Virtually all players would prefer (1) helmets to (2) no helmets, but will end up choosing (2) if left to their own devices, and so requiring helmets shifted the equilibrium from (2) to (1). Minimum wage laws can also be understood as a strategic intervention. Left to fend for themselves, it may be perfectly rational for many workers to accept a sub-minimum wage rather than remain unemployed. Yet it would be better for most (perhaps not all) if they were prevented from agreeing to sub-minimum wage proposals—if employers would then offer higher wages rather than not hiring them at all.

Strategic intervention bears some resemblance to paternalistic intervention because it interferes with the agent for her own good. It is, however, importantly different. Whereas paternalistic intervention overrides the individual's preferences, strategic intervention serves to help or enable a person get the result that she already prefers but cannot obtain without such intervention.

The strategic argument may apply to interference with exploitative transactions. Recall the payoff structure of *Rescue*, where A can make a credible threat to opt for (1) (no transaction) rather than (3) (fair transaction) and so get B to agree to (2) (unfair transaction). The strategic argument maintains that if the state *prohibits* A from entering into transaction (2) or announces that it will refuse to enforce its terms in *Cash Poor* on the grounds that it is an "unconscionable contract," then A will propose (3) rather than (1). After all, given that A benefits from (3), A has no reason to opt for (1) over (3) if the state effectively takes (2) off the table. In short, the strategic argument says that we may be justified in not allowing A to exploit B if preventing such exploitation will cause A to offer a fairer deal to B rather than refusing to transact with B.

The relevance of the strategic argument to a given case depends on the facts. It is an empirical question as to how potential contractors will react to such intervention. The strategic argument might justify interfering in cases such as *Rescue* where A is the only seller and B is the only buyer, but might *not* justify interfering in cases such as *Lumber* where there may be many potential buyers if B did not want to contract with A at A's proposed price. Whether barring "unconscionable contracts" in a case such as *Cash Poor* helps the exploitee, similarly depends on the likely outcomes of such intervention. My tentative conclusion is that the strategic argument provides an important and plausible rationale for interfering with mutually advantageous and consensual exploitation in clinical research. The empirical question is whether interference with such research actually works to the advantage of prospective subjects.

Epistemological Arguments

There may be situations where it is difficult to determine whether a transaction is a case of HNE or MACE. Given these epistemological difficulties, it may make sense to prohibit all transactions of a certain type because the expected harms associated with cases of HNE may be greater than the expected benefits associated with cases of MACE. Interfering with genuine cases of MACE is simply the price we have to pay for prohibiting HNE. As I argued in Chapter 2 with respect to group soft-paternalism, something like this may be true of situations such as *Psychotherapy*. Suppose that most cases of psychotherapist/patient sexual relations are harmful to the patient and not based on morally transformative consent, but that *some* cases have no harmful (or even beneficial) effects and are robustly consensual. It does *not* follow that it should be permissible for psychotherapists and patients to engage in such relations when they believe it is benign and consensual. For given that neither psychotherapists nor patients are well positioned to have confidence that their relationship is mutually advantageous or consensual (and perhaps not exploitative), it may be better to prohibit all psychotherapist/patient sexual relations.

As with the strategic argument, the force of the epistemological argument depends on facts. For example, although it is clear that some cases of commercial surrogacy work out badly for the surrogate mother (as in the case of Mary Beth Whitehead), it is possible that most cases work out reasonably well.[50] If so, we would not be justified in prohibiting *all* commercial surrogacy transactions by appeal to the epistemological argument. If the independent review of research protocols is working reasonably well, we do not need to trust investigators to determine whether a protocol is beneficial or consensual, so there is no reason to think that the epistemological argument would justify interfering with mutually advantageous and consensual research on the grounds that there is a high probability that we are mistaken about its advantageousness and consensuality.

A Brief Interlude: The Permitted Exploitation Principle (PEP)

Before considering three additional arguments for interfering with mutually advantageous and consensual transactions, it is worth noting that the previous four arguments are *person affecting arguments*. They attempt to justify interfering with transactions on the grounds that interference is better for *someone*. Paternalistic and strategic arguments claim that interference advances the interests of the exploitee. The externalities argument claims that interference may be good for others. The epistemological arguments claim that interference will be bad for those who are not harmed by the transaction, but will be good for those who are harmed.

But could we justify interfering with mutually advantageous and consensual transactions when interference is *better for no one*? To get a grip on the problem, let us make the following assumptions which might be true of a case such as *Rescue* or *Lecherous Millionaire,* and may also be true of some cases of clinical research.

1. A is under no obligation to transact with B on any terms.
2. A proposes to transact with B on unfair terms.

3. A's transaction with B on unfair terms is to A's benefit (*ex ante*)
   and also serves B's interests (*ex ante*), all things considered
   (setting aside paternalistic arguments).
4. A's transacting with B on unfair terms will not harm other
   persons (setting aside externalities).
5. B makes a voluntary, informed, and rational decision to transact
   with A on unfair terms and we can reliably determine that this is
   so (setting aside epistemological arguments).
6. If A is not allowed to transact with B on unfair terms, A will *not*
   choose to interact with B on fair terms that are more favorable
   to B (setting aside strategic arguments).

If such conditions 1-6 obtain, then we must ask whether we could justify
preventing a transaction that is good for the parties involved, to which the
parties consent, that is worse for no one else, and in which interference will
not improve the outcome for the disadvantaged party.

Let us refer to the claim that it would be wrong to interfere with such
transactions as *The Permitted Exploitation Principle* (PEP). The PEP does *not*
claim that it is *morally permissible* for A to exploit B. Rather, PEP claims that
it is wrong to prevent Pareto superior or win-win transactions on the grounds
that the terms of such transactions are unfair. The PEP refers to the *morality
of regulating transactions*, and not the *morality of transactions* themselves.

The distinction between the morality of an act and the morality of regulation or interference is, of course, at the heart of liberalism. Consider freedom
of speech. Although it is wrong to make a speech in which one denies that
the Holocaust occurred, it may also be wrong to interfere with such a speech.
Some cases are more difficult.

> *The Bigot's Will.* After many years, B's son has declared that he is
> gay. B asks his lawyer, A, to re-write his will such that B is
> disinherited.

If B has a right to leave his money to whomever he wishes, then it would be
wrong to *prevent* him from doing so. In addition, if B needs a lawyer's assistance to accomplish his aim, there is not much distinction between preventing B from rewriting his will and refusing to assist him in doing so. On that
somewhat uncomfortable view, it is not only sometimes right not to interfere
with another's wrongdoing, it is sometimes right to assist others in doing
wrong if they have a right to do wrong.

Justice

With this interlude behind us, there are at least three (arguably) non-person affecting arguments for rejecting PEP. A deontological or egalitarian argument might maintain that we are *prima facie* justified in prohibiting an exploitative transaction simply because it is unfair or unjust.[51] Because I consider this argument in more detail in Chapter 6, I shall be brief here. I do not think it *incoherent* to claim that there might be deontological reasons to reject PEP, but such a view is difficult to defend. Clearly, one cannot reject PEP by appealing to some of the traditional arguments against consequentialism. The PEP does not claim that we should allow transactions just in case they have better aggregate consequences, where the advantages to some outweigh the harm to others. The permitted exploitation principle says that we should allow transactions when it would be better for *all parties* to the transaction and *worse for no one else*. Moreover, because PEP precludes intervention only when the parties give valid consent to the transaction, one cannot easily reject PEP on the grounds that it allows A to use B as a mere means to his own ends. Although we can disagree as to the force of the "mere means" principle and whether B's valid consent completely blocks that charge, B's valid consent surely goes at least some (if not) all of the way towards defusing that charge.

A Symbolic Argument

A symbolic argument for intervention maintains that we are justified in prohibiting unfair but mutually advantageous transactions in order to symbolize the view that the exploiters are behaving wrongly. The symbolic argument concedes that interference will prevent some win-win transactions to the detriment of the parties involved, but maintains that doing so will encourage fairer transactions in the long run. As Seana Shiffrin puts it, "One should not underestimate the benefits of having an environment in which exploitation does not occur, or at least, in which the state forbears from facilitating clearly unfair treatment."[52]

Now to the extent that a policy of interfering with or refusing to uphold MACE transactions motivates people to transact more fairly, the symbolic argument turns out to be a person-affecting (externalities) argument. A *pure* symbolic argument would argue that it is justifiable to interfere even if the symbolization has no effect on anyone's behavior. I find this very difficult to believe.

Complicity

A final argument for interfering with exploitative agreements focuses on the "enablers." It may be thought that even if the parties themselves have a right to enter into an exploitative transaction such as *Rescue*, "others may reasonably feel that they may or even must not assist" such transactions, say by being prepared to enforce its terms.[53] It may be wrong for me to try to prevent a friend from smoking, but it does not follow that I have to buy her cigarettes (even with her money). On this view, we may have "a permission and perhaps a deontological commitment not to assist grossly unfair treatment" even if the exploited party prefers that we do so.

The complicity argument is of obvious relevance to clinical research given that IRBs must specifically approve a study if it is to go forward. If the argument can be sustained, then it might justify IRBs from refusing to approve exploitative research not because it is contrary to the interests of research subjects, but because it's wrong for IRBs to assist or enable immoral transactions.

I am not convinced that the complicity argument can be sustained. First, I believe that the complicity argument puts too much pressure on the distinction between the "prohibition" of a transaction and "non-enabling" or "non-enforcement" of a transaction. For example, it suggests that the state is *not* complicit with the unfair transaction in *Rescue* if it chooses not to prohibit it, but that the state is complicit in a case such as *Cash-Poor* if it chooses to enforce the terms of the transaction. Given that the transaction will not occur unless the state is prepared to enforce its terms, it is arguable that if the state should not lend its hand in *Cash-Poor*, then perhaps it should also prohibit the transaction in *Rescue*. Similarly, it is arguable that if the state should not prohibit in *Rescue,* then it should lend its enforcement powers in *Cash-Poor*.

Second, the complicity argument also seems to involve a paradoxical relation to the wrongness of a transaction. If an exploitative transaction is wrongful because it does not do enough for B, then its wrongness is a function of its effects on B. Yet the complicity argument is strangely indifferent to the interests of those who are treated wrongfully. To the extent that the "enablers" should be concerned with advancing the interests of those who are treated wrongfully and should also be concerned to respect their autonomy, then they should be prepared to hold their noses and assist A's wrongful exploitation of B if, *ex hypothesi,* the transaction will not occur without their assistance.

The Moral Force of MACE: A Problem of
Non-Ideal Theory

Where does this leave us? I have argued that exploitation is wrong even if the transaction or arrangement is mutually advantageous and consensual. I have also argued that there are often good reasons to adopt what I have called the Permitted Exploitation Principle (PEP). Although there is a plausible strategic argument for prohibiting or not facilitating such transactions (depending upon the facts), there are also moral reasons to permit and even to enable such exploitative transactions. As a general principle, the moral default position is that we should not prevent and we should positively enable transactions that are beneficial to the disadvantaged and to which they consent.

To put the point in different terms, PEP is a plausible principle of *non-ideal* moral theory. Roughly speaking, ideal moral theory aims to provide the principles for a just society and a just world. Ideal theory defines our moral aims. By contrast, non-ideal moral theory concerns what a person should do "in circumstances where at least some others are not doing what they are required to do."[54] Non-ideal theory seeks to provide the principles by which individuals should act under unjust or non-ideal moral conditions and the principles that should underlie social policies for regulating actions by individuals and organizations under non-ideal moral conditions. Whereas Rawls's *A Theory of Justice* is a project in ideal moral theory, Rawls himself acknowledges that the problems of non-ideal theory "are the pressing and urgent matters . . . that we are faced with in everyday life."[55] Ideal theory is *logically* prior to non-ideal theory because we need to know toward what we should aim. But we also need moral principles for the world in which we find ourselves, imperfect though it is.

It is, of course, a matter of some dispute as to what is the best ideal theory of a just society. It is even more debatable as to what people and societies owe each other. Rawls famously does not extend his principles of a just society to the world as a whole.[56] Be that as it may, the principles that define a just global distribution of wealth and income as a matter of ideal theory will *not* tell us what non-ideal principles apply to the unjust world in which we find ourselves.

The principles that define when we should allow or enable transactions are important elements in both ideal and non-ideal theory. The present point is this: just because a transaction would not occur under ideal or just conditions, it does not follow that it is wrong for it to occur under non-ideal conditions or that it would be better to disallow it or not enable it to happen. Given the non-ideal background conditions under which people find themselves, there should be a very strong presumption in favor of principles that would allow people to improve their situations if they give appropriately robust consent and if doing so has no negative effects on others. And this is so even if the transaction occurs only because the background conditions are unjust.

Exploitation in Clinical Research

Let us now return to the issue of clinical research in developing countries by focusing on the possible use of PCTs such as ST. As I noted at the outset, it is often claimed that clinical research must not be exploitative if it is to pass ethical muster. Commentators have implicitly advanced a version of what I called The *Exploitation Argument*. That argument maintains something like this:

(1) If a practice is exploitative, it should not be permitted.
(2) Placebo controlled trials (PCTs) that withhold proven effective treatment are exploitative.
(3) Therefore, IRBs or other relevant decision-makers should not permit PCTs such as ST.

This argument also applies, of course, to other ways in which clinical research is thought to be exploitative, such as the failure to provide post-trial treatment to those who received an intervention in the course of a trial. On closer inspection, and as evidenced by the quotations with which we began, those who claim that PCTs such as ST are exploitative actually make several different but related arguments and offer several different prescriptions for nullifying or reducing the alleged exploitation. In this section, I seek to apply the previous analysis of the concept of exploitation to these issues.

Three preliminary observations. First, it is not clear whether those who accept the exploitation argument regard trials such as ST as cases of HNE or MACE. They do not explicitly recognize the distinction or appreciate its potential significance. Second, if we assume that participation in such research is advantageous to the participant and consensual, I hope to have shown that (2) is more difficult to support than is often supposed because we lack a non-problematic theory of the fairness of transactions. Third, even if we assume that (2) is true, I hope to have shown that it is not at all obvious that we should accept (1) and (3). Indeed, it is arguable that (1) should be rejected unless one of the arguments for intervention can be sustained and is applicable to this context.

Is The Surfaxin Trial Exploitative?

As we have seen, some commentators have argued that a trial such as ST is exploitative because it would deliberately withhold standard treatment that is available in the home country of a sponsor such as DL. The Declaration of Helsinki states that "The benefits, risks, burdens and effectiveness of a new intervention must be tested against those of the best current proven intervention."[57] Call this *The Standard Care Principle*. ST certainly seems to be incompatible with this principle unless we follow Robert Levine and interpret "best proven current intervention" as "the *de facto* standard of care" that "would otherwise be available" to the subjects in their locale.[58] That would be a fudge. In any case, the issue here is not how best to understand the Declaration of Helsinki. The issue is whether a straightforward reading of the *Standard Care Principle* is a defensible principle for the non-ideal conditions where such care is not available and where investigators have no independent obligation to provide it. If DL is not required to provide any care at all to Bolivian infants, is it unfair to offer them a 50% chance of receiving surfactant therapy? If it is unfair, *why* is it unfair?

It is worth noting here that analogues to the standard care principle also arise in non-medical contexts.[59] Just as we can ask what constitutes fair treatment of research participants, we can ask what constitutes a fair wage to workers. Is Nike treating its workers in Thailand unfairly if it offers what are low wages by American standards but higher than the wages earned in comparable work in Thailand? The wages may well be too low, but few believe that fairness requires that Thai workers be paid the same as American workers.

It may be argued that the standard care principle does not reflect a general principle of fairness, but the view that physicians have special moral obligations to their patients that are not replicated in other contexts such as manufacturing. As Sonia Shah puts it, "If researchers know that one option is better than the other, they are ethically obligated to simply administer it: failing to do so puts subjects—*who are also their patients*—in harm's way"[60](emphasis added). Lurie and Wolfe argue that researchers are "obligated to provide the best scientifically proven intervention—independent of the economic status of the volunteers and regardless of where the study is conducted." Not to provide such interventions "is completely inconsistent with the Hippocratic oath. . ."[61] On this view, investigators exploit subjects when they fail to treat subjects as *patients*—however consensual their participation as subjects might be.

There are two major difficulties with this line of argument. First, if clinical researchers should regard their subjects as patients, then one needn't appeal to exploitation to criticize such studies. The claim that researchers exploit their patients would not be false, but it would be entirely otiose. Second, this argument for the standard care principle assumes what has to be shown, namely, that researchers are obligated to treat participants as if they were patients. The issue is not whether investigators have M.D. degrees. Even if the investigators are *not* physicians, it is possible that the principles of medical practice should govern the relationship of investigators with subjects. But assuming that the researchers *are* physicians, we cannot assume that the ethical principles that govern clinical research are identical with or entailed by the principles that apply to relations between physicians and patients. Surely, simply *referring* to participants as patients does not show that investigators must or should treat participants as patients.

One move won't work. If researchers should treat subjects as patients (or something close to that), they may not be able to avoid such obligations by seeking and receiving consent. Suppose a physician employed by DL says this to the parent of a prospective subject:

> Although I am trained as a doctor, it is important that you understand that I do not regard your child as my patient. I am conducting a trial. If you choose to enter the study, your baby will be placed on a ventilator in the hospital. Your baby may or may not receive what we hope will be shown to be a beneficial treatment. In effect, we will flip a coin. If it comes up heads, the air that is pumped into your baby's lungs will contain Surfaxin. If it comes up tails, the air that is pumped into your baby's lungs will have nothing else. If you agree to enroll your baby in the trial, your baby's chances of survival will be better than and certainly no worse than if you did not participate in the study. But my goal is to determine whether and how well Surfaxin works, and not to provide the best possible treatment for your baby. It is unfortunate that your baby is in this situation and that medical care is not

> otherwise available to you, but we are not responsible for that.
> If you don't want to participate with us on those terms, that's your choice.

In my view, uttering this statement does *not* suffice to get investigators off the moral hook. It is at least possible (although not obviously true) that some of the ethical obligations of researchers are *inalienable*, that is, they cannot avoid these obligations by announcing that they do not intend to fulfill them and receiving the subjects' consent to interact with them on those terms.

On the other hand, the statement reflects the plausible view that there is an important distinction between the obligations of physicians to patients in personalized medical *care* and the obligations of investigators to subjects in medical *research*.[62] Defending the precise contours of that distinction is an issue on which considerable ink has been spilt. But there must be some such distinction. Although the researcher may be *constrained* to avoid certain sorts of harms to subjects, the *aim* of research is to seek generalizable knowledge. By contrast, the *aim* of personalized medical care is to advance the health of the patient and setting aside certain complications (such as duties to warn third parties), the treating physician has an obligation to pursue that goal. Surely a researcher could not ethically adhere to a study protocol or administer study procedures not required for treatment if he were under an obligation to deliver personalized medical care.[63] In any case, the present point is that whereas one cannot claim that ST is *not* exploitative just because it involves medical research, one can't assume that it *is* exploitative simply by appeal to the ethics of personalized medical care.

And so we are back to the question as to whether ST is exploitative. I argued above that a transaction is exploitative only if B receives less from (or pays more for) the interaction than is required by a plausible principle of fairness. This raises several issues. First, I argued that A exploits B only when A gains or expects to gain from the transaction. In the present context, it is ambiguous as to precisely who are the beneficiaries on the side of the alleged exploiters. It is clear that DL is thought to be the principal agent of exploitation in ST, but it is worth noting that such research might be regarded as exploitative because citizens in the developed world, who risk nothing, stand to gain from trials conducted on citizens of underdeveloped societies. In other cases of alleged exploitation, such as SCAT, the study may be conducted by a not for profit institution, such as the National Institutes of Health. Who is *gaining* from the alleged exploitation? We might say that the scientists gain, but, in this case, the intended indirect beneficiaries are the infants born to HIV-positive mothers in developing countries.

Second, if a transaction is exploitative when the gains from the transaction are unfairly distributed, we must determine whether we should evaluate those gains from an *ex ante* or an *ex post* perspective, and whether we should adopt the same perspective for both parties. Angela Ballantyne argues that "both the benefits and burdens associated with trial sponsors are primarily *guaranteed*."[64] This is false. Although the costs to trial sponsors may be roughly guaranteed, the scientific and financial benefits are not. That is why the trial is done. Consider this case.

> *Oil.* A proposes to buy land from B in the hopes that he will find
> oil. On the basis of a geologist's analysis, A's *expected* profit
> from drilling will be $10 million. A offers to pay B $100,000.
> B accepts. A finds no oil and loses $1 million on this project.

I believe that A may have exploited B in *Oil* because A's *expected* gain may have been excessive relative to B's *actual* gain, even though A's *actual* gain was negative whereas B's *actual* gain was positive. Similarly, I believe that investigators can exploit trial participants even if, *ex post*, the participants gain whereas the investigators do not.

Ballantyne argues that an *ex ante* perspective is insufficient. She thinks that non-exploitative research should provide participants with a positive increase in *expected utility* and a fair *ex post* distribution of benefits.[65] It would seem that sauce for the goose should be sauce for the gander. If, as I have argued, we should evaluate the gains to "A" from an *ex ante* perspective, I do not see why we should evaluate the gains to "B" from both an *ex ante* perspective and an *ex post* perspective. The crucial question is whether investigators have offered a fair *ex ante* package of benefits to research participants. After all, even if A is offering *personalized medical care* to B, we do not evaluate the ethics of A's behavior by reference to its *ex post* effectiveness.

From an *ex ante* perspective, then, it is arguable that a PCT such as ST is actually beneficial to *all* participants, since all participants have a 50% chance of receiving beneficial treatment and, in the actual case of ST, even those not getting the drug would have profited from intubation and better all around care. This is not a conceptual trick. Consider standard medical treatments. If B has an illness for which the standard therapy works 50% of the time, A can expect to be paid even if the treatment does not work for B. I am not here claiming that it is unproblematic to conduct a PCT when standard treatment is available. I am claiming only that in asking whether ST is exploitative, we should evaluate the benefits to participants from an *ex ante* perspective.

Third, it is not clear how to measure the parties' relative benefits in a case such as ST. The critics of ST tend to emphasize that the participants might *not* receive surfactant therapy, but say little as to what they do receive. If we evaluate the participants' benefits in something like "utility gain" relative to the *status quo* in which they receive no medical care at all, the expected utility gain of participants in Bolivia—an increased probability of survival—is enormous.[66] Moreover, assuming that there is an adequate supply of potential participants, DL does not gain *that* much from the participation of any individual participant. I am not claiming that comparative utility gain is the best way to assess the fairness of a distribution of benefits. To the contrary. I suggested above that A can exploit B even if B gains much more from the transaction than A (as in *Unfair Surgery*). At the same time, the claim that a distribution of benefits is unfair or exploitative must also be defended. And setting aside an appeal to the "standard care" principle, it is not at all clear why the *ex ante* distribution of benefits between DL and the participants in ST is unfair. And *if* it is *not* unfair, then the claim that the subjects are exploited does not get going.

Fourth, some critics claim that trials such as ST are exploitative because they "serve the interests of those who live in wealthy nations."[67] We do well to remember that the indirect beneficiaries of research have genuine medical needs. More importantly, and as to whether the subjects are exploited, the issue is not the legitimacy of the interests that are being served, but whether those who serve those interests are being treated fairly. *If* those who knit oriental rugs are treated fairly—and I do say *if*—then they are not being exploited just because they are providing goods for affluent westerners.

A fifth point deserves more extensive discussion. Call it the *off-shoring objection*. Off-shoring and out-sourcing are often conflated. We outsource labor when a person or firm hires others to provide some service. And so a university might "outsource" its custodial work or landscaping to a private firm. We "off-shore" labor when we use persons from other nations—typically separated by oceans—to provide some service. Objections to off-shoring labor and services are often raised in non-medical contexts such as the manufacture of clothing in Asian sweatshops or the use of customer service agents in India. Still, it may be thought that there is something particularly obnoxious about a practice in which the affluent directly or indirectly entice poor people from LDCs to provide a medical service that will primarily benefit comparatively affluent people in developed societies, and it may seem particularly worrisome when the inducement to participate is the prospect of receiving life-saving medical treatment as in ST. And while the off-shoring of clinical research is a growth industry, it has been the target of considerable scholarly criticism. More to the point, I have not encountered any sustained attempt to *defend* the practice in the academic literature.

But what, precisely, is the ethical problem here? At a basic level, outsourcing or off-shoring is simply an extension of the division of labor and trade. We "outsource" labor whenever one party has a *comparative advantage* in producing a good or providing a service, and a party can have a comparative advantage over another even if one party is superior at both. The principle works within families. My wife may be a better cook and a better cleaner than I, but if she is *much* better at cooking and only a *little* better at cleaning then I have a comparative advantage in cleaning. It makes sense for her to outsource the cleaning to me and for me to outsource the cooking to her. Similarly so within firms. A lawyer may be able to type faster than her secretary, but her secretary has a *comparative* advantage with respect to typing nonetheless.[68] It is more efficient for her to "outsource" her typing to a secretary who is paid $20 per hour while she engages in legal work for which she is paid $200 per hour. The affluent hire nannies, gardeners, house cleaners, painters, or volunteer (professional) soldiers to perform tasks that they could but would prefer not to perform. This is the stuff of everyday life and as a general principle it is a desirable practice so long as such transactions are consensual, mutually advantageous, and fair. Moreover, we may think that we should not interfere with such transactions if they are consensual and mutually advantageous, even when they are not fair.

In principle, the off-shoring of labor across national boundaries is no different. If Britain has a comparative advantage over France as a producer of cotton, whereas France has a comparative advantage as a producer of wine (even if France is a more efficient producer of both cotton and wine), then it makes sense for France to produce wine for Britain and for Britain to produce cotton for France. Americans (and that includes low income Americans) benefit from the fact that goods are produced at lower cost in China than if they were produced in the United States.[69] As Adam Smith puts it,

> What is prudence in the conduct of every private family, can scarce
> be folly in a great kingdom. If a foreign country can supply us with
> a commodity cheaper than we ourselves can make it, better buy it

of them with some part of the prudence of our own industry, employed in a way in which we have some advantage.[70]

As with products, so too with services. American customers benefit from having telephone inquiries answered by persons in India rather than in Indiana, given that the Indians are paid substantially less than Indianans. We may object to and work to change the circumstances that render it reasonable for people to consent to work for low wages but, as a general principle, we do the people of LDCs no favor if we deny them the opportunity to produce goods and provide services that will mostly be consumed in the developed world.

It is, of course, an empirical question as to whether and how much people—and which people—in LDCs benefit from trade with the developed world. Even if there are aggregate gains from trade, there will certainly be individual losers from trade within every society. If the United States offshores the production of steel, the American users of steel may benefit, but steel workers will not. If kleptocratic rulers in LDCs capture much of the surplus of trade with the developed world, the majority of people in LDCs may not gain. All that said, it is certainly plausible to think that most workers in LDCs actually do benefit from trade. A moderate left-wing economist such as Paul Krugman writes that "while fat-cat capitalists might benefit from globalization, the biggest beneficiaries are, yes, Third World Workers."[71] Krugman adds that wherever "new export industries have grown, there has been measurable improvement in the lives of ordinary people."[72] Such industries typically offer higher wages than workers could receive elsewhere and developing the export sector typically has a positive "ripple effect throughout the economy." And, as Martin Wolf points out, this is particularly so for women, "whose status can be transformed in patriarchal societies by opportunities to earn incomes for themselves."[73]

I think it fair to say that philosophers and ethicists have shown little interest in the benefits of trade or globalization. As Teson and Klick have noted, "None of the major works on global justice draws on the relevant economic literature, the general consensus of which recommends free trade as a way to enhance global and national wealth and thus benefit the poor."[74] It is not clear why this is so. Teson and Klick speculate that philosophers may lose interest because the defense of free markets relies on empirical economic arguments that are not well understood and because the benefits of free trade, such as they are, flow from egoistic behavior rather than a commitment to global justice and the amelioration of deprivation—"Promoting trade . . . is not a sufficiently *lofty* way to discharge our duties based on justice."[75] There may also be a signaling issue. Given that the benefits of free trade are often touted by persons on a side of the political spectrum with which many do not wish to be associated, commentators might be concerned that sympathy for this approach may not convey the appropriate signals about their own political and moral sympathies.

Assuming that the general case for the benefits of free trade is roughly correct, the off-shoring of clinical research has the potential to be a win-win transaction. To put the point in admittedly crude terms, it could be argued that people—including infants—in LDCs have a "comparative advantage" in serving as research participants and that if we are concerned for *their* welfare, there should be no objection to off-shoring medical research in much the same way that we off-shore the manufacture of apparel or customer service support for computers. Distasteful as it might seem, it may be advantageous for the citizens of LDCs to be used as research subjects, and, if so, we should encourage its development.

I hear the groans. It might be thought that it is one thing to employ Indians to answer phones, and quite another to employ them as subjects in a trial of a new drug for Type-2 diabetes, whether they do it for money or for access to medical treatment that they would otherwise not receive. Shamoo and Resnik say that

> it is especially important to prevent pharmaceutical companies
> from using people in developing countries as cheap labor to test
> drugs that will only be used in the developed world, because this
> would constitute an egregious form of exploitation.[76]

They do not say why this practice is exploitative much less "egregious" exploitation. Moreover, if the egregious exploitation that they seek to prevent is a form of *mutually advantageous and consensual* exploitation, it is not clear why we should want to prevent it. Would they seek to prevent running shoe manufacturers from "using people in developing countries as cheap labor to manufacture shoes that will only be used in the developed world" if what is cheap labor to us are among the better jobs available in such societies? And if Shamoo and Resnik believe that we should not seek to prevent such transactions in the non-medical sphere, why should we seek to prevent such transactions in the medical sphere?

We have been assuming that the transaction between investigators and participants in ST is mutually advantageous. The question is whether investigators are *exploiting* subjects nonetheless when they conduct a placebo controlled trial if an efficacious intervention is available. I have argued that if we set aside direct appeals to the "standard of care" principle, the critics have advanced no independent arguments as to why the distribution of benefits between the parties is unfair—perhaps because they think it so obvious that ST is exploitative that an argument is not necessary. After all, the investigators would be "right there" and would be withholding potentially life-saving treatment from infants they are using to develop generalizable knowledge. If that's not exploitative, what is? Although I think the issue is more complicated than that, I want to assume, for the sake of argument, that ST is exploitative and that DL must do more for its subjects (or perhaps others) if it is to avoid the charge of exploitation.

As should now be clear, even if we assume that ST is exploitative, the question remains as to whether DL should be permitted to go forward with the trial if participation is both advantageous (*ex ante*) to the exploitee and consensual. Lurie and Wolfe say that "An unethical research study is an unethical research study even with informed consent."[77] This is clearly too quick, for the question is whether morally transformative consent is sufficient to transform a study that would otherwise be unethical into a study that is rendered ethical. But even if a subject's transformative consent does not render the *study* ethical, such consent might justify not *interfering* with the study. It is to the issue of consent that I now turn.

Consent

There are several questions that we can raise here: (1) do the participants (or their surrogates) in studies such as ST typically give morally transformative consent? (2) If not, is it possible that such participants *can* give morally transformative consent? (3) Is "community consent" necessary or sufficient to satisfy this dimension of ethical research?

Clearly, the answer to questions (1) and (2) will turn on our criteria for morally transformative consent (which I considered in Chapter 3) and the relevant empirical data. Although we cannot resolve that here, I am sure that the answer to (1) is at least sometimes no. There are no doubt numerous and egregious cases in which investigators have not met the requirements of any plausible view of morally transformative consent. They may have deceived or failed to give relevant information to prospective participants. There may be cases in which the participants are not competent to give morally transformative consent. Moreover, it is entirely possible that the parents will not fully understand that the researchers are prepared to withhold life-saving therapy from their infants.

It may or may not be feasible to resolve these sorts of cognitive mistakes. What then? As I argued in Chapter 2, a major function of the independent review process is to assure that it would be reasonable for the participant to give consent when she is not in a position to make such judgments. If prospective subjects (or surrogates) are not themselves capable of giving morally transformative consent because they lack the ability to comprehend what the research involves, there are two (compatible) options. First, an independent review process can determine that it is reasonable for the subject to consent and, in effect, ask the subject to give the functional equivalent of a child's "assent." Second, we can require that the participant's (or parent's) expressed consent be supplemented by the consent of a surrogate such as a representative of the government or a health official who can reliably determine that the participant's decision is consistent with her long term interests.

We should, however, distinguish between the sorts of *cognitive* deficiencies in a subject's consent that can be remedied by IRBs or surrogates and worries about the *voluntariness* of the subject's consent. It is sometimes argued that research such as ST is not based on morally transformative consent because the participants have no reasonable alternative but to consent to participate. On this view, impoverished parents who would ordinarily have no medical care available to treat their infants with respiratory distress syndrome do not give morally transformative consent to participate if that is their only *chance* of obtaining medical care for them. They are coerced by their circumstances as it were.

As I argued in Chapters 3 and 4, the fact that prospective subjects do not have viable alternatives to participation does not preclude their giving morally transformative consent. We do *not* say that a patient's consent to surgery is involuntary, coerced, or invalid just because her only alternative is to die, and if we do not think that the prospect of death undermines valid consent to treatment, there is no reason to think that the prospect of receiving no medical care undermines valid consent to participate in research. I have argued that A's proposal is coercive in a way that renders B's consent non-transformative only if A proposes to violate B's rights if B rejects A's proposal. And the central fact is that DL does not propose to violate a potential subject's rights in ST should a potential subject decide not to participate.

Annas and Grodin disagree. They argue that

> in the absence of health care, virtually any offer of medical assistance (even in the guise of research) will be accepted as 'better than nothing' and research will almost inevitably be *confused* with treatment, making informed consent difficult[78] (emphasis added).

But parents would not be *confusing* treatment with research in this case if participation represents their only access to treatment.

There may be other worries about consent. As I have argued, a proposal might constitute a *seductive offer* or *undue inducement* even if it is not coercive and, if so, it would compromise consent in a different way. CIOMS worries that the offer of medical care may "induce prospective subjects to consent to participate in the research against their better judgment."[79] But as I argue in Chapter 4, it is important to distinguish between two claims:

(1) an inducement constitutes a seductive offer that distorts the judgment of the subjects and motivates them to consent to participate when doing so does not advance their interests;

(2) given the subject's objective circumstances, the inducements make it rational for the subjects to participate.

When (1) is true, there is good reason to regard consent as not transformative, but there is no reason to regard consent as not transformative in (2).

The point, disturbing as it might be, is that although extreme poverty *can* give rise to the distorted judgments in (1), it can also lead to judgments that are crystal clear. As Shamoo and Resnik put it, "We should not equate economic vulnerability with lack of sound judgment."[80] And if (2) is true, we do not respect the subject's humanity or rationality by denying their capacity to make their lives less miserable than they already are. David Rothman writes that "abject poverty is harsh enough without people having to bear the additional *burdens* of serving as research subjects."[81] But if serving as a research subject is a benefit, all things considered, we might say that abject poverty is harsh enough without denying people the opportunity to make their lives somewhat less miserable by participating in biomedical research and receiving benefits that they would not otherwise receive.

Let us assume that the participants (or their surrogates) do or can give morally transformative consent to participate in ST. Some commentators have argued that medical research such as ST not only requires the consent of the participants (or their surrogates), but also requires the consent of the community. This view need not claim that a community's consent could *override* the absence of consent from an individual. After all, a major purpose of insisting on informed consent is so that an individual's interests cannot be involuntarily sacrificed for the interests of the community. It does say that the community's consent might also be necessary.

Broadly speaking, there seem to be at least four arguments for requiring community consent in LDCs. First, some commentators reject what they regard as a "highly individualistic" conception of rights and duties that underlies the significance of informed consent, one that allegedly assumes an "atomistic view of the person" that they find wanting or, perhaps, that is not accepted in some developing societies even if it is accepted here. This is a large topic that we cannot here pursue in depth. But suppose that a society believes that a woman should secure her husband's permission to enroll in a trial and that her own consent is not sufficient. It might make sense as a political or practical matter to accommodate such beliefs, but I am not prepared to grant that refusing to do so assumes an unjustifiable "atomistic view" of the person. Here I would prefer the company of the Universal Declaration of Human Rights, which also appears to regard individual rights as a universal value.

Second, it may be argued that a community's consent can be required because its present and future members have interests that are not identical with the interests of the individual subjects. A study might have genuine negative externalities for the community, and, if so, it is perfectly sensible for the community to demand that its consent is also necessary to protect its interests. For example, research might draw a community's medical personnel away from their traditional work to the detriment of the community (although, perhaps, to the advantage of the medical personnel). It is another question, however, as to what sorts of alleged or perceived interests justify denying the opportunity for individuals to participate in research if they consent. Charles Weijer observes that "Providing information on disease treatment may negatively affect beliefs regarding traditional healing."[82] No doubt true. But it is doubtful that a community's interest in preserving false beliefs about healing justifies preventing its citizens from receiving efficacious medical care to which they consent.

Third, a community may require that its consent be obtained so that it can leverage the individual's participation to promote the interests of other members of the community. I will not here assess the merits of this argument save to note that it has *absolutely nothing* to do with protecting the subject from exploitation.

Fourth, the community or its government may be well positioned to act as a proxy for the subject, given that the subjects may exhibit the sorts of cognitive deficiencies I noted above. As I argued in Chapter 2, there is nothing untoward in this form of "soft paternalism" if the community can and will make sensible decisions on behalf of persons whose competence is suspect. In this case, however, the community's consent is required not because it has its own interests to protect but because it is better positioned to protect the interests of the subject than the subjects themselves.

But this raises a difficulty with some of the arguments advanced by the critics of studies such as ST. If we take seriously the community's authority to *reject* ST on behalf of its members, then it is difficult to justify ignoring its *acceptance* of ST. There may be a strategic argument that justifies prohibiting a community from accepting such a trial if doing so will prevent a "race to the bottom" among the societies that might compete for being used for such studies and if so doing will result in studies that provide better care for the participants. But bracketing such reasons, it will be difficult to argue that a trial should not be permitted if both the prospective subjects and the community's representatives consent to it.

Reasonable Availability and Fair Benefits

As I noted at the outset of this chapter, those who claim that much multinational research is exploitative focus not solely on the trial design itself, but on the availability of benefits when the trial is completed. Annas and Grodin say

> Unless the interventions being tested will actually be made available to the *impoverished populations* that are being used as research subjects, developed countries are simply exploiting *them* in order to quickly use the knowledge gained from the clinical trials for the developed countries' own benefit[83] (emphasis added).

This and similar statements are ambiguous as to *who* has a claim to receive such benefits. If they are claiming that the research subjects themselves have a claim to receive benefits when the trial is over, then we must ask whether such benefits are required to render the package of benefits fair from an *ex ante* perspective. But that seems an unlikely interpretation of their view. For one thing, it is irrelevant to research such as ST. If the infants survive the trial, they will not need surfactant therapy in the post-trial environment.

It is more natural to regard "them" as referring to the community. On that view, if we are to avoid exploitation in multi-national research, the community whose members participate in a trial should somehow benefit from the research. On one view, there must be some reasonable assurance that products derived from the research will be available in that country. As CIOMS puts it, "As a general rule, the sponsoring agency should agree in advance of the research that any product developed through such research will be made reasonably available to the inhabitants of the host community or country at the completion of successful testing."[84]

Advocates of the "fair benefits" view take a more catholic approach to community benefit.[85] They argue that the *amount* and not the *type* of benefit is crucial to avoiding exploitation. They note that reasonable availability applies only to Phase III research of a successful product, and would have little bearing on Phase I and Phase II research, as well as Phase III research that did not yield a successful product. In addition, they point out that reasonable availability does not consider other potential benefits of research in developing countries, including training of health care or research personnel, and the development of the health care infrastructure. They also suggest that insisting on reasonable availability is condescending, as it "precludes the community's deciding which benefits it prefers."[86] I consider this issue in more detail in Chapter 6. The present question is whether and how the provision of benefits to the *larger population* would negate or mitigate exploitation of research subjects. Consider these four claims.

1. There is an intrinsic connection between the exploitation of the research subjects and the exploitation of the population, such that research that would otherwise not exploit the research subjects does exploit those subjects if the wider population is not treated fairly.
2. There is an intrinsic connection between the exploitation of research subjects and the exploitation of the population such that research that would otherwise exploit the research subjects

would not exploit the research subjects if the wider population is treated fairly.

3. Although the research may exploit the subjects, the moral weight of this exploitation would be offset if the community receives sufficient benefits such as to render the research permissible all things considered.

4. Although the provision of benefits to the larger population is entirely distinct from the exploitation of research subjects, ethical research requires (1) that the research subjects not be exploited and (2) that the larger population from which the subjects are drawn also benefit from the research.

I am inclined to reject (1) on conceptual grounds. I simply do not see why a participant is exploited because the community does not benefit. But perhaps that is too quick. Winston Chiong argues that

Subjecting a patient to the risks of clinical research, without making good faith efforts to ensure that the benefits provided by this research will be available in the patient's own community, suggests a lack of respect and concern for a patient's broad social circumstances that we would not reasonably want physicians to bear towards any of their patients.[87]

Chiong's claim rests on two questionable assumptions, namely that research subjects should be understood as "patients" and that participation is risky rather than (*ex ante*) beneficial. But setting that aside, Chiong is not actually arguing that there are *independent* reasons for providing benefits to the community in addition to the subject. He seems to be arguing that not providing those benefits to the community shows a lack of respect *for the subjects themselves*. It would seem, however, that the relevance of the investigator's respect for the "broad social circumstances" of the subject to showing respect for the subject would be for the *subject* to decide. If the mother of a child with respiratory distress syndrome is prepared to have her child participate in ST even if DL will not make Surfaxin available to other Bolivian infants, we can't bar her participation by reference to respect for *her or her child*.

I would similarly reject (2) on conceptual grounds. I do not see why the most generous provision of benefits to the community would negate or mitigate the exploitation of the subjects themselves. Suppose, for example, that football players at University X should receive a fair share of any surplus that X receives from their efforts, but that X uses that surplus to support money-losing athletic programs for women. Although the use of the surplus for those ends might *justify* the exploitation all things considered, it does not cancel or negate the exploitation itself.

Claim (3) is more plausible. From a consequentialist perspective, it is possible that the provision of benefits to the community might *justify* or override the wrongness inherent in the exploitation of subjects even if it does not remove or negate the wrongness of the exploitation. But to the extent that the principles of ethical research are primarily concerned with the interests and autonomy of *research subjects*, we should be loathe to tolerate such exploitation as a means by which to generate benefits to the community. So (3) is on shaky grounds.

On (4), research is ethically justifiable only if it is justifiable with respect to the subjects themselves *and* with respect to the larger populations from whom the subjects are drawn. As Ezekiel Emanuel puts it, "it is an ethical imperative that populations receive sufficient benefit from research in which *they* participate"[88] (emphasis added). Although this is a plausible view, I do not think it is persuasive. If "they" refers to the populations, it does not seem as if "they" participate in research at all. It is the subjects who participate, not populations. And if ST is beneficial to the participants and if they or their proxies give morally transformative consent, it seems *prima facie* wrong for the community to hold them hostage to DL's willingness to provide benefits to others. (Of course, communities may provide resources of various kinds—personnel, logistical support, infrastructure, etc.—that could have been used for other purposes. If so, communities can reasonably ask to be compensated for their investment. I consider that claim in more detail in Chapter 6.)[89]

Now the view that investigators should provide benefits to the community might not be justified by the goal of avoiding exploitation but, rather, by principles of beneficence or distributive justice that seek to provide more health care resources to the poorest areas of the world. That is plausible. And a more fully developed non-ideal theory than I have offered would provide principles for moving from our current non-ideal world to a world that is more just. Still, we must be careful not to conflate valid concerns about the distribution of medical resources in the world with concerns about the relationship among the participants or the nations involved in particular studies and with the exploitation of those participants.

In this connection, it is also important to distinguish between the claim that the distribution of resources in the world is unjust and the claim that the sponsor or the home country of the sponsor is *causally responsible* for the injustice. Crouch and Arras argue that the misery of people in underdeveloped societies "must be due in no small measure to the flagrantly unjust behavior of the former colonial powers, which plundered their natural resources and subjugated their peoples. . ."[90] Along similar lines, Thomas Pogge has argued that the affluent nations of the world have harmed—not merely failed to help—the worse off by upholding an institutional regime that, among other things, allows the rulers of many nations to enrich themselves by selling natural resources to wealthy nations while refusing to share the benefits with the population.[91] I am sure that this causal view is at least part of the truth, but I suspect that it is only partially correct. Some of the poorest societies of the world have had little economic contact with the highly industrialized nations. They have suffered not because imperialism has made them worse off, but because the affluent nations have "found too little there to be exploited."[92] Of course, even if the industrialized nations have not *caused* the poverty of the underdeveloped society, they may still have obligations of justice or beneficence to *ameliorate* that poverty. Moreover, it is arguable that given the special competencies of medical investigators and the resources available to their sponsors, they should do their part in this general effort through medical research. But the force of those arguments has little to do with exploitation.

The Permitted Exploitation Principle Revisited

I have argued that the claim that ST is wrongfully exploitative of the research subjects or the community is more difficult to sustain than is often supposed. But let us assume, for the sake of argument, that ST or some comparable trial is exploitative. If ST is harmful or non-consensual, then these are good reasons not to allow it to go forward, although we would not then need to invoke its exploitativeness as the rationale for interference. But if ST is a case of MACE, I have argued that there is good reason to endorse the *Permitted Exploitation Principle* as a default position. I considered several rationales for resisting PEP. The question is whether they apply in the present context and to what effect.

Remember that PEP is a claim about the ethics of *interference* and not a claim about the ethics of a *transaction* itself. In a commentary on ST,

Robert Temple confuses these two issues: "One must ask . . . why, if every-one in a trial is better off because of participation, and no one is denied anything otherwise available to them, the trial is not ethically acceptable."[93] I argued above that it is not ethically acceptable for A to exploit B in *Rescue* just because B is better off and is not denied anything otherwise available. And the same is true for clinical research. Temple may be right in thinking that ST should be permitted, but wrong to think that ST is ethically accept-able because it renders everyone better off (at least *ex ante*).

Alex John London makes a similar mistake. London refers to the essence of PEP as the "minimalist view" because it claims that we should permit a transaction so long as it does not worsen anyone's position and is consen-sual. Setting aside the derisive language (who would want to support a posi-tion described as "minimalist"?), London is mistaken as to what PEP claims.

> The minimalist view accepts the *status quo* in the host community
> as the appropriate "normative baseline" against which proposed
> research initiatives are evaluated – meaning that the *status quo* is
> treated as the threshold of a person's moral entitlements in this
> particular sphere.[94]

Not so. PEP does not "accept" the *status quo* in any deep moral sense. PEP need not deny that all Bolivian infants with RDS are morally entitled to sur-factant therapy. But it does not follow that DL, in particular, has an obligation to provide surfactant therapy to any or all Bolivian infants with RDS. It is important to note that London does not claim that DL has an obligation to conduct its research in Bolivia just so that it can make surfactant therapy available to those to whom it would not otherwise be available. London might claim that DL has an obligation to provide surfactant therapy to its subjects because the moral entitlement of research subjects shifts as soon as they become research subjects. But that is to presuppose precisely what is at issue.

London also maintains that PEP assumes that transactions are fair simply "because they provide mutually beneficial terms of cooperation that each party can freely accept."[95] Not so. PEP does claim that transactions are *fair* just because they are mutually advantageous. It claims that there is reason to permit such transactions even if they are *unfair*.

In addition to making questionable claims about the *content* of PEP, London also makes questionable claims about the consequences of *accept-ing* PEP.

. . . the minimalist position prevents one from assessing the extent to which individuals in the host community have a legitimate claim against their own government to better conditions. It also keeps one from assessing the influence of third parties, such as foreign governmental and corporate entities, on the community's basic social structure.[96]

Not quite. To accept the view that we should permit ST because it is advantageous to all concerned hardly "prevents" anyone from also asking whether the Bolivian government is doing all that it could or should for the children or from asking whether the decisions of third parties have harmed the basic social structure of Bolivia, and it is hard to see why anyone would think that it would.

Of course, even if the "minimalist" view does not "prevent" us from addressing other or larger issues, it is arguable that it "does little *to bring attention* to the root causes of the developing world populations' most pressing health needs" and that its acceptance would perpetuate "an ad hoc and piecemeal approach to the health needs of populations that already bear the greatest burden of disease and deprivation."[97] This is not a claim about the truth of the minimalist view, but an empirical claim about the effects of adopting that view. It is possible that the acceptance of a view that encourages mutually advantageous and consensual transactions within a context of injustice and deprivation does less to address those background conditions than a view that focuses on the background conditions themselves even if the latter view might lead to avoidable harm to those who would benefit from such transactions. On the other hand, it is also possible that precisely because acceptance of the "minimalist view" will permit studies such as ST, it will draw attention to the desperate background conditions that make it rational for parents to enroll their infants. It's hard to tell.

In any case, the present question is not whether accepting PEP represents the most effective mechanism of change, but whether PEP should be accepted on its own terms. The case for accepting PEP is simple and straightforward, although not less meritorious for that: if a transaction is better for the exploitee and if the exploitee consents to be exploited, then we should allow the transaction to go forward. I have argued, however, that even if we start with PEP as the default position, there is a plausible *strategic argument* for prohibiting exploitative transactions such as ST. If refusing to allow ST will result in a less exploitative or non-exploitative trial, then we can justify the prohibition with respect to the interests of the participants. Whether the strategic argument actually justifies a given prohibition depends on the counterfactual: what will happen if we do not allow the transaction? If refusing to allow the transaction will cause the exploiter to offer less exploitative terms, then such refusal makes sense. If refusing to allow the transaction will cause the exploiter to go elsewhere and not transact with *these* prospective participants, then the refusal does not advance the interests of *these* exploitees. It is an empirical question as to what the effects will actually be.

Consider two scenarios. In Scenario One, the costs of doing research in Bolivia are *greater* than the costs of doing research in the United States, say because it is necessary to provide the infrastructure that makes such research possible. In that case, DL would prefer to conduct its trial in the United States unless differences in the trial design made it less costly to do the research in Bolivia. The advantage of a PCT is that sample size can be smaller, the results can be obtained more quickly, and costs are lower because there is no need to purchase drugs produced by rival companies. On this scenario, DL might rank the options in this way:

1. PCT in United States
2. PCT in Bolivia
3. ACT in United States
4. ACT in Bolivia

Option (1) is a complete non-starter since such a trial would not be approved for nations where infants would normally receive surfactant therapy, and, even if it were approved, parents would never consent to participate. If (2) is also disallowed as exploitative, then DL will prefer to conduct an ACT in the United States (3) than to conduct an ACT in Bolivia (4). In this case, the strategic argument does not apply; intervention does not advance the interests of Bolivian infants.

In Scenario Two, however, the costs of doing research in Bolivia are *lower* than the costs of doing comparable research in the United States, perhaps because salaries are lower or because the prevalence of the condition under study is greater and it is possible to recruit a sufficient number of subjects at fewer sites, etc. In Scenario Two, DL's ranking is this:

2. PCT in Bolivia
1. PCT in U.S.
4. ACT in Bolivia
3. ACT in U.S.

As with Scenario One, a PCT in the U.S. (1) is off the table. But if DL is not allowed to choose option (2), on the grounds that it is exploitative or because, say, it is inconsistent with the principles incorporated in the Declaration of Helsinki, then given the choice between (3) and (4), DL will prefer (3). In this case, the strategic argument for prohibiting (2) serves to advance the interests of Bolivian infants.

It is an empirical question as to which scenario is closer to the truth in a given case. In the present context, it appears that Scenario One is closer to the truth. Robert Temple of the U.S. Food and Drug Administration conjectured that if DL were required to conduct an active controlled trial, it "almost surely would be conducted in the United States or another developed country" and there would be "no trial of any kind of a surfactant in Bolivia."[98] And this is precisely what happened. When DL's proposed protocol was widely criticized as exploitative, it abandoned the proposal for a PCT in less developed countries and conducted an ACT in the United States and other developed societies. This does not show conclusively that the standard care principle is wrong. It does suggest that advocacy of the principle can be self-defeating if its aim is to advance the welfare of prospective subjects.

Similar issues arise with respect to whether investigators should be required to provide post-trial treatment to participants in clinical trials, an issue that has been particularly salient with respect to the provision of anti-retroviral drugs to persons who become HIV positive in the course of an HIV-vaccine trial or who respond positively to anti-retroviral therapy (ART) in the course of a study of the ART. Using rather neutral language, The National Bioethics Advisory Committee says "It has been pointed out that expecting industrial sponsors to provide expensive drugs free of charge after a trial is over might curtail interest among companies in developing interventions specifically for diseases prevalent in developing countries."[99] But it's not just that this requirement might work to the detriment of the populations in developing countries; it might work to the detriment of the trial participants themselves. The NBAC does not say whether it thinks that this argument has merit or takes a position on its force. It says simply that this concern "has been pointed out" and that the unwelcome consequence "might" occur. But the point is arguably quite crucial. We must ask whether we want to endorse an ethical view that, if it is followed, motivates investigators to abandon research from which prospective participants can expect to benefit and to which they would consent.

Pogge's Challenge

In an important and insightful analysis of exploitation in international research, Thomas Pogge seems prepared to bite precisely that bullet.[100] He argues that to adopt the Pareto principle or what I have called PEP is, in effect, to encourage investigators to scour the earth in search of infants with RDS whom they can intubate but refuse to infuse their air with a surfactant. And, he adds, "It is hard to have confidence in a morality that encourages and rewards such predatorial behavior."[101] When put that way, it seems hard to disagree.

In developing his analysis, Pogge makes use of three standard moral categories: moral freedom, moral goodness and moral constraint (or requirement). Moral freedom refers to that which one is permitted to do. Moral goodness refers to the moral quality of the state of affairs one's actions bring about. Moral constraint refers to that which one is not permitted to do or that which one is required to do. Pogge accepts that DL has the moral freedom not to conduct its study in a poor country rather than the United States (or not at all). He also acknowledges that "It is morally bad . . . that many human beings . . . should die as a result of a drug company's decision to test a new treatment in its rich home country rather than among the poor abroad."[102] Nonetheless, Pogge argues that testing Surfaxin against a placebo when effective live-saving treatments are available is a violation of the operative moral constraint or requirement, namely, that physician-investigators should not deliberately withhold life saving treatment from those they are using as subjects when they could provide treatment without incurring extraordinary additional costs.

Now in arguing that ST is unethical, Pogge does *not* appeal to a *general duty to rescue* the infants that DL could save, in which case DL might lack the moral freedom to conduct its research in the United States. His point is that it is wrong for DL to *use* these infants as research subjects by not saving them.

In developing his argument, Pogge asks us to consider a provocative example (which I paraphrase)

> *The Filmmaker.* A filmmaker wishes to produce a documentary about behavior of fishermen whose boats are in distress. He believes that the film will help others avoid counterproductive panic-induced behavior. A successful film requires that the fishermen not be rescued until it is too late. The film crew flies to a location off the coast of a poor country and waits for a

radio signal of a ship in distress. When it receives a distress signal, the film maker radios back with the following proposal. If the fishermen agree, the filmmaker will flip a coin. If it comes up heads, the filmmaker's crew will fly by helicopter and save them. If it comes up tails, it will fly by helicopter and film them and make no effort to save them, but will remain in the area until another ship is in distress and it will then save those fishermen. Because the fishermen have no better option, they readily agree.

Pogge maintains that it would be wrong for the filmmakers not to save the fishermen given that they are in a position to do so, even though the fishermen consent to the arrangement, even though the fishermen clearly benefit *ex ante* from the arrangement, even though the filmmakers have a legitimate purpose in making the film, and, most importantly, *even though the filmmakers would have absolutely no reason to be in a position to save the fishermen if they would be obligated to save them once they found themselves in a position to do so.*

The italicized passage is crucial. One can deny that the filmmakers have an obligation to put themselves in a position where they *can* rescue the fishermen and yet also accept that one has a general duty to rescue when such occasions occur in the normal course of events (as when passing by Peter Singer's pond in which a child is drowning) and even when doing so imposes considerable costs.[103] Consider this example that Liam Murphy borrows from Shelly Kagan.

> *Astronomers.* For years some astronomers have been planning an observation that must take place at sea at a particular date and time; many hundreds of thousands of dollars have been spent in preparation. Just as they are about to take their readings, they receive a Mayday signal. If they rescue the sailors in distress, the project will come to nothing. But, as we intuitively think, rescue they must.[104]

There is an important distinction between the astronomers and the filmmakers. The astronomers have reason to be at sea even if there is a risk that they will have to scuttle their project in order to rescue the sailors. Given that they are in a position to rescue the sailors, it is arguable that they must do so. By contrast, the filmmaker would not put himself in a position to rescue the fishermen if he would be required to do so. As Pogge puts it, "The filmmaker has no earthly reason to be near the ocean with his radio equipment and helicopter if this can win him no exciting filming opportunity, but can only slap him with a moral rescue burden."[105] Pogge recognizes that acknowledging that the filmmakers have the relevant moral freedom not to make the film while insisting on compliance with the operative moral constraint not to let the fishermen perish may yield a world that is less morally good than it would have been in the absence of that constraint. No fishermen will be saved. But, as he puts it, "morality cannot plausibly be purged of such counterproductivity entirely."[106]

But even if morality cannot be purged of *all* counterproductivity, this is not the sort of counterproductivity that we have come to expect of a sensible morality. We expect that respect for one's "moral freedom" not to be maximally beneficent will result in deaths or harm that one could have prevented if one had been more beneficent. We also expect that acknowledging deontic moral constraints will result in preventable deaths when it prohibits us from sacrificing some for the sake of others. But we do *not* ordinarily expect deontic constraints (or requirements) to prohibit acts that would prevent harm to the persons *on whose behalf the deontic constraint or requirement is imposed.* In the case at hand, the moral requirement to save the fishermen does *not* serve to protect the fishermen from being sacrificed for the benefit of others; it leads to the preventable deaths of the fishermen themselves. If it is hard to have confidence in a morality that allows that allows filmmakers to deliberately refrain from rescuing fishermen in distress, it is also hard to have confidence in a morality that renders it certain that the fishermen will not be rescued.

In an essay that deserves more attention than it has received, Michael Lockwood says that

> If a project is a worthwhile one, harms no one and benefits many, then it may . . . be morally permissible, in pursuing the project, to let people die or otherwise omit to save them from harm—when one could do so with the greatest ease—*if doing so would be damaging to the project itself.*[107]

Lockwood's view applies more clearly to SCAT than to ST because the aim of SCAT is arguably more worthwhile and because whereas the scientific question posed in SCAT could not be answered without a placebo control, DL could have answered the scientific question while providing surfactant therapy to all participants. But the issue here is the principle. Is Lockwood correct? I find myself torn. It does seem wrong for the filmmakers to let the fishermen die. But it also seems wrong to impose a requirement (that the filmmaker rescue the fishermen) that is so demonstrably self-defeating given that the requirement will cause the fishermen not to be saved. Who is right? Pogge or Lockwood?

Let us assume that it would ordinarily be wrong or even "grotesque" for the filmmakers to offer the coin-flip deal once they are on site. That leaves open the question as to whether it would be wrong for the filmmakers to embark on their *plan* and, if so, whether the legitimacy of the *plan* alters the morality of the (otherwise wrongful) proposal. When put that way, Pogge's filmmaker example raises an issue for moral theory (somewhat) analogous to Gregory Kavka's famous problem about rationality—*The Toxin Puzzle*.

> [A billionaire] places before me a vial of toxin that, if I drink it, will make me painfully ill for a day, but will not threaten my life or have any lasting effects. . . . The billionaire will pay me one million dollars tomorrow morning if, at midnight tonight, I intend to drink the toxin tomorrow afternoon. He emphasizes that I need not drink the toxin to receive the money; in fact, the money will already be in my bank account hours before the time for drinking it arrives, if I succeed. . . . All I have to do is . . . intend at midnight tonight to drink the stuff tomorrow afternoon. I am perfectly free to change my mind after receiving the money and not drink the toxin.[108]

Kavka's puzzle is framed in terms of *intentions*: could one (rationally) intend today to drink the toxin tomorrow when one knows that it will be irrational to drink the toxin tomorrow? Is it possible to form an intention to perform a future act, given the foreknowledge that you will have a strong incentive not to perform that act? We could also frame the puzzle in terms of the rationality of forming and carrying out a *plan* to drink the toxin. One would want to be able to embark on such a plan. The question is whether it could be rational to drink the toxin as part of that plan after one has already received the money. Some believe that, having made the commitment, it would be mad to drink the toxin when the time comes. David Gauthier argues that it is perfectly rational to make such a commitment for prudential reasons, that it would be mad not to be the sort of person who would drink the toxin.[109]

Now I have no (rational!) intention to add to the considerable literature on this puzzle. My present point is that morality may present us with arguably analogous situations. If it is permissible for the filmmakers to embark on a plan that contains what would otherwise be an impermissible failure to rescue, there are two principal possibilities: (1) although the plan not to rescue is permissible, the filmmakers are morally required to rescue nonetheless; (2) the permissibility of the plan converts what would *otherwise* be an *impermissible* failure to rescue into a *permissible* failure to rescue. I have no original argument to make here, but if the failure to rescue is embedded in a permissible plan, then the failure to rescue may thereby become permissible.

One might try to defend the view that the filmmaker is morally required to rescue the fishermen by appeal to *non-person affecting moral principles*. On that view, not rescuing is wrong not because it is bad for the fishermen, but because it violates an abstract or impersonal moral principle. But Pogge does *not* take the *non-person affecting* tack. In acknowledging the potential untoward consequences of adopting his view, he notes that "There is a real danger . . . that the *very people in whose behalf morality imposes such constraints* end up worse off than they would have been without it."[110] And so it would seem that Pogge is stuck. On the one hand, he says that we cannot have confidence in a morality that encourages and rewards exploitative behavior. On the other hand, if we do not regard such behavior as permissible, there is a real danger that the persons we regard as the victims of exploitation will end-up worse off. Until convinced otherwise, I prefer principles under which people are not worse off.

The Consequences of Principles

This heading is slightly misleading. Principles don't have consequences, but the *acceptance* of principles does have consequences. I believe that we cannot determine whether we should promulgate certain principles such as the "standard of care principle" or PEP without considering the consequences of the acceptance of those principles, particularly given that the acceptance of or compliance with those principles can have unintended consequences. And that is an empirical matter. I am *not* claiming that we must be committed to an *aggregative* consequentialism. It is to claim that we should be reluctant to endorse moral principles that are self-defeating or counter-productive in terms of the values that motivate those principles.

Consider this analogy. The Federal Aviation Administration once proposed requiring that all infants have an assigned seat on a plane and that they be placed in a child restraint (car seat) during take-off and landing. The FAA argued that this would reduce injuries and fatalities to infants. On examination, it appeared that the proposal would actually lead to an increase in accidental deaths and injuries to infants. If parents are required to buy a separate ticket for their infants, some parents will choose to drive to their destination rather than fly. Given that flying is much safer than driving, an infant that is being held by an adult on a plane is still safer than an infant who is in a car seat in a car. So if the point of the regulation was to save lives of infants—not just the lives of infants on *planes*—the regulation was unwise if it would have the alleged "diversion effect." And it was withdrawn.[111]

There is an important lesson here for those who develop and analyze the principles of research ethics. I suspect that many of the well-established principles of research ethics have *not* been put to this sort of an empirical test. I doubt that those who draft documents such as The Declaration of Helsinki or The Belmont Report or the Common Rule have thought it necessary to examine the consequences of compliance with the principles that they advance.

In criticizing the "double standard" that would allow research in LDCs that would not be allowed in the United States, Lurie and Wolfe argue that the long term health of people in developing countries will be "better served by standards that protect all patients and set a higher standard."[112] Writing about a study of HIV transmission in Uganda, Dirceu Grego says this:

> Unfortunately, neither researchers nor the research they produce will solve the problem of global inequalities in health. But if researchers were committed to treating all people as equals in research involving human subjects, then this demonstration of equity might serve as a spearhead for more widespread change. For this reason, it is crucial that the ethical requirements set by an indisputable international reference such as the Declaration of Helsinki be applied uniformly everywhere.[113]

I do not see how Lurie and Wolfe can be quite so confident that the promulgation and acceptance of the "standard care" principle will advance the interests of people in LDCs. They provide no evidence for their claim and do not seem to recognize that it is a claim for which evidence is required. Similarly, although Grego is right that the demonstration of equity "might" serve as a spearhead for more widespread change—even if it meant forgoing research—it is not clear that it will. Given that much of the criticism of studies such as ST has been based on appeals to the negative consequences of accepting so-called "double standards" that would regard such studies as permissible, we should also consider the consequences of accepting standards that would regard such studies as *im*permissible.

Of course principles are not always accurately applied. Although few commentators have put their arguments in these terms, it is possible that those who reject PEP are implicitly appealing to a version of the *epistemological* argument I considered above. Let us suppose, *arguendo*, that a reasonably accurate application of PEP will have better consequences than its rejection. It is possible that the application of PEP will be seriously flawed and that the moral gains consequent to the correct application of PEP will be outweighed by the costs consequent to the erroneous application of PEP and to the general weakening of important ethical considerations. This line of argument would exemplify a well-known strategy of adopting relatively "absolute" rules ("never go through a red light") as a second-best strategy even when first best rules ("go through red lights when it is safe to do so") that allow for greater flexibility are likely to be misapplied. From that perspective, the framers of documents such as the Declaration of Helsinki might argue that while the first best ethical principles would actually allow for trials that its principles preclude, there is a great danger that those responsible for applying such principles would allow trials that should *not* be approved, and so, in the long run, it may be better not to permit trials such as ST, even if it would otherwise be better to permit it. Once again, it is an empirical issue as to whether this argument works in the present context, but it is important to note that this argument does not reject PEP on its own terms.

Exploitation and Double Standards

As I just noted, some critics have argued that to allow a *PCT* in an *LDC* that would not be permitted in a developed society is to countenance moral relativism or a double ethical standard—"Acceptance of a standard of care that does not conform to the standard in the sponsoring country results in a double standard in research."[114] If ST would not be permitted in the United States, then it should not be permitted in Bolivia; we should not use "the abominable state of health care in [impoverished] countries . . . to justify studies that could never pass ethical muster in the sponsoring country."[115]

As Marcia Angell puts it, we must avoid an "ethical relativism" that would allow for research programs in Third World populations that "could not be carried out in the sponsoring countries."[116]

Angell's point has little to do with ethical relativism as it is usually understood. No one is claiming that it would be acceptable to conduct ST in Bolivia if it does not violate Bolivian values to do so. We can agree that the same *fundamental ethical* principles should apply to research wherever it is conducted. The question is whether the right universal values might have different implications in different contexts. The principle "When in Rome, do as the Romans do" has nothing to do with relativism; it is a corollary of the universal principle that one should show respect for others' norms when in their midst. The principle "serve food that your guests will like" is a universal principle that will yield different results for different guests.[117]

Similarly, the principle of informed consent is a universal principle that will yield different results in different cases, given that some people will consent to interventions whereas others will not. Thus one can administer medically necessary blood transfusions to those who consent, but not to Jehovah's Witnesses who refuse to consent on religious grounds. There are no double standards here, just a consistent application of the principle of informed consent to medical treatment. In the context of medical research, if it would be irrational for Americans to consent to participate in a placebo controlled trial of Surfaxin, but it would not be irrational for a Bolivian to do so, insisting that only "rational" consent can be taken as morally transformative will have different implications in the two societies. Once again, there are no double standards at play.

Or consider the assessment of risks and benefits in research. As we have seen, The Common Rule states that the risks of participation must be "reasonable in relation to anticipated benefits, if any, to subjects, and the importance of the knowledge that may reasonably be expected to result." Although this provision implies that IRBs can approve research when the importance of the knowledge outweighs the risks to the subject, consider the implications of a *subject*-centered version of the principle that requires that risks to the *subject* are reasonable in relation to anticipated benefits to the *subject*.

A subject-centered version of the reasonable risk criterion could be understood as a universal principle that has different implications in different social settings. Given that the infants in Bolivia would receive no treatment in the absence of ST, the risks of participation are certainly reasonable in relation to the anticipated benefits of participation. By contrast, if we apply that principle in a developed society where subjects could expect to receive the surfactant therapy outside of the trial, then the risks of participation to the subjects are not reasonable in relation to the anticipated benefits. Once again, I am *not* arguing that the placebo-controlled version of the Surfaxin trial passes ethical muster. I am arguing that hyperbolic polemical appeals to the notion of double standards will not resolve that question.

Conclusion

I began by discussing what I called *The Exploitation Argument*. The crucial moral premise of that argument maintains that if a practice is exploitative, then it should not be permitted. I have not resolved the question as to whether research such as ST is properly described as exploitative. Among other things, this requires an account of unfair transactions that neither I nor those who advance the exploitation argument have produced. I have also argued that even if ST is properly described as exploitative, it does *not* follow that it should not be permitted. To the contrary. I have argued that we should generally permit mutually advantageous and consensual transactions to go forward, even if they are exploitative. At the same time, I have argued that there are plausible justifications for not allowing some mutually advantageous and consensual transactions, and thus we must go on to ask whether those reasons apply in a given case. That is largely an empirical question.

The most important lesson of this discussion is not to decide whether ST or similar studies should be approved. The most important lesson is one of tone and spirit. I believe that we will not resolve questions as to the justifiability of studies such as ST by appeal to the derisive language of exploitation, double standards, relativism, minimalism, and so forth. We will resolve them by the rigorous examination of arguments and by the development and study of the relevant empirical considerations. Interested parties should withdraw some of their heavy rhetorical artillery and begin the hard work of deliberating about the best ethical principles for the decidedly non-ideal conditions under which research does and can take place.

Having said that, we would do well to remember that the alleged exploitation of research subjects occupies only one corner in the larger landscape of the ethics of clinical research. And this in two ways. First, and on the micro level, there may be important ethical worries about the recruitment and use of research subjects that do not appeal to the need to avoid exploitation.

Even when we keep our eye focused on the dyadic relationship between researchers and subjects, we may think that considerations of beneficence require certain forms of treatment of research subjects even if they would not be otherwise exploited. I shall explore some of those considerations in the next chapter.

Second, and on the macro level, there are several ethical desiderata that concern the research that does and, perhaps more importantly, does not take place in LDCs. It may be argued that research is an important public health activity in LDCs and that the principal goal of such research is not to treat the subjects properly, but to use such research to address the health needs of the global poor.[118] I have not addressed the question as to who has what responsibilities to shape the research agenda in a way that will address those needs. As I said at the outset of the book, I will be concerned with the recruitment and use of research subjects. I did not argue and do not believe that these issues are more important than the global issues that I do not address. Indeed, I believe the opposite. At the same time, my argument may ease the path towards policies that address the health needs of the global poor. If I am right in thinking that at least *some* of the worries about the recruitment and use of research subjects are overdone, then my argument may help to clear the way to greater attention to these larger questions even though I have not done much to address them myself.

6 The Interaction Principle

The Problem

Clinical research typically involves an interaction between an investigator (A) and a subject (B). A seeks to obtain generalizable knowledge from his use of B. In the cases in which I am interested (which represent only a sub-set of cases of clinical research), B can reasonably expect to benefit from participation in A's study in much the same way that an employee expects to benefit from working for an employer. The subject may receive medical treatment or medical screening that is otherwise unavailable. And she may be paid. Such benefits notwithstanding, it is often suggested that the researchers' use of the subject or that the interaction between investigators and subjects generate ethical obligations for researchers that go beyond those to which the parties might reasonably agree. It is also sometimes argued that research should be permitted only if researchers are prepared to meet those obligations. Similar claims are often made about the interaction between researchers and the communities in which research takes place. In this chapter, I seek to explore the force of such claims.

The sorts of cases in which I am interested involve what we might call *package deals*. A proposes to provide benefits to B in return for obtaining something *from* B or being able to use B or do certain things *to* B. Consider *Lawn Mowing*.

> *Lawn Mowing.* A proposes to hire B to mow his lawn for a fee (X).
> B agrees to mow A's lawn for X. Call (X) "the contractual
> level" of benefits.

A has no independent obligation to interact with B. It is morally permissible for A to mow his own lawn even if A knows that hiring B for X would be to B's advantage. What I shall call *The Interaction Principle* (IP) maintains that one can have obligations or moral reasons to provide *super*-contractual benefits to those with whom one engages in mutually beneficial and consensual transactions. The Interaction Principle maintains, in effect, that even though A has no obligation to provide *any* benefits to B if A chooses not to interact with B, A nonetheless can acquire an obligation to provide benefits that go beyond that to which A and *B would otherwise have agreed* if A chooses to interact with B. I say "would otherwise have agreed." If the law requires A to pay a minimum wage of $7.50 per hour to B where A and B would otherwise have settled on $5.00 per hour, then the *actual* contract between A and B already incorporates super-contractual benefits. It may be thought that even if A would do nothing wrong if A were not to hire B, there is a minimum level of compensation that B should receive if A does hire B and thereby benefits from B's labor.

Just as Moliere's Monsieur Jourdain was speaking prose for forty years without knowing it, I believe that many of the canonical principles of research ethics and much of the writing by bioethicists on these issues tacitly assume something like IP. This would not be particularly worrisome if, like speaking prose, IP were unproblematic. It is not. Although IP might seem to be a natural and intuitively attractive feature of our moral outlook, it has some paradoxical implications and, at a minimum, its rationale, scope, and force are unclear.

In Chapter 5, I considered the argument that researchers must do more for participants or their communities if they are to avoid the charge of exploitation even when the research is mutually advantageous and consensual. Although some of the claims as to what researchers should do for participants or their communities can be couched in the procrustean bed of avoiding exploitation, the force of IP goes beyond what can sensibly be put in those terms and deserves a more thorough and focused discussion.

IP has two principal corollaries with which I shall be concerned. First, to accept IP is to *reject* what I will call *the nonworseness claim* (NWC).

Bracketing effects on third parties, NWC maintains that it *cannot* be morally worse for A to interact with B than not to interact with B if the interaction or package deal is beneficial to B and if B consents to the interaction. Second, to accept IP is to endorse the *greater obligation claim* (GOC). Simply stated, GOC claims that among the potential beneficiaries of A's actions or resources, A has greater obligations to provide super-contractual benefits to B than to others, even though B has *already* benefited from interaction with A whereas others have received no benefit from A.

We can locate the obligations generated by interactions within the traditional distinction between *general obligations* (or what Rawls calls "natural duties") which are owed to everyone and do not depend upon any prior relationship between the parties, and *special obligations* or what Samuel Scheffler calls "associative duties" that are owed to specific persons.[1] The duty not to harm others is a general obligation. So is the duty to rescue strangers in need, because that duty does not depend upon any prior relationship or voluntary undertaking between the parties. Some special obligations are rooted in voluntary actions or undertakings, such as the obligation to keep a promise or pay a debt. Other special obligations may be rooted in *non-voluntary* relationships, and so we may have special obligations or associative duties to members of our family or country even though we did not choose our family members or fellow citizens.

Given the distinction between general and special obligations, we can make two preliminary points. First, the obligations that derive from interactions are special obligations. Second, the moral questions raised by interactions are, I believe, distinct from the question as to whether we have greater obligations to "identifiable lives" than to "statistical lives"; whether, for example, the state has greater moral reason to spend resources to rescue five miners who are trapped in a coal mine than to spend those resources preventing a larger number of future deaths in mining accidents.[2] Although some of IP's intuitive appeal may be rooted in the identifiability of the persons with whom one interacts, much of its force seems to derive from the fact that A *benefits* from the interaction with or the use of B—and no one benefits from the fact that miners are trapped.

Now it might be objected that what I have described as *super*-contractual obligations are often merely *contractual* if, as often occurs, A interacts with B knowing that he thereby acquires obligations that go beyond that to which A and B would otherwise have agreed. For example, an employer may voluntarily and knowingly agree to pay the prescribed minimum wage, although the employer and employee would have agreed to a sub-minimum wage if left to their own devices. It would, however, be a mistake to regard the obligation to pay a minimum wage as deriving solely from contract, because the *terms* of that contract are not themselves fully subject to contract.

Now, given that the benefits of an interaction flow both ways, it is at least somewhat surprising that we rarely ask just who has super-contractual obligations to whom and why. Suppose that A hires B for $5.00 per hour to mow his lawn. Why should we assume that the super-contractual obligations— if any—run from A to B rather than from B to A? We might think that A should pay B more than $5.00 per hour, but we don't think that B should do A's laundry in exchange for the opportunity to mow B's lawn at $5.00 per hour. We may think that investigators should express their gratitude to research participants by providing super-contractual benefits to them, but it is rarely (*never?*) claimed that research interactions impose super-contractual obligations on *subjects*. We do not think that participants should express their gratitude for gaining access to an experimental drug or medical exam by agreeing to blood draws that are not required for the research but which may be useful to the investigators for other purposes. To simplify matters, I will simply assume that the super-contractual obligations at issue apply to researchers and not to subjects.

To set the stage, consider a (not so) hypothetical example.

> *Nike and Hike.* Two companies produce athletic shoes: Nike and Hike. Nike sets up factories in less developed countries (LDCs) in which it employs people for wages that are at or above typical local wages, but which do not provide what could reasonably be called a "living wage" at local prices, much less a living wage by American standards. The employees work long hours under "sweatshop" conditions that would be unacceptable in the United States. Hike believes that it cannot compete successfully with Nike if it had to pay higher wages or provide (much) better working conditions in LDCs, but it can compete by making big capital investments in automation and producing athletic shoes in the U.S. Observing that Nike has been subject to considerable criticism for its employment practices, or, perhaps because it believes that it is immoral to employ workers in sweatshops at low wages, Hike builds a highly automated plant in the U.S.

I assume for the sake of argument that the package deal offered by Nike is beneficial to the employees and consensual, although I certainly do *not* thereby claim that "sweatshop" employment in developing societies always meets that description.[3]

Now let us also suppose for the sake of argument what has decidedly *not* been said or demonstrated, namely, that Nike presents a case of mutually advantageous consensual *exploitation* because the terms of the transaction are unfair. As I argued in Chapter 5, the latter claim is more difficult to defend than is often supposed. It requires a principle of fair wages and employment practices, and it may also assume that it is feasible for Nike to provide better terms without losing its competitive place in the market. Nonetheless, bracketing the possibility that Nike's practices have negative externalities for the host society, it seems undeniable (given the stated assumptions) that Nike is doing more to advance the interests of people in LDCs than Hike even if Nike's motivations are entirely self-interested whereas Hike is concerned to avoid exploitation.

Faced with this analysis, some might alter their views. If one uses Hike as one's mental anchor and if Hike is doing nothing wrong by producing shoes in the U.S. without sweatshop labor, and if Nike's practices are better for poor people in LDCs than Hike's, then perhaps Nike's practices are not (so) morally objectionable, first appearances to the contrary notwithstanding. On the other hand, if one uses Nike as one's mental anchor and if Nike exploits its workers, and if Hike does less for poor people than Nike, then perhaps Hike's practices are indeed morally objectionable, first appearances to the contrary notwithstanding. Exploiting workers à la Nike may be bad, but not providing jobs for them à la Hike may be worse.

By contrast with these two views, IP implies that Nike's practices might actually be morally worse than Hike's because Nike is wrongfully using or interacting with its employees and Hike is not. As I indicated above, to accept IP is to *reject* the *non-worseness claim* (NWC). NWC maintains that it *cannot* be morally worse for A to interact with B than not to interact with B if: (1) the overall interaction or package deal is better for B than non-interaction, (2) B consents to the interaction, and (3) such interaction has no negative effects on others. By contrast, IP implies that precisely because Nike benefits from the labors of its employees, it may acquire obligations to provide super-contractual or "fair" benefits to its employees whereas, *ex hypothesi,* Hike is already treating its relatively few workers fairly and so has no super-contractual obligations to them.[4] Because Nike is violating its obligations whereas Hike is not, Nike's behavior is worse.

Now to say that Nike's actions are "morally worse" than Hike's is ambiguous as between an axiological moral evaluation of the *state of affairs* that results from its actions and a deontic moral evaluation of its *actions*. One might maintain that the state of affairs that results from Nike's actions is not morally worse than the state of affairs that results from Hike's actions, but that Nike is acting wrongly whereas Hike is not. I will return to this distinction below. For present purposes, I will rely on the undifferentiated claim that Nike's actions are morally worse than Hike's, for the intuitive appeal of IP does not seem to rest on a sophisticated distinction.

Let us now consider GOC. The IP claims that A may have a greater special obligation to provide super-contractual benefits to those who have already benefited from interaction with A than to provide benefits to those with whom A has not (yet) interacted. Suppose that Nike earns greater profits than it anticipated and is considering three options: (1) giving a bonus to its workers; (2) contributing to a fund for those who applied for jobs with Nike but who were not hired; (3) investing its profits in new factories that will expand the number of persons it can employ. A commitment to GOC suggests that Nike has reason (of undetermined weight) to choose (1) because it has a greater obligation to the workers from whose efforts it has made its profits than to those that it did not or might hire, even though its current workers have already benefited from their employment and are demonstrably better off than those who applied but were not hired (2) or would be hired if Nike built additional manufacturing plants (3).[5]

To use the language of economics, there will be opportunity costs to any super-contractual resources that A provides to B. Perhaps we need not worry much if Nike's only feasible alternative to (1) is (4) to give those profits to its rich investors. But not all cases have that structure. If (2) is a feasible alternative and Nike chooses (1) over (2) or (3), then the opportunity cost of (1) is that those who were not hired or will not be hired fare less well than they otherwise would.

All this is obvious and should not need stating. Nonetheless, I think it does need to be stated because many of the canonical statements of research ethics and much bioethics scholarship maintain, in effect, that researchers should provide super-contractual benefits to research participants without considering the opportunity costs of the policies they favor. For example, Marcia Angell writes that research "must hold human welfare above the interests of society and science."[6] This is misleading. The contrast between the personal-sounding "human welfare" and the impersonal-sounding "society" and "science" conceals the underlying tension between advancing the welfare of the human subjects of research and the welfare of other present and future persons who stand to benefit from research. Along similar lines, The Declaration of Helsinki says that "In medical research involving human subjects, the well-being of the individual research subject must take precedence over all other interests." Taken literally, this statement cannot be true. Research often requires asking subjects to undergo procedures that are not in their interests. It is certainly plausible to claim that research should not impose *nonconsensual* burdens on subjects in order to promote the interests of others. But it is far from clear that the *well-being* of subjects should have strong priority over the well-being of others if the package deal of participation is already beneficial to the subjects and if they consent to such participation. Yet this is precisely what GOC seems to claim.

Many critics of research in developed societies take special aim at pharmaceutical corporations that seek to profit financially by the use of poor persons in LDCs. But the opportunity costs entailed by a commitment to IP will be felt whoever sponsors the research. Although public or non profit sponsors of research, such as NIH, need not worry about generating profits, such institutions certainly have limited resources. If NIH-sponsored researchers are required to provide super-contractual benefits to research subjects or their communities, there will be fewer research projects or that projects will have smaller samples, and so forth. Here, as elsewhere, there are no free lunches.

With respect to the private realm, if we frame the choice as one between greater profits for the corporation and greater benefits for the research subjects we may think that morality should push us towards the latter and towards minimizing the former. Better to benefit the poor than the rich. But that would be too quick. Here as elsewhere, appearances can be deceiving. It is often a complex empirical question as to who benefits and who loses from a policy, tax, regulation, or the like. Consider the Tobacco Master Settlement Agreement (MSA) of 1998 that required a group of tobacco companies to make payments of $250 billion to the states over a 25 year period.[7] Although it may appear that the settlement will be paid out of the profits that would otherwise accrue to the owners and managers of the filthy and deceptive tobacco companies, the companies have shifted most of their burden to the disproportionately poor consumer in the form of higher prices. Similarly, it is a complex empirical question as to who does or would ultimately pay the price of requiring commercial researchers to provide super-contractual benefits to subjects. Does it inhibit the pace of innovation and the cure of disease? Does it reduce the number of studies that a company can conduct, thereby depriving others of the opportunity to benefit by participating in research? It is hard to know.

My plan is this. In the next section, I shall discuss several principles or arguments of research ethics that seem to be motivated by IP and which implicate NWC or GOC. Although the force of IP is certainly not limited to research in LDCs, the case for that principle is arguably strongest in that context, and so I will focus on principles of research ethics that are most at home there. I then revisit IP and its two corollaries (the rejection of NWC and the acceptance of GOC) and consider whether these positions can be defended.

IP and Research Ethics

Researchers have greater obligations than the rest of us.

If one doesn't interact directly with research subjects in LDCs, then one is subject to the general demands of justice and beneficence, about which views vary from the very demanding (e.g. Peter Singer) to the relatively demanding (e.g. Thomas Pogge) to the somewhat demanding (e.g. Rawls) to the non-demanding (lots).[8] Those of us who live in considerable affluence may have general obligations of beneficence to provide resources for medical care or medical research for those who live in LDCs, either as individuals or through our governments. In addition, if citizens and institutions in the developed world have benefited from *harms* imposed on the impoverished citizens of LDCs, then we would have arguably stronger obligations of compensation or rectification for harm.

But whatever the general obligations of beneficence, justice, or rectification that apply to citizens or governments of developed nations, it is commonly thought—or simply assumed—that medical researchers and their sponsors have greater obligations towards subjects and their communities than do citizens or the governments of the countries in which the sponsoring organizations are located. Many of the standard principles of research ethics of the sort that are found in the Declaration of Helsinki and CIOMS and many of the arguments advanced by prominent bioethicists explicitly or implicitly claim that because researchers benefit directly from the use of research subjects in LDCs whereas ordinary citizens of affluent nations do not, the researchers have special obligations of reciprocity towards the research subjects or their communities that go beyond the general obligations (large or small) of justice, respect, and beneficence that apply to everyone else. I state this view here in very general terms. As we shall see, it gets played out in several ways.

Responsiveness

It is accepted wisdom that clinical research in developing societies should be "responsive" to the health care needs of the community in which research takes place. Call this the "responsiveness principle" (RP). On most (not all) formulations, RP does not claim that researchers are under a positive moral requirement to conduct responsive research. It is generally not claimed, for example, that it would be wrong for NIH or Pfizer to conduct research on Alzheimer's disease in the United States because Alzheimer's is not a priority health need in LDCs. The main thrust of RP is negative: It is wrong to conduct research in LDCs that does *not* satisfy RP; the people of LDCs should not be used for research that will primarily benefit people in affluent nations. If the people of LDCs are to be used for research, that research must meet a super-contractual condition: it must address a research question that is responsive to the needs of the host society.

Versions of RP appear in many documents. Guideline 10 of CIOMS ethical guidelines for biomedical research states:

> Before undertaking research in a population or community *with*
> *limited resources*, the sponsor and the researcher must make every
> effort to ensure that the research is responsive to the health needs
> and the priorities of the population or community in which it is to
> be carried out[9] (emphasis added).

The Participants in the 2001 Conference on Ethical Aspects of Research in Developing Countries say that it is "widely accepted" that clinical research "should address a health problem of the developing country population."[10] Recommendation 1.3 of the National Bioethics Advisory Commission states: "Clinical trials conducted in developing countries should be limited to those studies that are responsive to the health needs of the host country."[11]

It is not clear what RP actually requires. If RP allows for research in LDCs on the full range of diseases that occur in an LDC, then the principle is relatively vacuous. Given that some, but relatively few, Ugandans reach the age at which they are likely to develop Alzheimer's, research in Uganda on Alzheimer's would be compatible with a broad version of RP. If RP is to have any bite, it must mean that research in a developing society must focus on a health *priority* of the host nation.

RP is sometimes wrongly conflated with the "reasonable availability" principle (RA) which maintains that researchers should assure that the product of their research is available to either participants or other members of the host society at the completion of a trial. This conflation is easy to understand in light of the Declaration of Helsinki's statement that

> Medical research involving a disadvantaged or vulnerable
> population or community is only justified if the research is
> responsive to the health needs and priorities of this population or
> community and if there is a reasonable likelihood that this
> population or community stands to benefit from the results of the
> research.[12]

Nonetheless, RP and RA are distinct. Whereas RA concerns the *fruits* of research in LDCs, RP is best understood as putting restrictions on the research *questions* that are permissibly investigated in LDCs. So whereas the proposed Surfaxin Trial fell short on RA, it was arguably compatible with RP, given that respiratory distress syndrome was a health priority in South America.

The standard formulation of RP is asymmetric as between the developed and less developed world. It is *not* claimed that it is morally problematic to conduct research in developed societies that is responsive to the health care needs of people in developing societies. Few would object on grounds of responsiveness to a recent proposal by U.S. investigators to conduct a Phase I infection-inducing challenge study of a malaria vaccine in which healthy volunteers would be exposed to malaria-infected mosquitoes, even though malaria is virtually unknown in the United States.[13] Indeed, I once saw (in the Washington, D.C. metro) a recruitment advertisement for a Johns Hopkins University study of immunization for dengue fever that proudly shows a composite picture of an American and Vietnamese face with the words— "I live in DC, but I'm helping save lives in Vietnam" (although the appeal to altruism is followed by the offer of over $2,000). At the same time, some would object on grounds of responsiveness to a study of treatments or diagnostic procedures for Alzheimer's in a developing society even if the participants were themselves treated fairly and were to consent to participation.

Despite its wide acceptance, RP is deeply puzzling. We do not appeal to anything like RP in standard economic contexts in which people in the developed world benefit from the labor of people in developed societies. There are numerous objections to the practice of off-shoring manufacturing and services, but few would argue that Nike should locate production plants only where there is a special need for athletic shoes or that it is important that athletic shoes be provided to the society in which they are produced. As Martin Wolf puts it, "Some critics [complain] that the workers in developing countries are unable to afford the goods they make. This complaint is demented. One works in order to buy not what one makes, but what one needs. . . ."[14] It might be thought that the moral force of the responsiveness principle is greater in the research context than in the standard production context, but if so, we need an explanation as to why this is so.

Note that RP seems to violate NWC. Consider a benign hypothetical case in which Pharma, a major U.S. drug company, proposes to conduct a randomized controlled superiority trial of a new hypertension drug, Q, in Uganda. The case is intentionally benign so that the force of RP is not affected by other variables. The trial enrolls subjects who exhibit hypertension, but who are not receiving medication. Half the participants would receive Q and half would receive an existing drug, R. Although Pharma offers to provide Q or R (whichever is more effective) to all participants when the trial is complete, Pharma intends to market Q in developed nations. Pharma could run an active controlled trial of Q in the United States, but it might prefer to conduct this trial in Uganda because Uganda has more "treatment naïve" subjects and because other research related costs are significantly lower.

It would appear that the proposed trial of Q would not be compatible with RP since hypertension is not a health priority in Uganda and, to make matters worse, the fruits of the research would not be available to the community if the trial should prove successful. But to forego this research on these grounds violates NWC, given that the participants would benefit from and consent to participation. It is surely paradoxical to claim that it would not be wrong to conduct this research in the United States, in which case *no* Ugandans benefit, but that it would be wrong to conduct this research in Uganda where *some* Ugandans benefit.

One might defend RP by arguing that non-responsive research typically has negative effects on the host societies or, perhaps, that barring non-responsive research will have positive effects. First, it might be argued that most research imposes health costs on the community—using resources for research rather than for medical care—and that insisting on responsiveness is a way to off-set or compensate the society for the burdens imposed by research. Second, it might be argued that non-responsive research uses Pharma's resources in a way that does little to contribute to the health of impoverished people in LDCs and, moreover, it displaces responsive research in a world in which 90% of research resources are spent on resources for 10% of the world's population. And so by putting road-blocks in the way of non-responsive research, it may be thought that RP will motivate or incentivize researchers to use their resources in ways that will help to close the 90-10 gap. By denying some people (e.g., Ugandans with hypertension) the opportunity to participate in research to their benefit, RP advances the interests of others at risk for higher priority diseases such as malaria.

These claims provide a plausible defense of RP, although it is an empirical question as to just whether such "blocking" strategies will have positive effects. But these claims about externalities do *not* rest on a rejection of NWC, for NWC assumes that the interaction has no adverse effect on others. They do not give us reason to bar non-responsive research that has *no* systematic negative effects on others.

Standard of Care

As we saw in Chapter 5, it is often claimed that it is ethically impermissible to withhold a proven effective therapy as part of a randomized placebo-controlled trial. I am not here concerned to revisit the worries about exploitation. Rather, I want to suggest that the *standard care principle* can be understood as relying on IP and is therefore vulnerable to the objections that can be raised against that more general principle.

The standard care principle might be defended on the grounds that research subjects should be regarded as "patients" toward whom investigators owe specific obligations *qua* physicians. For reasons we have considered elsewhere, that view must be rejected if we are to engage in research at all. For example, such a view would preclude many procedures designed to measure study outcomes but which provide no benefit to the subject. I think it more promising to assume that the standard care principle relies on the view that researchers have special obligations to those who they use in research that they do not have towards those who are not research subjects.

In condemning the *Surfaxin Trial*, Lurie and Wolfe argued that ". . . the provision of placebo . . . to the 325 infants in the control group will result in the preventable deaths of 16 infants," that is, those infants *included* in the study who died because they received sham air but would not have died if they had received traditional surfactant therapy.[15] Fair enough. But note that a decision to include, say, 650 subjects in the study (as contrasted, say, with 1,000) also results in preventable deaths to the infants who were *not included* in the study because of a decision about sample size. And, quite reasonably, Lurie and Wolfe do not maintain that the researchers had an obligation to expand the sample size *ad infinitum* in order to provide surfactant therapy to more infants. They implicitly acknowledge that the scope of the study is legitimately constrained by its scientific rationale. Lurie and Wolfe assume without argument that Discovery Labs would owe some form of surfactant therapy to the subjects *in* the research project whereas they owe nothing to other infants with RDS who are not a part of the study even though *all* of the infants in the study would have been prospectively better off than infants not in the study; and even those in the control group would have received a higher standard of care than is customary in the society. Why? The most plausible answer is that Discovery Labs seeks to benefit from the use of its subjects but does not interact with nor benefit from its non-use of non-subjects.

The previous point could be put more generally. Larry Gostin maintains that

> Once a person enters a research project, particularly if he or she is poor and lacks adequate access to medical care, the investigator assumes some duty of care to safeguard that person's health and welfare. Doctors involved in a trial cannot turn their backs on obvious illness and health care needs of trial participants.[16]

Why is this so? After all, there are millions of persons—most of whom are not research subjects—who lack "adequate access to medical care." If Gostin is appealing to the principle that investigators have physician-like duties to treat their subjects as patients, then everything turns on whether the physician-patient model applies to clinical research. But Gostin could be arguing that even if the physician-patient model does not apply, researchers still have special responsibilities to provide super-contractual care to those whom they use as research subjects as contrasted with those who are not research subjects. So stated, the argument rests on IP. Let me be clear. I am *not* here denying that researchers have these sorts of special obligations to research subjects, nor am I claiming that they would act more beneficently towards non-subjects if they did less for these subjects. I am claiming only that the view that researchers have these sorts of special obligations to research subjects needs defense.

Post-Trial Obligations to Research Subjects

If an intervention proves effective and superior to other interventions in clinical trials, it will typically be available (in time) as part of standard medical care in developed countries. In LDCs, things are strikingly different. Even if a *subject* benefits from participation in a trial, the intervention may not be provided as part of standard medical care upon completion of the trial. For that reason, it is frequently argued that if researchers use a subject to test the effectiveness of an intervention, then those subjects should—at a minimum—be provided with the intervention at the conclusion of a successful trial. Paragraph 30 of the Declaration of Helsinki states:

> At the conclusion of the study, patients entered into the study are
> entitled to be informed about the outcome of the study and to
> share any benefits that result from it, for example, access to
> interventions identified as beneficial in the study or to other
> appropriate care or benefits.[17]

Ruth Macklin says that "individuals who serve as research subjects should not be made worse off after a clinical trial is over than they were while the research was being carried out."[18] Zhiyong Zong writes,

> Once studies do yield beneficial interventions and trial participants
> can continue to benefit from them but have no alternative access
> such as through the regular health system, post-trial provision for
> participants from developing countries should be mandatory.[19]

Let us assume that many researchers would be able to enroll a sufficient number of prospective subjects if they did not offer post-trial treatment and that participation on those terms is in the interest of those subjects all things considered. Do researchers or sponsors have super-contractual obligations to provide such treatment?

In discussing an anti-retroviral therapy (ART) trial in Uganda, David Rothman argues that, "As compensation to their subjects for enrolling in the research, investigators who come to Uganda should be required to leave their subjects better off."[20] But compensation for what? If the subjects are likely to be harmed by participation, then it is arguable that they are owed compensation for the harm, not to mention that the validity of their consent is certainly questionable. But if the subjects can expect to benefit from and consent to participation, it would seem that compensation for *harm* is irrelevant. James Lavery acknowledges that subjects may benefit but argues that reciprocity may demand more:

> Justice as reciprocity . . . . involves a more holistic recognition that research participants represent a *sine qua non* of clinical research, and that the essential nature of their contribution warrants some special gratitude or recognition, over and above the potential benefits inherent in a given research design.[21]

But one cannot argue that investigators have super-contractual obligations to subjects simply by citing a principle of reciprocity or gratitude, because it is precisely the content and force of such principles that is at issue. After all, it could be argued that the benefits provided to the subjects by their participation in the trial already fulfill the requirements of reciprocity.

One objection to the claim that researchers have post-trial obligations should be set aside, namely, that such an obligation is inconsistent with the purposes of research. NIH policy states that since it is "statutorily authorized to support and conduct biomedical *research*" (emphasis added), it cannot use its resources for *treatment* following the completion of a trial.[22] The NIH statement is a plausible interpretation of the existing statutes but is a non-starter as a *justification* of that policy. We would laugh at a corporation that said, "Giving drugs away free is inconsistent with our goal, which is to maximize profit." If morality requires that such drugs be provided to research participants, then the pursuit of profit must be constrained by the relevant moral requirements. And the same holds true for public or not-for-profit organizations. If it is wrong *not* to provide post-trial treatment to trial participants, then the existing policy should be changed so as to require its provision even if doing so would consume resources that would otherwise be devoted to research.

Now some of the statements on post-trial treatments are ambiguous as to whether the principle is best understood as a *moral* duty of investigators or as an enforceable prerequisite for conducting a trial. And some statements are ambiguous as to who is responsible for the provision of the treatment. Some suggest that it is the sponsor's obligation, whereas others simply say that participants should be provided with post trial treatment but do not claim that this responsibility lies exclusively with the sponsor. If, however, it is the sponsor's responsibility to provide post-trial treatment, then this principle threatens to violate NWC, for then a sponsor could avoid wrongdoing by refusing to engage in the research even if subjects benefit from participation *without* post-trial treatment.

Let us return to the fundamental question: do sponsors have a super-contractual obligation to provide post-trial treatment or other benefits to research subjects? It depends on how we understand the relation between investigators and subjects. On a contractual model, participation could be understood as a form of temporary employment. On that view, researchers owe nothing to their subjects when the trial is completed if that is not part of a fair labor agreement. As a general rule, we simply do not believe that employers have an obligation to ensure that employees are no worse off when their employment ends than during the period of employment. This is particularly so when the employment is task specific, as when one hires someone to paint one's house, but this is also true of other temporary jobs. American retailers frequently hire temporary personnel for the holiday shopping season, but they have no special obligations towards these employees when the season is over.

There are (at least) two ways to resist this line of argument. The first objection is simply stated: Whereas ordinary employment is typically beneficial (all things considered), participation in research is a burden (all things considered). Although non-consensual and non-beneficial labor are still all too well known throughout the world, many workers believe that the compensations of employment outweigh the burdens and risks of work, considerable though they may be, as perhaps vividly demonstrated by the willingness of Mexicans to illegally migrate to the United States in order to take physically demanding and unpleasant jobs. By contrast, it may be argued that the (*ex ante*) benefits to the subjects from participation in research do *not* typically exceed the burdens, and thus reciprocity demands that investigators provide post-trial treatment to compensate participants for their willingness to expose themselves to risks or discomforts of participation.

I know of no systematic data as to whether research subjects typically benefit from participation, all things considered. Indeed, it is not clear by what metric to make such judgments. Although some subjects knowingly take on the risks and inconveniences of participation for altruistic reasons, many people consent to participate in research because they believe that the package deal of participation is better than non-participation. Even if they do not expect to receive a direct medical benefit from an intervention that is being studied, they may expect to benefit from the general level of care (compared with what they would otherwise receive). If the participant's expectation of benefit is misplaced because investigators actively deceive subjects or because the risks of participation are not adequately disclosed or because the subjects are in the grips of a therapeutic misconception, then their consent is arguably not transformative. But if participants give valid consent, then it seems reasonable to assume that they do *not* regard the package deal of participation as a burden, all things considered.

Of course, whether the package deal of participation in research is a benefit or a burden depends, in part, on what counts *as* a benefit of participation. As we have seen, there is considerable controversy as to how to count benefits such as financial payment (See Chapter 4). If the subjects can justifiably regard financial compensation as a benefit of research, then much research that is not now regarded as beneficial might be reclassified or could become reclassified if the payments were increased. In any case, *the present argument is limited to those who do give valid consent and who can reasonably expect to benefit from participation, all things considered, whatever the appropriate metric of benefits.* So, one cannot resist the analogy between temporary employment and participation on the ground that participation is a net burden whereas temporary employment is not.

The second way to resist a contractual or employment model is to grant that participation in research is (*ex ante*) beneficial, all things considered, but then argue that the obligation of investigators to provide post-trial benefits to participants is greater than the obligation of ordinary employers to provide post-employment benefits to employees. As Macklin puts it: "[I]f we view health care, medical benefits, and the research that yields these goods and services as a special sort of social good, we can readily reject the idea that research involving human subjects should be treated no differently from other activities driven by market forces."[23] But it is not sufficient to say that "if" we view research as a "special sort of good" then we *can* reject the view that serving as a research subject is like being a temporary employee. For it must be shown that (1) we *should* view health care and research as a special sort of social good and (2) that, once we do, there are good reasons for thinking that research is not only distinguishable from ordinary employment, but that the distinction supports the claim that researchers have greater post-interaction obligations than employers.

Although Macklin provides a defense of (1) the distinction between the good of health care and some discretionary goods, her argument does not distinguish health care from other basic needs such as food, shelter, and clothing. In any case, even if we accept (1), Macklin provides no argument for (2) and it is precisely such an argument that is necessary here. After all, it is not as if providing post-trial treatment to research subjects is of monumental moral significance, whereas providing the money that people need for basic needs and which they will lose when temporary employment ends, is a morally trivial activity that is, to use Macklin's (derisive?) phrase, "driven by market forces."

Even if there is no argument for the general claim that researchers have greater post-interaction obligations than employers, it may be argued that the cessation of treatment is a greater *loss* than the cessation of employment and researchers have a responsibility to mitigate that harm. First, it is possible that given the ways in which the body responds to an intervention, the cessation of treatment might leave the research subject medically worse off than if she had never received treatment. If so, then there is probably a defect in the subject's consent: why *should* she agree to participate without a guarantee of post-trial treatment if she will end up worse off? So this objection does not provide independent reason for the provision of post-trial treatment when consent is valid. Second, and as a psychological phenomenon, the loss of a good may feel much worse than never having received it all, and, as Lavery suggests, is likely to involve "a range of dignitary harms . . . including grief, frustration, and disappointment."[24] Here, once again, we can raise a question about consent. For if a subject does not have the information or competence to anticipate these feelings, the validity of her consent is problematic. In any case, although Lavery asserts that "the psychology of this loss is also important ethically," it is an open question as to whether and to what extent allocation decisions should be strongly responsive to such emotional phenomena. The fact that the *cessation* of treatment will reduce B's psychic welfare more than the *commencement* of treatment will increase C's psychic welfare is not, in itself, a decisive argument for favoring B over C.

It might be thought that researchers have a special obligation not to *abandon* trial participants that they do not have towards non-participants. Such a view is implied by Gostin's remark that "Doctors involved in a trial cannot turn their backs on obvious illness and health care needs of trial participants." By itself, the claim that one shouldn't abandon trial participants doesn't do any moral work, for we cannot properly describe the cessation of a relationship or interaction as wrongful abandonment unless we assume that there is an obligation to continue the relationship. One does not "abandon" the person who paints one's house when the job is done. The interaction simply stops. If the "abandonment" argument rests on an appeal to the norms of medical care, as implied by Gostin's reference to the responsibility of "doctors," then, once again, this move begs the question by presupposing that investigators have an obligation to regard their subjects as patients.

Gostin's argument might be understood as a claim about virtue or character or moral psychology rather than a claim about obligation. Perhaps it is or should be psychologically difficult for investigators to "turn their backs" on those with whom they have been so intimately involved, from whom they have obtained private information, into whom they have stuck needles, whose illnesses they have observed, and who they know will benefit from further treatment. The disposition to want to help those with whom we have interacted to our benefit is one that we should want to encourage and support if it does not seriously compromise the enterprise of research itself or have other untoward consequences.

Unfortunately, the disposition to treat subjects as patients may pose serious problems if it is not well contained. The pursuit of generalized knowledge often requires that investigators *not* respond to the needs of individual subjects, but to adhere to a predetermined protocol. Much research also requires study procedures such as blood draws and biopsies that pose little risk but are of no medical benefit to the subject, even when participation is beneficial, all things considered.

In addition, there can be significant opportunity costs to the use of fungible resources to provide for the needs of subjects when those resources could be devoted to additional or higher quality research. The desirability of using resources for *other* research projects must gain weight when subjects have, *ex hypothesi, already benefited* from participation, whereas other non-subjects are receiving no help at all for the variety of crippling diseases from which they suffer and which might benefit from research or treatment. As Merritt and Grady remark, "[I]n a country where only a fraction of HIV-infected people who need ART are able to get it, and rationing is inescapable, why should the fact that someone participated in ART research confer priority for continued ART . . . while their needy compatriots go without?"[25]

We have been considering whether researchers have greater obligations to subjects than to others. That issue concerns the ethics of research. I now want to revisit the question as to whether researchers should be *required* to assure that post-trial treatment will be provided as a condition for approval of a trial. That issue concerns the ethics of *regulation*. Requiring researchers to provide post-trial treatment increases the cost of doing research and increasing costs may motivate researchers not to undertake the research or to conduct the research in a developed society. True, some research projects would be undertaken anyway and those research subjects may benefit from the requirement to provide post trial treatment such as antiretroviral therapies. But, at the margin, increasing the cost of research will deter at least *some* research from being undertaken at all, and, in still other cases, it is likely to cause sponsors to shift the location of research from LDCs to developed societies where participants have (public or private) insurance that would pay for such treatment. And so on the assumption that subjects benefit from participation *without* post-trial treatment, requiring the provision of post-trial treatment to subjects would make some potential subjects worse-off if such requirements have a diversion effect.

At least one group of prospective subjects made precisely this claim. In 1997, the rate of HIV infection in South Africa was extraordinarily high and ARTs were not provided by the South African public health services. Multinational drug companies wanted to conduct research in South Africa because of its combination of a "large infected population and proven medical expertise."[26] Research Ethics Committees (the equivalent of IRBs) in South Africa were considering whether to approve ART protocols for combinations of experimental drugs with approved drugs. The sponsors said that they would provide the "cocktail" free for two to three years, but without any guarantee that the treatment would be continued at the conclusion of the trial, in part because the continuation of treatment would require the sponsor to buy expensive drugs produced by other companies. One ethics committee maintained that "it is not ethical" to do such research unless post-trial treatment is assured and that it had the responsibility "to ensure that patients are not exploited."[27]

In response to these worries, AIDS activists argued that, *for them*, the trials "are seen as treatment rather than research—and are often the only way in which [they] have any access to treatment . . ." No therapeutic misconception here. From their perspective, "access to limited and potentially beneficial treatment is better than no treatment at all."[28] In effect, they appealed to NWC. If the researchers have no independent obligation to conduct the research and would not engage in the research if they were required to provide post-trial treatment, and if there are no important ethical objections to the design of the trial itself on grounds of safety or scientific validity, then it seems problematic for the REC to argue that *if* the researchers conduct a study in which participants benefit and to which they consent, then they must offer such treatment to the subjects.

Interestingly, and importantly, a close reading of the views of the Research Ethics Committee demonstrates considerable sympathy with that view. In response to the claim that "informed consent" by the participants would nullify the force of their concerns about exploitation, the committee granted that "in theory this is correct" but worried that too many participants were "insufficiently educated to understand the implications of what they are consenting to."[29] Similarly, Zong considers the argument that respect for the subject's autonomy implies that the subject should be able to consent to a protocol that does *not* guarantee post-trial treatment. He also avers that such consent is likely to be defective.

> . . . the informed consent procedure for trial participants from
> developing countries is significantly undermined by their
> inadequate understanding of the implications of what they are
> consenting to and the inability of many investigators to explain the
> trial effectively. Therefore, the informed consent procedure should
> not be taken as an excuse to deprive participants from developing
> countries of the right to access post-trial interventions.[30]

Here I would make four points. First, Zong assumes that subjects have a "right" to post-trial treatment and that claim must be defended. Second, even if we assume that subjects start with a right to post-trial treatment, it is simply not evident that researchers cannot or will not effectively explain the terms of participation or that participants do not or cannot understand those terms. Certainly, the AIDS activists thought that most HIV-positive subjects understood the benefits and limitations of participation. Third, if there were insurmountable deficiencies in consent, it is not clear why the same persons could give valid consent to participation *with* the guarantee of post-trial treatment, for there would no doubt still be issues that they do not understand. Fourth, even if the participants cannot reach a level of understanding necessary for morally transformative consent, there is still a problem in justifying preventing them from participating in research. For if participation without the guarantee of post-trial treatment is *beneficial* to the participants, one can hardly justify barring participation on soft-paternalist grounds in order to protect the subjects from harm.

Ancillary Care

Consider two cases introduced by Henry Richardson and Leah Belsky in their seminal article on ancillary care.

> *Schistosomiasis.* In the course of conducting research on malaria in Africa, investigators may find that some participants have schistosomiasis, a parasitic disease that is caused by drinking contaminated water. Although schistosomiasis has a low mortality rate, it is a serious and debilitating chronic illness that can cause liver and intestinal damage.
>
> *Ectopic Pregnancy.* In the course of research studying vaginal microbicides, researchers discovered an ectopic pregnancy in one of the participants, a condition that called for immediate surgery that was not available at the trial location.[31]

As with other issues we have examined, we can pose two questions here: (1) are investigators obligated to provide ancillary care in such cases? (2) Should a commitment to provide such care be a condition of approval of the research? Richardson and Belsky argue that the answer to (1) is a limited yes. Although they do not sharply distinguish between these questions, I think they would argue that the answer to (2) is a yes whenever the answer to (1) is a yes.

Richardson and Belsky argue for a "limited entrustment" model on which investigators have an obligation to provide ancillary care if it would not unduly strain the research effort.[32] As they define it, ancillary care refers to treatments that are "beyond what is necessary to implement a study's design safely and validly," and is also beyond any (contractual) treatments that investigators may offer in order to recruit and enroll a sufficient number of participants. Unlike other arguments in this territory, Richardson and Belsky's entrustment model is explicitly based on the view that obligations stem from the interaction between investigators and subjects.

To amplify the previous point, note that Richardson and Belsky explicitly set aside two strategies for supporting ancillary care obligations (ACOs). First, they do *not* appeal to a general duty to rescue those in need. Although they believe that moral agents do have a duty to help people in need "when one can provide the help without serious sacrifice or risk," a general duty to rescue would not distinguish the obligations of investigators to subjects from their obligations to non-subjects who are similarly proximate and needy.[33] Second, the entrustment model does *not* appeal to the medical care model that holds that investigators must treat their subjects as patients. Richardson and Belsky accept the view that research is a distinct and morally worthy enterprise, and so researcher/physicians (as contrasted with non-physician researchers) do not confront their subjects simply as patients. At the same time, Richardson and Belsky also explicitly reject the "researcher as pure scientist" or "contractual" model on which the investigators' obligations are limited to those to which they agreed.[34] They argue that the interaction between investigators and subjects generate ACOs *independent* of any agreement between them. Moreover, and crucially, they maintain that investigators cannot permissibly ask subjects to waive any claim they might have to ancillary care as a condition of their participation. On Richardson's and Belsky's view, the right to ancillary care is inalienable.

Richardson's and Belsky's use of the term "entrustment" may mislead. The entrustment relationship is moral, and not psychological. Under appropriate conditions, the investigator is morally entrusted with responsibilities toward his subjects even if he or the subject herself does not regard the investigator as having acquired those responsibilities. By soliciting permission to receive private information from vulnerable subjects, investigators become entrusted "with special responsibilities pertaining to the information thus gathered."[35] The entrustment responsibilities of investigators are triggered by obligations of compassion, engagement, and gratitude. I will focus here on the appeal to gratitude or reciprocity because reciprocity has played a prominent role in discussions of the obligations of investigators and sponsors to the subjects of research, and because it reflects the thought that researchers have these obligations precisely because they *benefit* from the interaction.

So what does reciprocity require? Despite frequent appeals to the notion of reciprocity in bioethics, there are precious few theoretical accounts on offer, a situation that reflects a similar vacuum in political and moral philosophy. More than a century ago, Henry Sidgwick complained that he could find "no clear accepted principle" by which to determine how much one party owes another and there has been precious little progress since then. In some contexts we may opt for a "pure procedural" account and let the market or contractual agreements dictate the answer.[36] We do not think that I should pay more than the market price for a good just because I expect to benefit more than other buyers or because I benefit more than the seller. In other contexts we may think of reciprocity as a case of "imperfect procedural" justice, where there is a (to be determined) independent criterion of what one party owes to each other. So we may think that A owes B more than $5.00 per hour in *Lawn Mowing* even if they agree on that wage.

Intuitions about reciprocity appear to reflect at least three factors: (1) the degree to which A benefits from the interaction with B; (2) the degree to which B has sacrificed or benefited from the interaction; (3) A's capacity to reciprocate. Sidgwick offers this example.

> [I]f a poor man [B] sees a rich one [A] drowning and pulls him out of the water, we do not think that the latter is bound to give as a reward what he would have been willing to give for his life. Still, we should think him niggardly if he only gave his preserver half-a-crown: which might, however, be profuse repayment for the cost of the exertion. Something between the two seems to suit our moral taste: but I find no clear accepted principle upon which the amount can be decided (1874, 234).[37]

This is a hard case. B's efforts have generated a massive benefit for A, and A has the capacity to offer a significant reward. These two factors would suggest that A should give B a hefty amount. If A had been poor, then the benefit to A (his life) might have been equivalently great but a smaller expression of gratitude would seem to be fair.

Of course, B's benefit or sacrifice also matters to what A owes B. In Sidgwick's case, B did not have to sacrifice much in order to generate this benefit, which would imply that reciprocity requires a less generous reward. And in the research contexts on which we have been focusing, we are assuming that participants do *not* sacrifice their interests, but actually benefit. Consider the following case.

> *Red Cross.* B and C come into the local blood donation center to give blood. B is self-employed. C's employer gives employees 2 hours off from work to give blood. C gives blood because he finds the process and time off less burdensome than his time at work.

Should A (The Red Cross representative) express less gratitude to C, who has benefitted from the process than to B, who has made a moderate sacrifice of time? Politeness may require that A treat both B and C the same, but it would not be surprising if, when A says "Thanks for coming in" to C, that C would respond, "No, you don't understand. Thank *You!* You gave me the opportunity to get off from work." If this is right, then the issue as to how much investigators owe to participants will depend on the extent to which (1) researchers benefit from a subject's participation and (2) how much the subject *already* benefits from participation.

If we focus on specific obligations of reciprocity, the contributions of participants to a research project raise an issue of moral arithmetic that is generally ignored. In Sidgwick's drowning case, A benefits directly from B's sacrifice. By contrast, each participant in research may be making but a small contribution—one data point—to the overall project. Suppose that A needs 10 people to pull on a rope to get his car out of a ditch and that rescuing his car is worth $10,000. Although the marginal value created by each puller is $10,000 (nine pullers can't get the job done), we are inclined to say that each generated the equivalent of $1,000 for A. So if we are trying to assess the contributions of an individual research participant to a large research project, we will need to make a comparable adjustment. Given all this, we cannot assume that obligations of reciprocity support the provision of ancillary care.

Even if we assume that investigators do acquire ACOs in the course of research, there is another issue that must be joined. If we assume as a default position that malaria researchers have an obligation to provide care for schistosomiasis and that microbicide researchers have an obligation to provide surgery for an ectopic pregnancy, the following question arises: Can researchers and subjects "contract around" such obligations, say, in the way that potential spouses can sign a pre-nuptial agreement that alters what would otherwise be their obligation with respect to the division of property if they were to divorce? Assuming that the researchers are not required to engage in the research in the first place, and assuming that they would prefer not to saddle themselves with additional ACOs that are not related to their research aims, can they justify asking prospective participants to waive claims on ancillary care as a condition of participation?

Richardson says no. On his view, ACOs are "non-waivable" or inalienable constraints on the obligations of researchers. He understands that subjects must be able to waive their rights to privacy, for otherwise research would be impossible. But they will not be adequately protected unless these waivers are "backed up by non-waivable, special duties of beneficence suited to mitigating the potential ill effects of this waiver."[38]

But why must these rights be non-waivable? As a general proposition, respect for an agent's autonomy entails that she has the ability to waive her rights, particularly if the ability to waive a right is necessary to obtain a good or achieve an aim or goal that is otherwise unattainable. One may have a right to freedom of speech, but one can sign a confidentiality agreement under which one agrees not to speak about certain matters in order to secure a job or a legal settlement.

Judith Thomson believes that no rights are intrinsically inalienable. Indeed and, *pace* Mill, she maintains that one has the right to sell oneself into slavery if one could give valid consent to do so. At the same time, and as a practical matter, she thinks it unlikely that anyone would actually voluntarily and knowingly consent to be enslaved, and so a "person who seems to be selling such a right is likely to be either not doing so freely or not doing so wittingly or both."[39] Thus, Thomson maintains that it may be best to *treat* some rights as inalienable on epistemological grounds even if, as a matter of fundamental principle, they are not inalienable.

It's not clear whether Richardson would regard (probable) defects in consent as the *only* reason to treat a right as inalienable, but he does argue we cannot assume that consent to waive a right to ancillary care would be sufficiently voluntary or informed because of the great inequality of bargaining power between investigators and subjects. Unfortunately, and despite frequent references to inequality of bargaining power, it is not clear just how such inequalities compromise the voluntariness or the validity of consent, worrisome though they sometimes may be.[40]

> *House Sale.* B has taken a job in another city and must sell her house before she goes. If B had ample time, she would probably receive $300,000 for the house. A is aware of B's predicament and offers $250,000. B accepts

Although A has B "over a barrel," it does seem as if B's agreement is valid. She could hardly seek to undo the contract (should a better offer come along) on the grounds that the inequality in bargaining power rendered her agreement involuntary.

There are other cases in which Richardson's claim seems more plausible.

> *Gynecologist.* A gynecologist requires patients to waive their right to sue and to accept binding arbitration to settle any potential disputes or she will not treat them. Nearly all gynecologists in the area have a similar policy.

Although no individual gynecologist has sufficient bargaining power to compromise the voluntariness of the waiver, the gynecology "cartel" might be able to do so. Under such conditions, what I called the *strategic argument* for interfering with mutually advantageous transactions might justify treating a woman's right to sue as inalienable if doing so would strengthen the hand of the individual patient.[41] Similarly, it might strengthen the hand of prospective subjects if we treat any waivers of claims on ancillary care as having no moral force. Here as well, the force of the strategic argument turns on empirical considerations: does treating the right as inalienable renders prospective subjects better off?

Richardson also suggests that the inequalities between investigators and subjects create an informational asymmetry that compromises consent. The investigators understand the care that the prospective subjects might need, but prospective subjects do not: "How can we possibly suppose that [subjects] would have any grasp on what they would be giving away if they waived rights to care that they might, in the course of the research be found to need?"[42] Richardson is concerned that prospective subjects are inclined to act myopically and that they will make a decision at Time-1 that they will reasonably regret at Time-2. Suppose, for example, that malaria researchers were to say that they will enroll subjects in a trial from which they can expect to benefit only if they waive their right to ancillary care.

> For many in rural Africa, this would be a good bargain. Note, however, that a divergence arises between the *ex ante* and the *ex post* perspectives. *Knowing* that he or she has malaria or schistosomiasis . . . the individual might come to see things differently, such that, from that later perspective, the initial choice would not be reckoned a reasonable or rational one.[43]

Richardson's worries may prove too much. After all, if subjects do not have the information to grasp what participation involves, then they cannot give valid consent to participate in research *independent* of any worries about ancillary care. Moreover, we might be able to correct for these sorts of informational deficiencies. If waivers were *otherwise* permissible, IRBs could require a process in which subjects are explicitly told that they would be waiving any claim on medical care that they might be found to need and even tested to ensure that they understand. It might still be wrong to approve such an agreement, but not on grounds of an informational deficiency or the validity of consent.

Upon analysis, I think Richardson is less concerned with the asymmetry of information than with "decisional myopia," that is, a person's tendency to discount the long-term costs of their decision.[44] Richardson is concerned that a subject would make a decision at Time-1 that does not serve her interest at Time-2 and beyond. Here, we must be careful. It certainly does *not* follow that just because one regrets a Time-1 decision at Time-2 that the Time-1 decision should be viewed as unreasonable or irrational or without moral force. It might be perfectly reasonable for a healthy 20-year-old to choose a medical insurance policy with a high deductible at Time-1 even though, at Time-2, she is saddled with medical expenses and reasonably regrets her Time-1 choice. Second, it is not at all clear that a subject who requires ancillary care, at Time-2, should regret her Time-1 decision to waive a right to ancillary care. If a prospective subject were not likely to receive treatment for diseases discovered during research but would otherwise benefit from participation, it is not unreasonable for the subject to accept what is offered. Indeed, Richardson concedes as much when he says that waiving a right to ancillary care in order to gain a spot as a participant might be a "good bargain." To be clear, I do not claim to have shown that investigators should be permitted to ask prospective subjects to waive a right to ancillary care if they have such a right. The strategic argument may justify treating the right as inalienable. But it is difficult to sustain the view that a right to ancillary care is inalienable on the grounds that a subject could not give valid consent to waiving such a right.

This is not just a hypothetical or philosophical matter. It may be in the interests of many prospective subjects that they be able to waive claims on ancillary care. If researchers have a reciprocity-based obligation to provide ancillary care to those who are research subjects that cannot be waived, then researchers have a strong incentive to exclude prospective subjects who are likely to require ancillary care. Consider a trial of malaria treatments where participants are screened for malaria and HIV. If malaria researchers have reciprocity-based ACOs to provide ARTs to *participants* who are HIV-positive but not to non-participants, they could easily exclude HIV-positive persons from the study even though all prospective subjects can expect to benefit from participation in the malaria study and even if there is no scientific need to exclude HIV-positive persons. Now it is not clear what Richardson's and Belsky's limited entrustment model requires with respect to potential participants that are screened but excluded. But given their view that the strength of the investigator's entrustment responsibilities is a function of the risks that subjects are asked to bear and the overall intensity of the interaction, it would seem that investigators cannot owe much to those who are excluded from a trial.

If investigators have few ACOs to prospective subjects that are excluded, then insisting that investigators have non-waivable ACOs gives them a strong incentive to control their costs by excluding those who are likely to need substantial ancillary care. Once again, NWC rears its head. If it is not wrong to exclude a prospective subject and provide no additional care to her, it seems odd to claim that it is wrong to include that prospective subject and provide no ancillary care if inclusion in research is otherwise beneficial.

The case for ACOs also raises questions for GOC similar to those that we discussed in the context of post-trial treatment. Richardson and Belsky argue that the strength of the investigator's ACO is a function of the degree to which the provision of ancillary care will divert human and financial resources from the research effort. And so they argue that if the ability to carry out a malaria study would not be compromised if researchers were to treat the 10% of children infected with schistosomiasis, then they probably ought to be treated. If provision of ancillary care were to require a great deal more, then the limits entailed by the limited entrustment model may come into play.

Of course, even when those limits are not reached and even where investigators can use modest resources to provide ancillary care to research subjects, there is a question as to whether they should do more for research subjects that are already benefiting from their project than for others who are not benefiting. Suppose, given limited resources, that investigators face a choice between a reasonably solid malaria study with N subjects who are provided with ancillary care for schistosomiasis and a more statistically reliable study with N+ subjects who are provided with no ancillary care. Suppose as well that the expected benefits to other and future persons from a more reliable study (with N+ subjects) outweigh the expected benefits of providing ancillary care to the N participants. Richardson seems to prefer the smaller study. He argues that "refusing to aid" to subjects who need ancillary care is morally worse than omitting to provide comparable treatment or benefits to non-subjects.[45] As a matter of moral phenomenology, it is surely more difficult to say "no" to those with whom one has established a relationship than not to establish such a relationship in the first place. The question—which I will consider in more detail below—is to what extent this intuition can be defended.

Fair Benefits

It is often said that researchers have post-trial obligations to the host community. The core idea is that whereas researchers have no independent obligation to conduct research in an LDC, they acquire an obligation to provide benefits to the host community if they conduct research. An early and still popular version of this was to insist on "reasonable availability." On this view, research is ethical and, perhaps, should be permitted only if the therapy under investigation were made reasonably available in the host community if the trial proves successful. Although that principle still has its supporters, others have argued that it should be replaced by a "fair benefits" principle.[46] Its proponents argue that while "targeted populations in developing countries ought to benefit when clinical research is performed in their community," the researchers and the community should have the flexibility to negotiate a different package of benefits so long as that overall package is fair.

The fair benefits approach has important advantages. Some research (e.g., pathophysiology) does not involve the study of an intervention, and so "reasonable availability" would not require that the researchers provide any benefits to the community post-trial. Even when a trial involves the study of a potentially efficacious intervention, "reasonable availability" would offer nothing to the community if the trial is not successful. In addition, the community may sensibly prefer a different package of benefits that generates more health care bang for the buck. For present purposes, however, the differences between "reasonable availability" and "fair benefits" are mostly irrelevant. The crucial point is that *both* approaches maintain that researchers owe *some* benefits to the host communities, and that is the view I want to examine. So for convenience sake, I will regard the "fair benefits" approach as the target of the analysis.

At its core, the fair benefits approach appears to rest on a variation of IP. Because investigators interact with the community as well as with the subjects, reciprocity demands that investigators provide benefits to the community as well. But unlike the previous cases in which we asked whether the fact of interactions between investigators and subjects generate obligations of reciprocity, here we have to ask whether there is a fact of interaction between investigators and the community that *could* give rise to obligations of reciprocity.

To say that "impoverished populations . . . are being used as research subjects" is ambiguous as between two claims: (1) researchers use impoverished subjects drawn from an impoverished population; (2) researchers use the *impoverished population* from which the subjects are drawn.⁴⁷ But what does (2) mean? Certainly the mere fact that research subjects are *from* a nation or community (1) does not mean that the researchers interact *with* or use a population (2) in a way that could generate obligations to the community. To see this, consider *Fly In*.

> *Fly In*. NIH is studying a treatment for a disease which is found predominantly in Nation N. It can do a higher quality study if it flies subjects from N to an academic medical center in the United States. The study pays all expenses for the subjects and one member of each subject's family.

Although the subjects are drawn *from* the population of N, the study is not performed *in* N, and it does not seem as if the "impoverished *population*" of N is being "used as research subjects." The subjects themselves are used— even if they benefit. But the wider population of the community is not used at all. I suggest, then, that research typically does not "use" the population from which research subjects are drawn in a way that *could* give rise to obligations of reciprocity unless the project has adverse effects on the community. Researchers may have obligations to provide benefits to the community for other reasons, but such obligations would not be obligations of reciprocity.

If we assume that the conduct of research has effects on the non-participant members of the community in which it takes place, we can ask two questions: (1) does the conduct of research have adverse (or insufficiently positive?) effects? (2) If so, does generating such adverse effects obligate the researchers to provide benefits to the community? Let us take these in reverse order. If an interaction between A and B has harmful effects on other members of the community, then it is arguable that they are owed compensation. But this is not always so. We sometimes think that the negative externalities of consensual and mutually advantageous transactions should lie where they fall. For example, if A hires B away from C (her previous employer), we do *not* generally think that A needs to compensate C. If Borders opens a store and its interactions with customers drive a local bookshop into bankruptcy, we do not think that Borders must compensate the local bookshop owner. We could not have a well functioning market if actors were required to compensate in such cases. In other contexts, however, we take a different view. If A, an electricity company in Ohio, sells power to

Ohioans but pollutes the air of people in New Hampshire, we may require the company to compensate its victims. Consider a less direct externality. American hospitals recruit nurses from the Philippines. Given that these mutually beneficial and consensual interactions between the *parties* reduce the number of nurses available in the Philippines, it is plausible to maintain that the American employer or the United States government should somehow attempt to mitigate such harmful effects on Filipinos. Similarly, it is plausible (although not self-evident) to claim that researchers have obligations to mitigate for any adverse effects on the community that result from their research.

And that brings us back to the first question. The argument that researchers are obligated to provide "fair benefits" to the community assumes that the community has been *burdened* by the research. That may not be true. If the research effort brings resources to the community that generate net benefits, it is hard to see why reciprocity demands that researchers provide benefits to the community above and beyond what it is already doing. Consider *Movie*.

> *Movie*. A movie company makes a film in a small Vermont town. It hires some local residents as "extras" for some scenes. It also uses local hotels, restaurants, caterers, construction workers, and drivers.

A movie production will typically generate both negative and positive externalities. Rooms in hotels will be harder to find. The police department may have to provide extra security. The community may experience its first traffic jam. Nonetheless, cities often compete for the privilege of being used for movie productions because of the infusion of demand for goods and employees. Such cities indicate that they do not think that they are due additional compensation beyond the benefits they derived from being "used."

So when it is said that the results of a clinical trial or other benefits should be made available "to study participants and *other inhabitants of a host country*," it is not clear on what basis the "other inhabitants" have a claim on the benefits generated by the contributions of their compatriots. Indeed, it is arguable that the provision of benefits to members of the community who have not put themselves at risk allows them to free ride on the participation of those who did serve as research subjects.

We might understand the "fair benefits" principle as a version of a morally justified hold-up (Robin Hood) operation. On this view, impoverished societies (or their advocates) attempt to extract resources from the affluent societies and thereby move the world towards reducing injustice and inequality. In effect, the fair benefits principle holds the prospective research *subjects* as hostages and demands a price or side-payment for letting them go. All things considered, this may be justifiable, particularly if investigators or sponsors are likely to pay the price. But this argument has nothing to do with reciprocity.

In this connection, although it certainly could be argued that all of us affluent *people* should do more to promote a more just distribution of health care resources in the world, we return to the concern raised above: why should that burden be placed on researchers or their sponsors? Suppose we believe that Americans who work full time should have enough money to live adequately.[48] On one model, the burden of providing a livable wage should rest on the employer, even if the value of the employee's labor is less than the cost of providing a livable wage, in which case the person probably won't be hired. On another model, each employer is allowed to pay a market wage, but the society should supplement the wage (through a policy such as the Earned Income Tax Credit) to bring the employee's net income up to the requisite level. On that view, the goal of providing workers with an adequate income is shared by the entire society and is not the sole responsibility of the employers. If something like the second model is preferable, as I believe, there is no reason to place the burden of promoting a more just distribution of health care resources on clinical researchers.

The Interaction Principle Reconsidered

In the previous section, I suggested that a commitment to IP underlies some of the common wisdom of research ethics. I also suggested we have some reason to be skeptical about the merits of two corollaries of IP: the rejection of NWC and the endorsement of GOC. Despite the concerns that I have raised, it is entirely possible that (some version of) IP is basically correct. To properly evaluate the viability of these principles of ethical research, we need to consider IP at a more theoretical level.

Even if IP or its corollaries is defensible with respect to *some* interactions, there is no reason to suppose that *every* mutually beneficial interaction gives rise to super-contractual obligations. There must be considerable space in our lives for parties to reach agreement on whatever terms they please (perhaps within broad limits) and without being morally required to do more than fulfill the terms of the agreement. But some interactions may strike us as different, depending on the duration and intensity of the interaction, the level of benefits the parties have received, the relative position of the parties, and the surplus available for providing additional benefits. Consider these cases.

> *Sweatshop.* A employs B for wages that are above average in B's LDC, but low by American standards. A makes a reasonable but not super-competitive profit on the goods that B helps to produce.
>
> *Teller.* A, a bank customer, transacts with B, a bank teller, thereby benefiting from her services. Although B is better off working as a bank teller than being unemployed, B's salary does not provide for a decent living.
>
> *Housekeeper.* A employs B as a full-time housekeeper for a minimum wage. B does not earn enough to live adequately. B has no other job opportunities and would be worse off if she were not employed by A.
>
> *Surgery.* B performs life-saving surgery on A for a normal fee.

I suspect that intuitions will vary with respect to these cases (not to mention that different individuals will have different intuitions about the same case). If interactions can generate special obligations, the duration and intensity of the interaction in *Sweatshop* may generate a special obligation although the price competition among employers may be such that A may not be able to pay B a higher wage. Although I believe that the interaction in *Teller* is so low on duration and depth as not to raise moral worries, Ruth Sample suggests that A exploits or wrongfully uses B because A effectively "tolerates" B's inadequate wages while benefitting from her interaction.[49]

Surgery raises an important and neglected issue. If we view *Surgery* as a case in which the *patient* employs the surgeon (rather than one in which the surgeon performs surgery on the patient), few would say that patient B owes surgeon A more than a normal fee out of gratitude or reciprocity even though this is a high intensity (short duration) interaction from which B has benefited much more than A. Here the contractual model seems at home. But why? Perhaps it is because we calculate B's gain not by comparison with the no surgery baseline but by comparison with B's having the surgery performed by *someone else*, in which case B's *marginal* gain from having the surgery performed by A is not all that great and so the normal fee applies. But why is the normal fee so low given the relative gains? Perhaps it is because we assume that A is already well off and our moral evaluation of the transaction takes place against this background. Perhaps it is because A's professional actions *typically* generate much greater utility for his patients than he obtains from his fee.

Of these four examples, I believe that the intensity and proximity of the interaction in *Housekeeper* represents the case in which IP has the most force and is also most analogous to the interaction between researcher and subject. Suppose that A has two applicants for the job: B and C. A judges them to be equally qualified, so she flips a coin, and B wins the lottery. Suppose as well that, in principle, A has four options: (1) not hire B (or C) and do the housework herself; (2) hire B for the minimum wage of $200 per week, which is not sufficient to provide for B's needs; (3) pay B $240 per week, which is sufficient to provide for B's needs; (4) pay $200 per week to B and give $40 per week to C, who is worse off than B and who would gladly have taken B's job if it had been offered to her. I have said that IP rejects NWC and supports GOC. NWC concerns the comparison of (1) and (2); GOC concerns the comparison of (3) and (4). Using *Housekeeper* as our framework, let us consider both.

Table 6.1

Option	B	C
1	$0	$0
2	$200	$0
3	$240	$0
4	$200	$40

NWC

NWC maintains that it cannot be worse for A to offer (2) than (1) because it is Pareto superior to (1) if we bracket effects on third parties. To think otherwise is to violate a principle that Christopher Boorse refers to as the "moral montonocity" of benefit. That principle maintains that "as to effects on one person only, it must be morally superior to benefit that person more rather than less" to which I would add as a friendly amendment—if that person consents to the interaction.[50] By contrast, those who endorse IP claim that it could be worse for A to employ B but not provide adequately for her needs

(2) than for A not to employ B at all (1) even though B benefits from such employment and consents to its terms.

When I reflect on the *principles* involved in *Housekeeper*, I find myself believing that (2) cannot be morally worse than (1) if it's better for B and if B consents to it. And thus it would seem that if A does nothing wrong in (1), then A is not acting wrongly in (2). By contrast, when I reflect on the case itself, I feel that A's action in (2) is (or might be) worse than (1) or, to put it somewhat differently, (2) might be wrong even though (1) is not wrong. It seems that a *package deal* that contains a wrongful element is not necessarily morally preferable to no deal or that it may be wrong for A to carry out the terms of part of the package even though A has no obligation to offer any package at all, even though B is better off accepting the package and even though B consents to accept the package. The question is whether that view can be defended.

Deontological Objections to NWC

It might be thought that NWC is a consequentialist principle and that it is therefore open to the standard deontological objections to consequentialism. Not quite. NWC is consequentialist in the minimal sense that it maintains that if the consequences of A's choosing (2) are Pareto superior to A's choosing (1), then it cannot be morally worse for A to choose (2) than (1) if B consents to (2). But NWC makes *no* appeal to the aggregate consequences of A's choice. NWC does *not* say that it is permissible to harm B or use B without B's consent if doing so has better *aggregate* consequences for others. NWC does not allow us to kill one person to redistribute her organs to save five others or push the fat man off the bridge in order to stop the trolley from killing five others.

There may be other sorts of deontological wrongs that can occur only when there is an interaction between A and B. Consider Derek Parfit's case in which A could choose between:

(1) not helping B at all
(2) saving 1 arm of B at some risk to A
(3) saving both arms of B at no additional risk to A.[51]

Parfit argues that if (1) and (2) were the only options, it would not be wrong for A to choose (1) and that it would be supererogatory for A to choose (2).

But, as Parfit also argues, if (3) were a viable option, it would be *perverse* for A to choose (2). Does this mean that (2) is both supererogatory *and* perverse or does it mean that (2) is now *wrong*? To say that it would be "perverse" for A to choose (2) over (3) might be to make a claim about A's psychology— why would anyone who is prepared to choose (2) over (1) also choose (2) over (3)? It seems *crazy*. But on the assumption that perversity constitutes a moral objection to (2), there is at least *a* moral reason to criticize (2) in the presence of (3) that does not apply to (1). Even so, it would not follow that (2) is morally worse than (1) in the presence of (3). For the way in which (2) is better than (1) may always outweigh the force of any moral criticism of (2).

Indeed, it might be argued that to think that (2) *could* be worse than (1) in the presence of (3) but would *not* be worse than (1) if (3) were not a viable option would be to violate a basic axiom of decision theory—"the independence of irrelevant alternatives." Under one common formulation, the axiom states that: "If (2) is preferred to (1) out of the choice set {(1),(2)}, then introducing a third alternative (3), thus expanding the choice set to {(1), (2), (3)}, must not make (1) preferred to (2)."[52] If we assume that it is *not wrong* for A to choose (1) and if we assume that (2) is *not worse* than (1), could it nonetheless be *wrong*—not just crazy—for A to perversely choose (2) in the presence of (3)? Could it be wrong to perform an act that yields a state of affairs that is morally better or, more accurately, is part of a package deal that is morally better?

I will return to these questions below, but first note that Parfit's example captures the *structure* of claims that are sometimes made about exploitation, unfairness, or the wrongful use of persons. If A does not hire B in *Housekeeper* (1), there is simply no question as to the fairness of B's compensation or whether A exploits B or wrongfully uses B. So if it is wrong to treat people unfairly or to exploit them, there is a moral reason to criticize (2) that does not and could not occur in (1). And it might be argued that the unfairness in (2) renders it worse than (1) which is not unfair.

I do not think that the wrongness of unfairness works this way. Even if the package deal in (2) is unfair, it is a better state of affairs than (1) when evaluated by *the reasons that we care about fairness*. Setting aside retributive justice, where fairness may require that we impose a deprivation, we should treat people fairly because doing so is better for those persons than treating them unfairly and not because we are trying to promote some abstract ideal.

Of course, people may reject deals that they believe to be unfair even though they expect to be better off if they accept them. As G.A. Cohen observes:

> It is not necessarily irrational (and it is sometimes felt to be morally imperative) to refuse to deal with a person who wields power in an untoward way even if, should you accede to the proposal he makes, you would be materially better off. That is not necessarily irrational both because how well off you are is not a matter of your material situation alone, and because how well off you are is not the only matter it is rational for you to care about.[53]

I agree. But if B decides to reject A's proposal because it is unfair, there will be no interaction between A and B and thus there will be no issue as to whether such an interaction is worse than no interaction. The question is what to say if B accepts A's proposal.

Somewhat paradoxically, the disposition to reject unfair but beneficial proposals may work to the long-run advantage of those who would otherwise benefit from such proposals. Consider the "ultimatum games" developed by behavioral economists.[54] In one version of these games, A is given, say, $20 and told to allocate that sum between A and (an anonymous) B. If B accepts A's proposal, each receives what A proposes; if B rejects A's proposal, both A and B receive nothing. Now if A and B are not anonymous or if these are repeat games, there are numerous reasons why A should be inclined—for self-interested reasons—to make a decent offer and B should be inclined to reject unfair proposals. But if A and B are playing an anonymous "one-off" game and so neither has the opportunity to garner any reputational advantage or influence each other's future behavior, it would seem that a self-interested A should propose, say, $19 for A and $1 for B, since it would be irrational for B to refuse A's proposal ($1 is better than $0) and A should know this. But the studies suggest that even under such conditions, B will, in fact, often refuse proposals that she regards as unfair (at least when large amounts are not at stake) for moral or emotional reasons ("I'm not going to let you treat me this way") and, because A predicts that B may reject such proposals, A makes a more equal proposal in the first place. Here the moral and the prudential are intertwined. The predictable psychological disposition to reject what is in one's interest on grounds of fairness tends to serves one's interest.

It's not clear what to draw from this. B will not consent to an unfair interaction if B prefers non-interaction to a beneficial unfair interaction. But it hardly follows that it is worse for A to treat B unfairly than not to interact with B if B *agrees* to the interaction. Recall *Housekeeper*. It may be sensible for B to try to convince A that she will reject (2) if that will move A to choose (3), but it doesn't follow that NWC *is* false about the comparison between (1) and (2) or that B believes that it is.

Still, it is arguable that NWC should be rejected on a different type of deontological view. Ruth Sample argues that "exploitation involves interacting with another being for the sake of advantage in a way that degrades or fails to respect the inherent value in that being."[55] And, she suggests, because her account of exploitation is non-consequentialist, "it explains why we often regard exploitation as worse than neglect, even when the consequences of neglect are worse [for the exploited]."[56]

This won't do. First, we can't simply help ourselves to this quasi-Kantian principle as if the principle itself were uncontroversial. After all, it would seem that we are sometimes justified in treating others merely as means or in a way that fails to respect that person's inherent value or even violates her rights. As Amartya Sen has argued, if A could prevent a serious harm to C only by taking B's car without B's consent, say by driving to the scene of the crime, A may be justifiably treating B (or B's property) merely as a means and failing to respect B's choices in the matter.[57] Second, it is not clear if and when a mutually advantageous consensual transaction is actually vulnerable to the Kantian deontological charge that the exploiter fails to respect the "inherent value" of the exploitee if *the exploiter regards the exploitee's valid consent as a necessary condition of interaction.*

Even valid or robust consent may not remove the deontological sting from such transactions. If so, it is not clear what is necessary to remove that sting. It may be thought that to respect others or to treat others as ends in themselves requires us to adopt a certain attitude towards others or to treat others with compassion, kindness, and benevolence. Not so. As Barbara Herman has argued, treating another as a person "is not a matter of attitude or feeling. Regarding you as a person is accepting a set of constraints on my actions."[58] As Kant himself argues, we treat wrongdoers as ends in themselves when they are given the punishment they deserve—and that includes their death if they have committed murder—although he would argue (and others would deny) that such punishment is compatible with respecting their inherent value.

Showing genuine respect for another may involve taking steps to meet the basic needs of other persons—the needs that must be met in order for them to function as agents. But it is not clear whether that duty should fall disproportionately on those who interact with such persons or falls more generally on all those in a position to provide for those needs. For the sticking point is this: *if it is permissible on Kantian grounds for A not to interact with B, does A violate the relevant Kantian maxim if A interacts with B to B's benefit and with B's consent?*

Actually, that's not quite right. The present question is not whether mutually advantageous and consensual interactions can fail to respect the inherent value in another person but whether they can do so in ways that are *worse than neglect* or non-interaction given the possibility of mutually advantageous and consensual interaction. It is true that A can't treat B "merely as a means" by neglecting B, but that does not resolve the question as to whether neglect might fail to show appropriate respect. A can treat B as a mere "thing" or "object" by not interacting with B and then the question is whether treating B as a "means" is worse than treating B as a "thing." Moreover, even if our intuitive commitment to non-consequentialist principles can "explain *why we often regard* exploitation as worse than neglect" as a matter of descriptive psychology, this does not show that mutually advantageous consensual and exploitative interactions *are* worse than neglect.

If we assume, *arguendo*, that Sample is right to claim that people generally regard exploitation as worse than neglect, that fact would hardly resolve the moral question. If, as I suspect, the word "exploitation" is generally associated with the thought that the interaction is harmful or nonconsensual, then the tendency to "often regard" exploitation as worse than neglect may not reflect the moral reality when the exploitation at issue is mutually advantageous and consensual. Our intuitions may involve an unacknowledged "transfer" of intuitions associated with harmful nonconsensual exploitation to mutually advantageous consensual transactions that are correctly regarded as exploitative. Second, the wrongful elements of interactions (such as unfairness) may simply be more salient than the badness of non-interactions. As Sample observes, "it is easier to lose sight of the value of other valuable beings when we do not interact with them."[59] This may be so, but the fact that one is more likely to "lose sight" of the value of others when we do not interact with them does not show that not interacting with them respects their value more than an exploitative interaction. "Out of sight, out of mind" may be a psychological fact (more so than "absence makes the heart grow fonder") but it is not a moral argument.

There are several additional reasons for thinking that an appeal to deontology won't justify rejecting NWC. Sample thinks that a maxim that would permit A to engage in a mutually beneficial transaction with B that ignores B's basic needs (as in *Housekeeper*) would not pass the test of Kant's categorical imperative.[60] Determining what passes that test is notoriously difficult, but even if Sample is right, it hardly follows that a maxim of permissible *non-interaction* that ignores the other party's basic needs would pass that test and Sample does not claim that it would.

More generally, appeals to deontology seem somewhat out of place with respect to the morality of mutually beneficial consensual interaction. Deontological principles are normally advanced as *side-constraints* on agents that serve to protect the targets of actions against *harms* or *rights violations* that could otherwise be justified on consequentialist grounds. We can't kill one person to redistribute her organs to save five others. But such constraints have no bearing on the case at hand, which concerns an interaction from which the target benefits and to which she consents. It might be objected that fairness is also a moral constraint. But we do not observe the constraint of fairness for the sake of the constraint. We observe it for the *person's* sake. Indeed, it is arguable that to observe or enforce a constraint—"don't allow others to act unfairly"—for the sake of the constraint itself "would arguably fail to treat the person as an end in himself" and so violate the deontologist's most fundamental commitment.[61]

It might be argued that it is morally impermissible for a person to treat *herself* in ways that are incompatible with appropriate self-respect. In *Housekeeper,* it may be argued that B does not demonstrate appropriate respect for herself if she allows herself to be exploited. Similarly, it may be thought that research subjects do not show sufficient self-respect if they allow themselves to be wrongfully used even if it is in their non-moral interests to do so.

I am not sure how to assess the force of this strategy. Although Kant thought that suicide fails to show respect for the value of a human life, others think that a life has value only if "the person whose life it is has reason to go on living or wants to live."[62] Similarly, although some might think that B is showing disrespect for herself if she agrees to work for inadequate pay, B might well think that providing for her family is a central value in her life. But even if this self-respect strategy suggests that Pareto-superior consensual transactions can be morally worse than non-interaction, I know of *no* defense of the principles of research ethics that appeals to this line of argument and so I set it aside.

Kamm's Disturbed Visitor

Frances Kamm also seems to rejects NWC.[63]

> *The Disturbed Visitor.* Suppose I wish to avoid helping someone
> with his severe emotional problems, and so arrange
> (permissibly) to leave town when he comes to visit. He will be
> totally lost in all respects in my absence, and I will be
> inconvenienced by leaving. It is in both our interests to agree
> to my staying in town to provide him with travel directions but
> also agree to my being relieved of the obligation to help him
> with his other problems—my being relieved, that is, of the
> ordinary obligation that anyone has to help someone nearby
> with severe problems. If I stay, and I alone am present when
> he is in trouble, does the agreement make it all right for me to
> ignore his plight? I think not. The situation and the obligation
> it would ordinarily give rise to dominate any agreement.

On Kamm's story, A has three options.

1. Leave town in order to avoid helping B with his emotional
   problems.
2. Remain in town and help B with his emotional problems.
3. Remain in town and reach an agreement with B such that A will
   provide B with directional help but will not help B with his
   emotional problems.

With respect to these options, Kamm takes the following position.

1'. It is permissible for A to choose (1).
2'. If A remains in town, A has an obligation to choose (2).
3'. It is impermissible for A to choose (3).

Now assuming that Kamm is right about (2'), it is not clear why she thinks
that it *is permissible* for A to leave town (1'). Kamm *asserts* (parenthetically)
that it is permissible for A to leave, but she does not *argue* for that claim and
most persons with whom I have discussed this case do not share her intuitions about the compatibility of (1') and (2'); they think that *if* one has an
obligation to help the visitor with his emotional problems if one is in town
(2'), then it is not permissible to leave town in order to avoid having to help
B with his emotional problems (1').

But let us assume that Kamm is right about (1'). Kamm maintains that a Pareto superior agreement (to help only with travel directions) such as (3) is morally unacceptable: "This is a case in which morality stands in the way of individuals' maximizing the promotion of their individual material interests." I'm not sure why Kamm uses the modifier "material" here, but how does Kamm propose to justify (3)? She suggests that it is "possible" that the agreement would fail to value certain sorts of relations between people— a value that is not compromised if A leaves, as in (1), but is compromised in (3). And it is also "possible," she says, that a "person's choice cannot override his nature or the nature of a situation, and those 'natures' may demand certain behavior." I agree that this is *"possible"* and that the situations "may" demand certain behavior, but I don't see here any argument for that view.

Kamm's set of claims ((1'), (2'), and (3')) about *The Disturbed Visitor* could be explained by the principle that one should not cause others unnecessary distress. By proposing (3), A conveys a lack of concern for B by proposing (3) that is not conveyed by (1). After all, assuming that B does not know why A has left town in (1), A's decision does not *convey* a lack of concern (even if it *reflects* a lack of concern) and does not cause any additional distress beyond the distress that B will experience because A is not able to help B with his emotional problems. On this view, it's not that (2') is true because A *is* in town, but because B *knows* that A is in town and would be distressed by A's refusal to help. And thus whereas (3) *appears* to be Pareto-superior to (1), the consequences of (3) for B may actually be worse than the consequences of (1) once we take account of its psychological effects and so would not be a counter-example to NWC. This is, no doubt, a more consequentialist and less intricate defense of (3') than Kamm would favor, but it is compatible with the intuitions to which she appeals.

Given all this, I do not think that Kamm's analysis of *The Disturbed Visitor* gives us much reason to reject NWC or the "contracting around" alternative in those cases where one clearly has no obligation to be in a position to render aid (as when researchers have no obligation to conduct research in the first place) and where "contracting around" what might otherwise appear to be one's obligations does *not* cause *additional* harm. Given the shakiness of the intuition that Kamm's "possible" principles are meant to support, *The Disturbed Visitor* does not give us reason to think that *if* it *would* be permissible for one to avoid one's obligation by not appearing on the scene, that it is worse or would *then* be impermissible to agree to do more than one was originally obligated to do if the agreement were truly Pareto-superior and consensual.

It is useful to consider Kamm's strategy in light of the distinction between an *agent-focused* moral theory and what philosophers call a *patient-focused* moral theory ("patient" refers to the persons affected by one's actions—not medical patients). Roughly stated, an agent-focused view claims that A may have moral reasons for action that are independent of the effects of his actions on others. A patient-focused view claims that A's reasons for action are dependent upon their effects on others "who endure and are acted upon."[64] Kamm's take on *The Disturbed Visitor* is fundamentally *agent-focused*. The question is not whether the disturbed visitor (patient) might have reason to reject A's proposal, but whether A's proposal violates some agent-focused principle of morality independent of its effect on the patient.

Yet Kamm is patient-focused when it comes to harm. In defending the "principle of secondary permissibility," she maintains that if A is allowed to cause harm to B and is physically able to do so, then it is morally permissible for A to substitute a lesser harm that would otherwise be prohibited. She asks us to assume that it is normally *im*permissible to push an innocent bystander (B) in front of a trolley that will crush his leg in order to save five other people from the trolley's killing them (I'm less sure about this). If, however, the alternative is to redirect the trolley away from the five and toward B, thereby killing him, and if redirecting the trolley *is* permissible, then, according to the principle of secondary permissibility, it becomes permissible to push B in front of the trolley, thereby crushing his leg.[65] Why? Because it is in B's interest to be pushed in front of the trolley rather than have the trolley redirected, thereby killing him. If Kamm adopts a patient-focused point of view in the context of "lesser harm," it would seem that she ought to adopt a patient-focus with respect to "greater good." If it is permissible for A not to interact with B, thereby providing no benefits to B, it should become permissible to perform an act—thereby providing some benefit—that would otherwise be wrong. Why? Because it is in the interest of B for A to do so. Getting half a loaf rather than none is the functional equivalent of having one's leg crushed rather than losing one's life.

Contractualism

As I suggested in Chapter 3, contractualism is probably the most important contemporary version of deontological theory. We can distinguish contractualism from contractarianism. Contractarianism, which has its roots in Hobbes, argues that morality is based on mutual self-interest. Contractualism, which is based on a commitment to the equal worth of persons, claims that morality is based on the principles to which parties would agree in a suitably defined choice situation. Contractualism reflects a commitment to impartiality, but that commitment can be realized in different ways. Rawlsian contractualism claims that the principles of justice are those to which people would agree from behind the "veil of ignorance." Although Rawlsian decision-makers are self-interested, the veil of ignorance assures that their choices reflect impartiality (just as the "you cut, I'll choose" procedure for dividing a cake assures that self-interested cake-cutters will try to cut equal size pieces). T.M. Scanlon's version of contractualism maintains that "An act is wrong if its performance under the circumstances would be disallowed by any set of principles for the general regulation of behavior that no one could reasonably reject as a basic for informed, unforced general agreement."[66] Unlike Rawlsian contractualism, agents know who they are. Morality emerges not from ignorance, but from each person's moral motivation to justify herself to everyone else and to the conditions for acceptance of such principles.[67] Moreover, unlike Rawlsian contractualism, which is limited to establishing the principles of justice for the basic structure of society, Scanlon's contractualism seeks to identify general principles of morality and is thus closer to the heart of the relationship between investigators and subjects.

Let us consider whether it provides a perspective from which to reject NWC. One might adopt a "complaint model" in attempting to determine those principles that could not reasonably be rejected.

> On this view, an individual's complaint against a proposed
> principle is the extent to which she would suffer loss or foregone
> gain if the principle is adopted, compared to what she would get
> under some alternative principle. According to the Complaint
> Model, a principle is reasonably rejectable only if the person
> whose complaint against this principle is greatest has a greater
> complaint than anyone would have if an alternative principle were
> adopted.[68]

Scanlon rejects the Complaint Model so understood because he does not claim that a person's complaints must be limited to concerns about his *well-being*. One can reasonably reject a principle that did not recognize, say, the value of basic rights, fairness, and reciprocity. At the same time, it seems that contractualism is fundamentally "patient-focused," even though it resists the aggregative features of some versions of patient-focused consequentialism.[69]

Contractualism asks whether any patient affected by a proposed rule would have an agent-relative reason to reject it. In some cases these reasons derive from the extent to which the rule would diminish the patient's welfare. In other cases the reasons do not concern welfare. For example, the rule treats the patient unfairly, or sends a message authorizing her mistreatment, or permits her to be misused. In any case, for contractualists, whether or not someone has a reason to reject a rule is always a function of her agent-relative reasons.[70]

If contractualism is patient-focused and if contractualism endorses principles of moral freedom that that allow for A *not* to interact with B under certain circumstances, it would appear that contractualism would support principles that allow mutually advantageous and consensual agreements relative to the baseline established by that moral freedom. And so contrary to Sample's claim, this version of deontological theory does not give us reason to regard unfair or exploitative interaction as necessarily worse than neglect.

Temkin's Teleology. I have suggested that it is not easy to reject NWC on deontological grounds, although I will consider a (quasi)-deontological strategy below. Before doing so, I want to consider Larry Temkin's strategy of resisting NWC by appeal to the notion of impersonal goods.[71] In his important work on inequality, Temkin argues that a situation which is better for every *person* might not be *morally* better because there are objective moral values such as equality and proportional justice that do not supervene on what is good for persons. On Temkin's view, it is morally bad that some people fare less well than others for reasons beyond their control. Not necessarily bad *for people*. Just bad. Consider two possible worlds where the numbers are measures of overall well-being:

Assuming that the inequalities between A and B are undeserved, Temkin argues that there is one crucial way in which World 1 is morally preferable to World 2. World 1 is more equal. And it's not that B is actually worse off in World 2 than World 1, say because B's envy (at A's 10) reduces her

Table 6.2

	World 1	World 2
A	5	10
B	4	5

well-being from the purported 5 to less than 4. *Ex hypothesi*, these numbers already include such psychological adjustments. Rather, World 1 is objectively better on one dimension simply because it is more equal.

Temkin's claim about the badness of inequality is meant to illustrate that we should not accept what he calls "The Slogan," to wit, that "One situation *cannot* be worse (or better) than another *in any respect* if there is *no one* for whom it *is* worse (or better) *in any respect*."[72] Temkin argues that there are situations in which non-person affecting values should be included in the overall assessment of a state of affairs. Interestingly, most of the examples Temkin uses to argue against "The Slogan" are ones in which there appear to be independent moral reasons of desert to think that someone *should not fare well* or as well as someone else. So there "would be *something* morally bad about the evilest mass murderers faring better than the most benign saints, even if there was *no one* for whom it was worse."[73] Less dramatically, we might think there is something bad about a situation in which an ordinary criminal fares as well as a law-abiding citizen even if his faring as well was better for him and worse for no one.

Assuming that we share Temkin's intuitions about such cases, there is a genuine question as to what the intuition shows. As is well known, the retributive intuition that criminals should fare less well than law-abiding citizens can easily be explained on a person-affecting approach that is consistent with "the slogan." Consider Bentham's view of punishment. Bentham regarded all punishment as inherently evil because punishment adds suffering to the world. On this view, the world in which the criminal fares as well as the ordinary citizen is, *ceteris paribus*, superior to the world in which the criminal is made to suffer. But Bentham understood that all things are not equal. If we want to deter people from committing crimes and imposing suffering on others, then we may have to impose suffering on the criminal in order to prevent more suffering.[74] And while Bentham did not say this, our willingness to impose such suffering may be enhanced by acquiring or not resisting (it may be natural) the retributive belief that such suffering is deserved. Similarly, if we want to deter people from sinning, then it is best to believe that sinners should fare less well than saints. On this two-tiered view, it is a good thing that we believe that sinners should fare less well than saints, even if their faring less well than saints is intrinsically not good. Temkin may think that this two-tiered explanation of the intuition that he uses to attach the slogan does not properly account for the intuition. But, at a minimum, this explanation does show that the intuitions to which Temkin appeals—if we accept them—do not offer decisive support for rejecting "The Slogan."

In addition, even if we accept Temkin's view about cases in which we might have reason to want some people *not* to fare well (or as well as others), "The Slogan" may still be roughly accurate in contexts in which we have no desert-based reason not to want people to fare well. Reconsider *Housekeeper*. It is difficult to see why Temkin's approach gives us any reason to prefer that that A not hire B as a housekeeper (1) to hiring her for an inadequate wage (2) on grounds of fairness or to believe that (2) is less *good* than (1). Moreover, even Temkin suggests that while non-person affecting moral principles might give us *a* reason to reject The Slogan, the Pareto-superior package deal might be morally better *all things considered*. So whereas Temkin thinks that a world in which all are blind is *in one way better* than a world in which only half are blind—because the world is more equal—he acknowledges that the latter might be better, all things considered. For equality is not all that matters. Similarly, even if there is *a* reason to think that it is worse (because unfair) to hire the housekeeper at an inadequate wage than not to hire her at all, Temkin's line of argument gives us little reason to think it is likely to be worse *all things considered*.

Expressive Arguments and Externalities

There are two additional related ways in which one might reject NWC. Derek Parfit argues that "some things are worth doing for their own sake," such as "acts that express respect for people, or some act of loyalty to some dead friend."[75] Similarly, some acts may be bad to do because they express callousness or indifference towards others. So it might be thought that A's decision not to hire anyone as a housekeeper is not bad because not hiring does not *express* indifference towards B's welfare, whereas paying B an inadequate wage is bad because it does express indifference or callousness.

I am not sure what to make of the force or relevance of this argument to our concern with the principles of research ethics. On the one hand, I feel the pull of the intuition that an act of loyalty to a dead friend is worth doing "for its own sake" even if it is better for no one, although the intuition may best be explained on other grounds. In any case, the advocates of the principles of research ethics do not claim that we should insist, say, on the standard of care or post-trial treatment for their own sake as a way to "express respect" for people even if it is not better for them. Rather, they claim that compliance with those principles will be *better* for people and thus this expressive argument, whatever its merits, does not support rejecting NWC in the present context.

Apart from any moral considerations having to do with the parties to the transaction, it is possible that a policy or attitude of not condemning the expression of indifference, callousness, or unfairness in choosing (2) in cases such as *Housekeeper* would have adverse consequences for the moral environment in which we live that are not possessed by the choice of (1), and that this environment will have genuine negative effects on human well-being. We have seen this appeal to "soft externalities" before.[76] It is to be taken seriously and might justify a policy that precludes (2). But as I have already noted, this argument does not actually reject NWC as it has been defined, for NWC assumes that a transaction does not have negative externalities.

Where does all this leave us? Despite the intuitive appeal of IP, we have not yet found a persuasive argument for rejecting NWC. If we assume that NWC is roughly correct, what follows? There are at least three possibilities. First, if non-interaction is not (seriously) wrong, it is possible that some interactions such as (2) in *Housekeeper* or some cases of allegedly unethical clinical research are indeed *less* wrong than some are inclined to think. Second, if an interaction is wrong and if non-interaction is worse than the interaction, then the non-interaction such as (1) in *Housekeeper* may be *more* wrong than we were otherwise inclined to think.

Actions and States of Affairs

There is another possibility. It is possible that NWC may be roughly correct with respect to the axiological moral ranking of *states of affairs*, but not with respect to the deontic moral ranking of *actions*. On this view, the state of affairs in which A pays B an inadequate wage (2) in *Housekeeper* is morally preferable to the state of affairs in which A does not hire B (1), but A acts wrongly in (2) because A treats B unfairly even though it is not wrong for A to choose (1). There is no reason to assume that wrongness tracks even a non-aggregative conception of moral worseness.

To examine the plausibility of this view, let us return to the concept of a package deal that is better, all things considered, than no deal but which contains a harmful component or provides inadequate benefits. In some package deals, the undesirable component is unavoidable.

Chemotherapy. A proposes to administer chemotherapy to B.
    The treatment is expected to extend B's life by several years
    but has unpleasant side effects. B consents to the
    treatment.

A's action in *Chemotherapy* is morally unproblematic. The package deal is beneficial all things considered and A cannot arrange things such that the undesirable side effects can be avoided.

In other cases, a package deal contains a component which would be wrong outside of the arrangement but which is a necessary part of the package.

Sparring. A is a prize fighter. A hires B as a sparring partner. B is
    paid to be punched by B and is instructed not to attempt to
    punch A with force.

Assuming no general objection to prize fighting, it seems that A does nothing wrong in hitting B if B gives robust consent to being so employed, as A would have no reason to employ or interact with B if A could not hit B. B's right not to be punched is *not inalienable.*

By contrast, there are package deals that contain what would otherwise and may continue to be wrongful action. Consider *Abusive Marriage.*

Abusive Marriage. A is considering marrying B. A is an abusive
    person, has abused B in the past and knows he is likely to
    abuse B in the future. B knows this as well, but believes that
    marrying A is her best alternative. B consents to marry A under
    these conditions.

I want to advance the following claims with respect to this case:

(1) It is permissible for A not to propose to marry B.
(2) The state of affairs represented by the package deal is morally
    preferable to the state of affairs in which there is no marriage
    because it is better for B and B consents.
(3) A state of affairs in which A marries B but does not act
    abusively is better than the state of affairs in which A marries B
    and acts abusively.
(4) It is wrong for A to act abusively even though B has consented
    to the package that contains the abuse.

There is nothing particularly controversial about (1) and (3). I have argued that (2) may also be true. The task is to show why (4) might be correct given (1) and (2). It's easy enough to say that deontic prescriptions are not a direct function of the evaluation of states of affairs when those states of affairs involve *different* persons. And so we can't kill one person to redistribute her organs to save five others even if the state of affairs in which we kill and redistribute is morally preferable to the state of affairs in which we do not. The task is to show that deontic prescriptions such as (4) are not a direct function of the evaluation of states of affairs when those states involve the *same* persons and when they have *consented* as in (1) and (2). Given that it is not wrong for A to offer no package deal to B, how can it be wrong for A to offer and act consistently with a package deal that is better for B than no package and to which B consents? Put somewhat differently, given that the right not to be hit is not inalienable in *Sparring,* why should we regard it as inalienable in *Abusive Marriage?*

If A's abusive behavior in *Abusive Marriage* were an uncontrollable feature of A's personality such that (3) is not a viable option, then it might *not* be wrong for A to propose the package deal and then engage in behavior that would otherwise constitute abuse. In that case, A's "hitting behavior" would be similar to the side effects in *Chemotherapy.* To see this more clearly, consider

> *Tourette's.* B owns a restaurant and needs to hire a chef. The restaurant has an open kitchen. A, an excellent chef, has Tourette's syndrome and regularly shouts obscenities. A informs B of his condition. B hires A.[77]

The undesirable behavior in *Tourette's* is comparable to the side-effects in *Chemotherapy.* B may reasonably refuse to hire A, but given that A cannot avoid his behavior, we would not criticize him for shouting obscenities and we would not think that such behavior violated the rights of the employer.

But what about *Abusive Marriage?* If the principles that govern the morality of package deals are meant to advance the well-being of patients such as B, it might be reasonable to adopt a prescription that regards some mutually beneficial interactions as wrong. The principle would say that it is wrong for A to enter into *Abusive Marriage* even though it is better for B than no marriage. The correct principles about the evaluation of action need not directly track the state of affairs that provides its ultimate justification. From a practical point of view, moral principles are meant to guide behavior, "to make claims about what we have reason *to do.*"

On the view just described, the moral evaluation of *actions* thus replicates the structure of the "strategic argument" for prohibiting unfair but mutually beneficial transactions such as rescues at an unconscionable price or jobs at less than a minimum wage. Although the strategic argument does not or certainly need not deny that an unfair mutually beneficial transaction is a better state of affairs than no transaction, it supports condemning such transactions *if* such condemnations typically motivate people to engage in fairer mutually beneficial transactions rather than not to transact at all.

On this view, we may justifiably accept claim (4) above, namely, that it is *wrong* for A to abuse B in *Abusive Marriage* even though she has consented to the package deal that contains the abuse and even though (1) A has no obligation to offer a package that involves marrying B and not abusing her, and (2) marrying A under these conditions is a morally preferable state of affairs to no marriage. But we do *not* accept claim (4) in a vacuum. We assume that A's abusive behavior in *Abusive Marriage* is not like the undesirable dimensions of *Tourette's* or *Chemotherapy*, neither of which is avoidable. We assume that men can control their behavior and will generally want to continue to marry even if they cannot abuse their wives, and so condemning such abuse will generally work to the advantage of women.

Contrast *Sparring* and *Abusive Marriage*. To regard hitting as impermissible in *Sparring* will not give rise to a better version of *Sparring*. It will lead to no deal. So we do not treat the right not to be hit as inalienable here. By contrast, we believe that if we regard hitting as impermissible in marriages, then that principle will not bar most marriages but will, instead, lead to less abusive marriages. And so we treat the right of a person not to be hit by her spouse as inalienable. But what if the world of *Abusive Marriage* were actually like the world of *Sparring?* Here I am prepared to bite the bullet. *If* the world in which we regard A's behavior as wrong in *Abusive Marriage* causes men to make choices that are *worse* for women—no marriage—then the package deal of *Abusive Marriage* might not be wrongful in that world. Hitting would be permissible in that world just as it is in *Sparring*.

What would such a world be like? It would be a world in which men get considerable psychic satisfaction from hitting their wives and relatively little benefit from the other dimensions of marriage and procreation. In that world, getting married and not hitting would be like hiring a sparring partner but not be able to hit him. Fortunately, that is not the world that we know.

We can now return to *Housekeeper*. Faced with a choice between (1), (2), and (3), A would choose (2), which is better for B than (1). But if the relevant set of moral principles presents A with a choice that is limited to (1) and (3), A is likely to choose (3) which is better for B than (2). If we say that (2) is wrong, thereby taking it off the off the moral table, then the expected result is *not* worse for B, given a sufficient likelihood that A will choose (3) rather than (1). Thus it is arguably better to regard certain types of interaction as wrong even when they yield a morally superior state of affairs in a particular case. And the same might apply with respect to the principles of ethical research. It may be best to regard certain research interactions as wrong even if they yield a better state of affairs than non-interaction in a particular case.

It might be objected that this strategic or two-tiered line of argument erroneously collapses the distinction between the claim that an action *is* wrong and the claim that there are good reasons to *regard it as wrong*. It might be said that even if the strategic argument can explain why it makes sense to act *as if* it is wrong for A to abuse B in *Abusive Marriage,* it does not explain the intuition that A's behavior in *Abusive Marriage is* wrong independent of the expected results. I concede that this is possible. But there is no reason to think that intuitions have to be explained or justified on their own terms. If we can adequately explain why it makes sense to regard A's behavior as wrong, that should be sufficient.

From this "practical" perspective of the moral evaluations of actions, we can extend the analogy between legal intervention and moral evaluation of actions. Our willingness to legally punish an activity need not and does not correlate perfectly with the comparative moral wrongness of respective actions. Suppose, for example, that "driving while tired" is just as dangerous as driving while intoxicated. If, for the sake of argument, we should prohibit driving while intoxicated, it does *not* follow that we should also prohibit driving while drowsy. Given that it is relatively easy to monitor alcohol levels but virtually impossible to monitor drowsiness, the law sensibly focuses and punishes that which it can monitor at an acceptable cost.

Given its practical purposes, our moral judgments may reflect a similar perspective. Reconsider Nike and Hike. It is much easier to turn our moral monitors on interactions à la Nike than non-interactions à la Hike. Interactions are finite in number and observable. By contrast, non-interactions are hard to monitor and it is often difficult if not impossible to identify those who would (counterfactually) benefit from interaction. Whereas our moral evaluation of Nike can reflect a clear counterfactual to—"You could have paid them *this* amount or provided *these* working conditions,"—it is less clear what we would want Hike to do to escape moral condemnation. Moreover, just as Mill thought there are good reasons to allow people to lead the lives they see fit to live even when individuals make bad choices, there are good economic reason to provide a legal, institutional, and moral background that allows manufacturers such as Hike the freedom to make investments as they see fit even when they make non-optimal decisions from an economic or moral perspective. If this is right, it might make sense to claim that Nike is acting wrongly even if its actions produce a better state of affairs than Hike's if this moves Nike in a better direction. Similarly, it might make sense to claim that some cases of clinical research in underdeveloped societies are wrong and perhaps should not be allowed even if the state of affairs they yield are morally superior to the state of affairs in which such research does not occur.

It *might.* Here I want to make a theoretical point and an empirical point. First, whether or not my "practical" account of the moral evaluation of actions is on the right track as a general proposition of ethical theory, it is clear that the relevant principles of research ethics are meant to serve a practical purpose, namely, to promote valuable research consistent with protecting the interests and autonomy of research subjects. These norms are embedded in laws and codes which are meant to be followed by regulatory and administrative bodies as well as investigators and their sponsors. If those norms do not serve to advance the interests of research subjects, then they should probably be rejected.

Second, it is an empirical question as to whether and which norms of research ethics serve the aims which justify those norms. If they do so, then, that is a reason in their favor. If, however, the regulations or norms deter research from which subjects will benefit and which does not compromise their autonomy, then we should probably reject the norm or regulation. Of course, a norm or regulation could have *both* effects. Minimum wage laws may raise the income of some employees while deterring the employment of others (when an employer believes that the value of a potential employee's work is less than the minimum wage) to the detriment of the non-employed. What then? We have to choose. If minimum wage legislation causes a significant increase in non-employment, then such laws would be hard to justify even if it helped some workers. On the other hand, if the principal effect of minimum wage laws is to raise the income of employees without significantly reducing employment, then such laws are much easier to justify.

A similar point applies to research. We cannot assume that good intentions and intuitively attractive principles should rule the day. The effect of the ethical principles that we enshrine in our regulations is an empirical question, not to be settled by arm-chair psychology or *a priori* philosophical analysis. If, for example, insisting on the standard care principle that would bar placebo controlled trials advances the interests of research subjects, then we have at least a very strong reason to defend it. But if the principle has the opposite effect, as was arguably the case in the *Surfaxin Trial,* then there is much less reason to defend it. Much the same can be said for the principle that researchers should provide post-trial treatment or ancillary care to research subjects or provide benefits to the host community.

But even if requiring researchers to devote greater resources to research subjects will not deter them from doing research, the question remains as to whether we should push them in that direction given the opportunity costs of doing so. Suppose, for example, that we favor principles that require Pfizer and Merck to devote greater resources to research subjects in the form of choosing active controlled trials over placebo controlled trials, providing post-trial treatment, and providing ancillary care, etc. Because the requirement affects both companies, these requirements will not weaken either company's competitive position, and so it will not deter them from conducting research. Nonetheless, such requirements will mean that both Pfizer and Merck will have to devote more resources to each research project, leaving fewer resources for additional projects or resulting in higher prices. Given the opportunity costs of requiring researchers to devote greater resources to research subjects rather than the potential beneficiaries of additional or better research, it is an open question as to whether that is the direction in which we want to push them. And, as I noted above, although there may be some important distinctions between research sponsored by private corporations and research sponsored by non-profits such as NIH, the same concerns can be raised there as well.

The Greater Obligation Claim (GOC)

GOC says that if A interacts with B to both A and B's benefit, A may have a special obligation to provide additional benefits to B as opposed to other persons. The issue is *not* whether A might have special obligations that arise from *commitments* that A has made to B. If A borrows $10 from B, then, *ceteris paribus,* A has greater reason to give $10 to B than to C even if C would derive a greater benefit from the $10. The question is whether A might have special obligations to B to which A has *not* agreed or whether it is morally permissible for A to undertake certain interactions with B only if A takes on (super-contractual) obligations to which A and B would not otherwise agree. It is important to stress, once again, that GOC cannot be justified by an appeal to beneficence, for the question is whether A should extend his beneficence towards B, who has already benefited from A or to others who have not. Rather, the question is whether reasons of reciprocity (or similar notions) can justify the claim that A should provide benefits to the persons he has used to his benefit rather than to persons that he has not so used.

There is a relationship between rejecting NWC and endorsing GOC that we have not explored in detail. Consider *Housekeeper* once again (see Table 6.1). I argued in the previous section that A may act wrongly in *Housekeeper* in choosing (2) if A would prefer (3) to (1). But even if A is prepared to pay a total of $240 (3) if it were wrong for him to pay $200 to B (2), the question remains as to whether A's super-contractual obligations should take the form of paying $240 to B (3) rather than distributing the $240 between B and C (4).

GOC maintains that because A derives benefits from his interaction with B, A has greater moral reason to provide super-contractual benefits to *B* as in (3) than to use those resources to benefit others with whom A has not interacted as in (4). If A employs B to clean her house, then A has greater moral reason to provide for B's needs than to provide for C's needs even if A is aware of C's needs, even though C is *worse* off than B, even though C applied for and would have taken B's position if it had been offered, and even if it was simply a matter of the flip of a coin that B got the job rather than C. For, according to GOC, the fact is that A benefits from B's work, not C's, and so A has obligations of reciprocity to B that A does not have to C.

Here we have principles and intuitions that pull us in different directions. While proximity, feelings of compassion and a commitment to reciprocity pull us towards (3), our concern for impartiality and for assisting the worse off pulls us towards (4). The tension here is importantly distinct from the well-known conundrum as to whether we have greater moral reason to help an identifiable life than a statistical life. Some cases raised by GOC may exhibit that tension; A could propose to pay $200 to B and use the extra $40 to pay for malaria nets in Africa. But other cases raised by GOC involve a choice among identifiable lives. In *Housekeeper* A must choose between B and a specific C. In some cases of medical research, A must choose between the identifiable lives of research subjects and the identifiable lives of those who are excluded from the research project.

Although GOC is hardly unproblematic, it is easier to defend than NWC. Whereas it is paradoxical to claim that it is worse or wrong for A to choose (2) than (1) in *Housekeeper* given that (2) is better for both A and B, there is nothing *paradoxical* about thinking that (3) is morally superior to (4). Indeed, the general trust of GOC is quite familiar. As Scheffler puts it:

> . . . . the importance of special obligations in common-sense moral thought seems undeniable. By any measure, they serve to define a large portion of the territory of morality as it is ordinarily understood. The willingness to make sacrifices for one's family, one's community, one's friends, and one's comrades is seen as one of the marks of a good or virtuous person, and the demands of morality, as ordinarily interpreted, have less to do with abstractions like the overall good than with the specific web of roles and relationships that serve to situate a person in social space.[78]

So the question is not whether we have special obligations. The question is whether and why such obligations emerge from interactions between researchers and subjects.

We can set aside one possible objection to GOC. It might be argued that we must reject GOC *if* we are committed to the equal worth of persons. But there is no fundamental incompatibility between a commitment to the equal worth of persons and the view that one has special responsibilities to particular people. I do not believe that my children have greater worth than my neighbor's children (O.K., I confess that I might believe this!), but it is perfectly reasonable for me to prefer the interests of my children over the interests of my neighbor's children (and for her to prefer the interests of her children over mine). There is a well-known and long-standing controversy as to whether the legitimacy of such preferences is a brute feature of our moral life or whether legitimate partiality must itself be justified from an impartial point of view.[79] Either way, the legitimacy of such preferences seems relatively unquestioned. Similarly, it is arguably reasonable (not necessarily right) for A to give preference to the interests of her housekeeper to the interests of a stranger. If so, we must determine whether the relationship between researchers and subjects is the sort of relationship that justifies such partiality and, if so, to what extent.

It might be thought that the case for GOC is stronger with respect to clinical research than in *Housekeeper* on the grounds that physician-investigators have special responsibilities to their patient-subjects. A physician cannot ethically withhold medical treatment from his patient just because he thinks that the treatment might do more good for others, although a physician may have to withhold treatment from *one* patient in a triage situation in order to provide treatment for another patient. And so it may be thought that physician/investigators cannot fail to provide for their subjects simply because their resources might be used to better effect for others. To do so is incompatible with the obligations of medical practice.

As I have argued at several points, even if the training and socialization of physician\investigators have encouraged many to think about themselves precisely this way, they do not have *physician*-like fiduciary obligations to their subjects, even if they have weaker and different fiduciary obligations. I would go further. To invoke Lon Fuller's distinction, it's not just that the model of medical care fails to reflect the investigator's *morality of duty;* the model of medical care does not represent an attractive *morality of aspiration*—on the assumption that clinical research is a morally worthy enterprise.[80] Even if A's ultimate goals or intentions are to advance his career or to generate profits through medical research, A does so by engaging in an enterprise that seeks to develop generalizable knowledge. The pursuit of that goal may be appropriately tempered by principles of respect for autonomy, compensation, fairness, and reciprocity. But the weight of those constraints will have to be determined on their own grounds and in competition with the value of clinical research, and not simply by appeal to the norms that govern the practice of medicine.

To press this point a bit further, suppose that the Bill and Melinda Gates foundation is supporting clinical research on AIDS in sub-Saharan Africa. Even a very wealthy foundation has limited resources. They are considering the following possible uses of a pool of funds:

(1) provide ARTs as post-trial treatment to participants in a successful ART trial (all subjects have AIDS), as seems to be required by The Declaration of Helsinki.[81]

(2) provide ARTs to those who are *excluded* from an AIDS vaccine trial when screening determines that they are HIV-positive.

(3) provide ARTs to those (previously) HIV-negative subjects who are *included* in an AIDS vaccine trial, but who sero-convert during the trial.

I do not have a firm idea as to which option is morally superior. I would note, however, that the participants in (1) are the *only* persons who have received a direct medical benefit from participation, although the subjects in (3) may benefit *ex ante*, if there were good reason to think that the vaccine would be effective, and may also benefit from various collateral benefits such as risk reduction counseling, free condoms, medical exams, and financial compensation. If the decision among these options were left to investigators, they would probably feel inclined towards (1) as they have witnessed the improvement of these subjects during the trial. Moreover, it is no doubt psychologically more difficult to remove or stop a therapy than not to begin one, even if the therapy will produce comparable benefits in both cases. Nonetheless, the mere fact that the scientific benefits of the ART trial (1) will come from the use of *those* participants does not, in my view, give them a weightier claim to resources that could otherwise be provided to persons who seroconvert during an AIDS vaccine trial, where the vaccine clearly failed them (setting aside the possibility that the subjects bear some responsibility for becoming infected).

As I have stressed, there are genuine opportunity costs to accepting the principles of research ethics that instantiate GOC. Insofar as the researcher's resources will not disappear into a black hole if they are not used to provide super-contractual benefits to subjects, but, rather, will be used in ways that will directly or indirectly generate greater medical benefit to others, we must confront what Scheffler calls the *distributive objection* to special obligations: why should A's relationship with B work to the disadvantage of C?[82] Do not say that these special obligations do not weaken one's general duties of beneficence but simply add such obligations to the mix, for "part of what it is to have such responsibilities to one's associates is to be required, within limits, to give their interests priority over the interests of non-associates, in cases in which the two conflict."[83]

So the issue before us is not whether we *can* have greater obligations to some than to others, but whether the interactions that occur in research generate these special obligations. As I have suggested, everyday life contains a wide range of contexts—including most commercial interactions—in which interactions do not generate obligations beyond those to which the parties agree. And this includes trade relations between affluent countries and poor countries. As Matthias Risse has argued, there is nothing morally special about a trade relation with those who produce what we consume.[84] We may have duties to the poor with whom we trade because they are poor, or because we benefit from interactions that are harmful to them or because we are in a position to rescue. And we may have duties to treat each other fairly and decently. But the fact that we benefit from the use of each other does not create additional obligations.

The likely negative response by bioethicists to the contrary notwithstanding, I believe that the "economic" or "trade" or "employment" perspective is a valuable and underutilized model for understanding the relationship between researchers and subjects. As I have argued, we can't simply assert that "medical research is different" as a justification for refusing to seriously consider the normative implications of that perspective. We must show participation in medical research differs from other contexts in ways that are morally relevant to the issue at hand.

Although the precise moral force of these differences between employment and medical research is not clear, there are several features of medical research that may be of moral relevance. First, the relationship is more intimate. It involves access to the body and the revelation of private information. Although I am inclined to think access to the body is less morally freighted than many, I concede that such access may give rise to obligations of reciprocity that go beyond what would obtain in ordinary employment relations into which people entered because of unfortunate background conditions. Second, the expectations of subjects as to what researchers will do for them are likely to be markedly different from the expectations of workers. Nike's employees do not think that Nike is in business to help *them*. By contrast, even when investigators clearly inform subjects that they are participating in medical research as opposed to receiving personalized medical care, it is predictable that many subjects will assume that those with medical training will not disregard their medical needs. Third, whereas employees incur risks and burdens as part of the package of employment, they are being paid for productive labor. They are not paid simply to be a (relatively) passive target of risks. By contrast, medical researchers directly impose risks on subjects. Even when the acceptance of risks is part of a beneficial package of participation, this feature of the relationship may also give rise to a special moral relationship. It is not clear how much force we should attribute to these and other dimensions of research, particularly if the researchers have clearly explained their aims and if the benefits of participation are actually quite considerable. Nonetheless, these (and other) factors may go somewhat towards justifying super-contractual obligations, even if they do not go very far.

The view or intuition that researchers have greater obligations toward subjects than to non-subjects may reflect deep features of human psychology rather than any special moral principle. Consider what behavioral economists call "the endowment effect," namely, that people value an object more once they own it. In one experiment, half the participants were *given* a mug. They had made no investment in acquiring it.[85] They were then asked to indicate the price for which they would sell it (willingness to accept (WTA)). Other participants were asked how much they would be willing to pay for it (WTP). On standard economic theory, WTA and WPT should be roughly equal. If the mug is worth, say, $5.00, the sellers should be willing to sell it for anything more than $5.00 and the buyers should be willing to buy it for anything less than $5.00. In fact, the owners demanded *much* more to sell than the non-owners were willing to pay. The arbitrary assignment of a property right in the mug changed its valuation.

If such a trivial ownership relation can affect the value we place on a mug, it is hardly surprising that investigators come to value the interests of sick or (otherwise) needy persons with whom they interact in intimate ways more than the interests of nameless or future persons. We can of course ask whether they *should* value those persons more. But that is not the only question. In addition to asking what researchers should *do,* we can ask what sorts of persons we want researchers to *be?* What constitutes a *virtuous* investigator? Do we want investigators to be the sorts of persons who will keep an eye on the persons before them or do we think that virtuous researchers and their sponsors will keep both eyes riveted on the pursuit of generalizable knowledge?

This question cannot be answered simply by reference to the virtues of compassion and sensitivity. Proper performance in some professions may require a "tunnel vision" that renders people insensitive to some consequences of their actions that would normally be relevant. We want emergency room physicians to be able to turn their backs on patients in need so that they can attend to even needier patients. We want lawyers to be psychologically able to zealously represent their clients even when this involves what would seem to be cruelty to witnesses or indifference to public safety or defending a client from a meritorious suit such that the plaintiff does not receive just compensation for his injury. We may want professors to grade students on their merits without considering the effects of the grades on their psychic well-being or their prospects for admission to graduate school. Consider Judge Lois Forer's view of sentencing:

> It is not easy to look any human being in the eye and say, "I am placing you behind bars for two years or ten years, sending you to a place where you will not be able to see your spouse and family except under degrading circumstances, a place which may not be physically safe, where you may be beaten or sexually abused, where most of your time will be spent in idleness or performing boring routine tasks . . ."[86]

It is not clear what we should conclude from this observation. Judge Forer concluded that we should find alternatives to imprisonment. But if sentencing criminals to prison is justified on retributive grounds or if it has a significant deterrent effect (on others) or incapacitation effect (because it keeps dangerous persons off the street), then we might want judges who are less sensitive than Judge Forer or we might want to make it easier for psychologically sensitive judges to impose socially beneficial sentences, say, by enacting strict guidelines that constrain their decisions.

The virtuous researcher is not a virtuous (treating) physician delivering personalized medical care. At the same time, it is unlikely that virtuous researchers need or should have the "tunnel vision" of a criminal defense lawyer. Even if we think that the demands of GOC are modest, we may want researchers to be people who cannot easily turn their back on the needs of subjects. Moreover, the demands of morality must be adjusted to the natural and otherwise desirable psychological tendencies of people. Compassion and sensitivity to those with whom we interact generally has desirable consequences and it is a disposition that cannot be easily turned off when doing so would otherwise be justified (do lawyers disprove this?). So even if it were otherwise morally preferable for researchers to reject GOC and act as if they were insensitive to the welfare of their subjects, such a demand may create excessive psychic strain.

After all this, I find that I am unable to reach a firm conclusion about the force of GOC with regard to issues such as the standard of care or the provision of post-trial treatment or ancillary care. There may not be a decisive case in its favor, but the case for special obligations is strong enough to render it permissible or reasonable for researchers or sponsors to use their resources in a way that is consistent with GOC, even if it would be morally preferable from an impartial perspective if they were to do *less* for subjects who have already benefited from participation and more for other present or future persons. On the other hand, I also do not think it unreasonable to move towards a "contractual" model of the obligations that investigators have towards subjects *if* that would actually move them to use research resources in ways that would do more to reduce human suffering subject to the demands of immediacy and urgency of suffering that no person could easily or reasonably refuse.

The italicized "if" in the previous sentence is important. As a *practical principle* for guiding the actions of investigators, the case for GOC and the principles of research ethics that it supports may be stronger than would be warranted on its (pure) philosophical merits. Sometimes the ideal or first-best solution to a problem is infeasible or is just not going to happen, and so it makes sense to opt for the second-best alternative, lest a third or fourth best alternative occur. GOC may exemplify the reasonable choice of the *second-best*. Suppose we assume that the first-best use of an investigator's resources is to use them for additional research projects that will benefit impoverished persons rather than on the relatively few lucky persons who have been fortunate enough to participate in research. But suppose as well that if we do not adopt a principle such as post-trial access, these resources are not likely to be used in this way. Rather, the resources may be used for research on diseases of the rich or given to the owners of the corporation as profits. Given that the resources available to researchers would not be put to first best uses (in pursuit of generalizable knowledge for the benefit of others) were they *not* used for the benefit of research subjects, the principles supported by GOC might represent the best feasible use of those resources.

To recall an earlier example, suppose that the government were considering whether to use a fixed level of resources to save five trapped coal miners (identifiable lives) or to prevent a larger number of coal miners from becoming trapped in the future (statistical lives), say, by devoting more resources to safety regulation. Even if (and I say *if*) there were a solid first-best moral argument for using those resources to prevent disasters in the future rather than using them to save those now trapped—and that is far from clear—there may be good reason to think that the resources will not be put to such benevolent use if the miners are not saved, and so it is better to simply go ahead and save the trapped miners. Similarly, even if there were a first-best moral argument for shifting resources from ancillary care or post-trial treatment to other research projects, it might still be better to use those resources in a manner consistent with GOC if those resources would probably not be put to such uses.

Conclusion

I have argued that at least some of the standard principles of research ethics assume that the mutually beneficial and consensual interaction between researchers and subjects or their communities generate super-contractual obligations. In some cases, it is thought that research interactions constrain the sorts of protocols that are permissible. And so it might be thought that it is impermissible for investigators to conduct a placebo controlled trial in violation of the standard care principle. Although the investigators would have no obligation to provide standard care to the prospective subjects if the prospective subjects did not become actual subjects, investigators acquire an obligation to provide such care once the prospective subjects become actual subjects. In other cases, it is thought that the interaction between investigators and subjects imposes additional obligations on investigators to provide post-trial treatment or ancillary care. In some cases, such as the concern with responsiveness and fair benefits, it is thought that interaction with the *community* either constrains the sorts of research questions that it is permissible to investigate or imposes obligations on researchers to provide benefits to communities beyond compensating the communities for harms imposed by the research. And it is thought that investigators should be required to provide such benefits as a condition of conducting research even if requiring them to provide such benefits leads them to abandon the research or move the research to another location and thus provide no benefits at all. Or, perhaps more accurately, the advocates of these principles have not considered whether their principles will have these consequences.

I have argued that its intuitive appeal notwithstanding, IP is more difficult to defend than is commonly supposed. As a matter of ethical theory, it is difficult, although not impossible, to defend the view that mutually advantageous and consensual transactions are wrong or otherwise problematic if they are better for all than non-interactions that we would not regard as wrong. It is even more difficult to defend a *policy* that would preclude or deter mutually advantageous and consensual transactions between researchers and subjects if such a policy did not yield compensating gains. If I am right, it is important to establish whether research interactions have these worrisome moral implications.

With respect to GOC, I have argued that some partiality towards research subjects may be defensible on grounds of reciprocity, but there may be sharp limits to its force. Although it is true that research subjects are often quite vulnerable and needy, they are often selected from a pool of potential applicants, many or all of whom are vulnerable and needy. Given this, and given that many subjects participate precisely because they reasonably expect to benefit (all things considered), it is not easy to argue that researchers have special responsibilities to those who have *already* had the good fortune to participate in research when researchers could choose to benefit others who are also disadvantaged and could benefit from participation in research or from the fruits of research.

I do *not* claim to have shown that the principles of research ethics that receive support from IP should be abandoned. There are at least two ways in which the thrust of my argument might be resisted. First, and as a matter of ethical theory, it is possible that that the case for IP is stronger than I allow. I have defended one line of argument for claiming that it can be wrong to engage in a mutually beneficial and consensual interaction when it would not be wrong to not interact. But it is possible that NWC can be successfully resisted along lines that I have criticized or along lines that I did not consider. And while I believe that the case for GOC and reciprocity is considerably weaker than is often supposed, I may have underestimated its strength even in the face of the opportunity costs that it entails. Second, and as an empirical and contingent matter, it is possible that the opportunity costs of complying with the standard principles of research ethics are less than I fear. It is possible that requiring researchers to provide super-contractual benefits will not deter valuable research or will not shift it to other locations to the detriment of people in LDCs. And it is possible that requiring researchers to provide super-contractual benefits to research subjects will simultaneously benefit those subjects but will not seriously deprive other impoverished people of the benefits of the fruits of research or the opportunity to participate in research, if only because those resources would not likely be put to such uses.

A final cautionary reminder. The argument in this chapter is limited to medical research to which subjects give morally transformative consent and from which subjects can expect to benefit (setting aside what counts *as* a benefit). I have no doubt but that there is *much* research that does not fit this description. But as morally objectionable as such research may be, it does not present difficult theoretical issues. The task there is not to determine what is morally required. The task is to see that the uncontroversial moral requirements are met. By contrast, I hope to have shown that it is much less clear what is required when subjects do give morally transformative consent and can reasonably expect to benefit from the package deal of participation. At a minimum, I hope to have shown that what I have called the interaction principle needs a more sustained defense than has been provided, and, less minimally, that to the extent that some standard principles of research ethics are justified by the interaction principle, those principles may have to be abandoned or substantially revised.

Notes

Preface

1. H. Jonas, "Philosophical reflections on experimenting with human subjects," *Daedalus* 98 (1969):219–47, 220.

Chapter 1

1. H. Jonas, "Philosophical reflections on experimenting with human subjects," *Daedalus* 98 (Spring 1969):219–47, 224.
2. U. Veronesi, et al. "Twenty year follow-up of a randomized study comparing breast-conserving surgery with radical mastectomy for early breast cancer," *New England Journal of Medicine* 347 (2002): 1227–1232. B. Fisher, et al., "Twenty year follow-up of a randomized trial comparing total mastectomy, lumpectomy, and lumpectomy plus irradiation for the treatment of invasive breast cancer," *New England Journal of Medicine* 347 (2002): 1233–1241.
3. D. Grady, et al., "Cardiovascular disease outcomes during 6–8 years of hormone therapy: Heart and Estrogen/Progestin Replacement Study follow-up (HERS II)," *Journal of American Medical Association* 288 (2002):49–57.
4. See J. Groopman, "Superbugs," *The New Yorker* August 11, 2008, 46.

5. See E.A. Stadtmauer, et al. "Conventional-dose chemotherapy compared with high-dose chemotherapy plus autologous hematopoietic stem-cell transplantation for metastatic breast cancer," *New England Journal of Medicine* 342 (2000): 1069–76.

6. J. B. Moseley, et al. "A controlled trial of arthroscopic surgery for osteoarthritis of the knee," *New England Journal of Medicine* 347 (2002): 81–8.

7. See The Global Forum for Health Research, http://www.globalforumhealth.org/About/10-90-gap.

8. See "Operating Profit," *The Economist* (August 16, 2008), 74.

9. See Open house on drug trials in India" http://infochangeindia.org/20051110275/Health/Features/Open-house-on-drug-trials-in-India.html.

10. S. Shah, "The Constant Gardener: What the movie missed," *The Nation* (August 30, 2005).

11. My colleagues at NIH have argued that there are seven criteria by which to evaluate the ethics of research. I believe that the two criteria noted here are the most important. See E. Emanuel, et al. "What makes clinical research ethical?" *Journal of American Medical Association* 283 (2000): 2701–2711.

12. I believe that some of those additional criteria (e.g. social value and scientific validity) could be subsumed under the reasonable risk criterion.

13. See the description of these cases in E. Emanuel, et al, *The Oxford textbook of clinical research ethics* (New York: Oxford University Press, 2008). Also see H. Beecher, "Ethics and clinical research," *The New England Journal of Medicine* 274 (1966): 1354–1360.

14. "*What the doctor didn't say*" (New York: Oxford University Press, 2006).

15. Jonas, "Philosophical reflections," 233.

16. *Ibid.* 238.

17. D. Heyd, "Experimentation in trial: Why should one take part in medical research," *Jahrbuch für Recht und Ethik* 4 (1996) 189–204. Reprinted in E. Emanuel, et al. (eds.) *Ethical and regulatory aspects of clinical research* (Baltimore: Johns Hopkins University Press, 2003), 162.

18. Shah, "The Constant Gardener"

19. L. Eisenberg, "The social imperatives of medicine," *Science* 198 (December, 1977): 1106.

20. See, for example, C. Elliott, "Guinea-pigging" *The New Yorker* January 7, 2008.

21. See *Exploitation* (Princeton: Princeton University Press, 1987).

22. World Medical Association, Declaration of Helsinki, as amended in 2008. Paragraph 32 states: "The benefits, risks, burdens and effectiveness of a new intervention must be tested against those of the best current proven intervention, except in the following circumstances:

- The use of placebo, or no treatment, is acceptable in studies where no current proven intervention exists; or
- Where for compelling and scientifically sound methodological reasons the use of placebo is necessary to determine the efficacy or safety of an intervention and the patients who receive placebo or no treatment will not be subject to any risk of serious or irreversible harm. Extreme care must be taken to avoid abuse of this option.

23. *Hard heads, soft hearts: Tough-minded economics for a just society* (Reading, MA: Addison-Wesley Pub. Co. 1987).

Chapter 2

1 This chapter is a revised version of Franklin Miller and Alan Wertheimer, "Facing up to paternalism in research ethics," *Hastings Center Report* 37 3 (2007): 24–34.

2. Department of Health and Human Services. Protection of Human Subjects. Code of Federal Regulations. 45CFR46, 1991.

3. E.J. Emanuel, D. Wendler, and C. Grady, "What makes clinical research ethical?" *JAMA* 283 (2000): 2701–2711.

4. I thank an anonymous reviewer for pressing me on this point.

5. See A. Wertheimer, "Liberty, coercion, and the limits of the state" in Robert Simon (ed.) *The Blackwell guide to social and political philosophy* (Oxford: Blackwell, 2002).

6. S. Shiffrin, "Paternalism, unconscionability doctrine, and accommodation," *Philosophy & Public Affairs* 29 (2000) 205–50.

7. See J. Feinberg, *Harm to Self* (New York: Oxford University Press, 1986), 12.

8. *Ibid.* 12.

9. R. Arneson, "Paternalism, utility, and fairness," in G. Dworkin (ed) *J.S. Mill's On liberty: Critical essays* (Lanham, MD: Rowman and Littlefield, 1997): 82–112.

10. Shiffrin, "Paternalism, unconscionability doctrine, and accommodation," 220.

11. J. S. Mill, *On liberty,* (Indianapolis: Hackett Publishing Co., 1978) Ch. 1, originally published in 1859, 9.

12. *Ibid.* Ch. 5, 95

13. *Ibid.*

14. Feinberg, *Harm to self*, 119.

15. Feinberg, *Harm to self*, 12.

16. Beauchamp and Childress state that "Reasons exist to doubt that [soft] paternalism qualifies as a form of paternalism that needs a defense." T.L. Beauchamp

and J.F. Childress, *Principles of biomedical ethics,* 5th edition (New York: Oxford University Press, 2001):181.

17. I thank an anonymous reviewer for pressing this point.

18. See "Is more choice better than less?" in G. Dworkin, *The theory and practice of autonomy* (Cambridge: Cambridge University Press, 1988).

19. R. Arneson, "Paternalism, utility, and fairness," 82–112.

20. See the discussion of the Belmont Report in Emanuel, et al (eds) *The Oxford textbook of clinical research ethics,* pp. 149–155. Also see the discussion of the International Ethical Guidance from the Council for International Organizations of Medical Sciences (CIOMS) in the same book, 168–73.

21. Code of Federal Regulations, 45CFR46.302.

22. Emanuel, et al. "What makes research ethical?"

23. I thank an anonymous reviewer for pressing me on this point.

24. T.L. Beauchamp, et al. "Pharmaceutical research involving the homeless," *Journal of Medicine and Philosophy* 27 (2002): 547–64, 555.

25. H. Beecher, "Ethics and clinical research," *New England Journal of Medicine* 274 (1966):1354–60, 1360.

26. See D. Wendler, "The assent requirement in pediatric research" in E. Emanuel, et al. (eds.) *The Oxford textbook of clinical research ethics,* 661–668.

27. Special Ethical Protections for Pediatric Research Participants: Subpart D and Assent http://www.fda.gov/oc/opt/presentations/SubpartD.html.

28. J.B. Moseley, et al. "A controlled trial of arthroscopic surgery for osteoarthritis of the knee," *New England Journal of Medicine* 347 (2002):81–88.

29. Emanuel, et al. "What makes clinical research ethical?" 2; Also see F.G. Miller and H. Brody, "A critique of clinical equipoise: Therapeutic misconception in the ethics of clinical trials," *Hastings Center Report* 33 (2003):19–28.

30. Department of Health and Human Services. Protection of Human Subjects. Code of Federal Regulations. 45CFR46, 1991.

31. G.J. Annas and M.A. Grodin, *The Nazi doctors and the Nuremberg Code* (New York: Oxford University Press, 1992): 2.

32. See S. Lederer, "Walter Reed and the yellow fever experiments," in Emanuel, et al. (eds) *The Oxford textbook of clinical research ethics,* 9–17.

33. http://en.wikipedia.org/wiki/Wesley_Autrey.

34. F.G. Miller and D.L. Rosenstein, "The therapeutic orientation to clinical trials," *New England Journal of Medicine* 348 (2003):1383–86.

35. T. Nagel, "War and massacre," *Philosophy & Public Affairs* 1, no. 2 (1972): 123–44, 132.

36. J. Rawls, *A theory of justice,* revised edition (Cambridge: Harvard University Press, 1999): 219.

Chapter 3

1. This chapter is an expanded and revised version of F. Miller and A. Wertheimer, "Preface to a theory of consent transactions: Beyond valid consent," in Franklin Miller and Alan Wertheimer (eds.) *The ethics of consent* (New York: Oxford University Press, 2009).
2. The Nuremberg Code. See http://ohsr.od.nih.gov/guidelines/nuremberg.html.
3. In addition to thousands of articles, it is discussed in depth in many prominent books. See, for example, J. Katz, *The silent world of doctor and patient* (New York: The Free Press, 1984); R. Faden and T. Beauchamp, *A history and theory of informed consent* (New York: Oxford University Press, 1986); J. Berg, et al. *Informed consent* (New York: Oxford University Press, 2001).
4. E.J. Emanuel, D. Wendler, and C. Grady, "What makes clinical research ethical?" *JAMA* 283 (2000):2701–2711.
5. See Baruch Brody., "New perspectives on emergency room research," *Hastings Center Report* 27, 1 (1997): 7–9.
6. R. Truog, et al, "Is informed consent always necessary for randomized, controlled trials?" *New England Journal of Medicine* 1999; 340(10):804–807. A cluster randomized trial involves randomizing social units or clusters of individuals rather than the individuals themselves. For example, a study might randomize among hospitals; all persons in a given hospital receive the same intervention.
7. *Groundwork of the metaphysics of morals* in I. Kant, *Practical philosophy*, ed. and trans. M. J. Gregory (Cambridge: Cambridge University Press, 1996), 429.
8. See A. Sen, "Rights & agency," *Philosophy and Public Affairs* (1982) 11: 3–39.
9. *On what matters*, Chapter 8 (Oxford: Oxford University Press, forthcoming)
10. *Ibid.*
11. R. Arneson, "The shape of Lockean rights; fairness, Pareto, moderation, and consent," *Philosophy and Social Policy* 22 (2005): 255–285, 264.
12. In a non-anonymous review of a draft of this book for Oxford University Press.
13. Hans Jonas, "Philosophical reflections on experimenting with human subjects," *Daedalus*, 98 (1969): 219–47, 223.
14. *Ibid.* 239.
15. C. Fethe, "Beyond voluntary consent: Hans Jonas on the moral requirements of human experimentation," *Journal of Medical Ethics* 19 (1993): 99–103, 99–100.
16. Jonas, "Philosophical reflections," 234.
17. Fethe, "Beyond voluntary consent," 100.
18. G. O. Schaefer; E. J. Emanuel; A. Wertheimer, "The obligation to participate in biomedical research," *Journal of American Medical Association* 302 (2009): 67–72.

19. L. Jaffe, "Law as a system of control," *Daedalus* 89, Spring, 1969: 406–26, at 424.

20. See "When a spoonful of sugar won't do," *The Economist* December 6, 2007.

21. A. Dula, "Bearing the brunt of the new regulations: Minority populations," *Hastings Center Report* 27, 1997.

22. A. Donagan, "Informed consent in therapy and experimentation," *Journal of Medicine and Philosophy* 2 (1977): 307–329.

23. *Harm to others* (New York: Oxford University Press, 1984).

24. Ibid., p. 6 (original emphasis).

25. K. Lippert-Rasmussen. "Against self-ownership: There are no fact-insensitive ownership rights over one's body," *Philosophy & Public Affairs* 36 (2008): 86–118.

26. J. Griffin, "Virtue ethics and environs," *Social Philosophy and Policy* 15 (1998): 56–70 (emphasis added).

27. C. Fabre. *Whose body is it anyway?* (Oxford: Clarendon Press, 2006) 113.

28. Fethe, "Beyond voluntary consent," 100.

29. R. Dworkin. "Comment on Narveson: In defense of equality," *Social Philosophy and Policy,* 1, (1983): 31–35.

30. N. Eyal, "Is the body special? Review of Cécile Fabre, 'Whose body is it anyway?' Justice and the integrity of the person," *Utilitas* 21(2009): 233–245.

31. "Against self ownership," 101.

32. *Ibid.* 105.

33. See Kelo v City of New London, 545 *U.S.* 469 (2005).

34. J. S. Mill, *On Liberty,* Ch 1.

35. *Ibid.*

36. "A person may cause evil to others not only by his actions but by his inaction, and in either case he is justly accountable to them for the injury." *Ibid.*

37. A. Ripstein, "Three duties to rescue: Moral, civil, and criminal," *Law and Philosophy* 19 (2000): 751–779.

38. "Philosophical reflections," 238.

39. H. Trachtman, "Does Uncle Sam really want you? A response to "Rethinking research ethics" by Rosamind Rhodes", *American Journal of Bioethics* 5, 1 (2005): W22.

40. R. Wachbroit and D. Wasserman, "Research participation: Are we subject to a duty?" *American Journal of Bioethics* 5 (2005): 48–49.

41. *On Liberty,* Ch V.

42. See F. Schauer, *Playing by the rules* (Oxford: Clarendon Press, 1991).

43. H. Beecher. "Ethics and clinical research," *New England Journal of Medicine* 174 (1966) 1354–60.

44. D. Schmidtz, "Islands in a sea of obligation," *Law and Philosophy* 19 (2000): 683–705, 695.

45. *Ibid.*

46. A. Spital, "Conscription of cadaveric organs for transplantation: A stimulating idea whose time has not yet come," *Cambridge Quarterly of Healthcare Ethics* 14 (2005): 107–112.

47. See the discussion of these cases in E. Emanuel, et al. (eds) *The Oxford textbook of clinical research ethics* (New York: Oxford University Press, 2008).

48. See L. Jansen, "The problem with optimism in clinical trials," *IRB* 28 (2006): 13–19.

49. See P. Appelbaum and C. Lidz, "The therapeutic misconception," in *The Oxford Textbook,* 633–44.

50. G. Sreennivasan, "Does informed consent to research require comprehension?" *Lancet* 362 (2003): 2016–18.

51. B. Brody, "Making informed consent meaningful," *IRB* 23, No. 5 (Sep–Oct, 2001): 1–5.

52. Faden and Beauchamp, *"History and Theory,"* 286.

53. In previous work, I relied on the concept of "valid consent." See A. Wertheimer, *Consent to Sexual Relations* (Cambridge: Cambridge University Press, 2003).

54. Faden and Beauchamp, *History and Theory.*

55. T. M. Scanlon, "The significance of choice," in *Tanner lectures on human values* Vol. 8 (Salt Lake City: University of Utah Press, 1989).

56. J. Kleinig, "Consent," in Lawrence Becker and Charlotte Becker (eds.) *Encyclopedia of ethics* (New York: Routledge, 2001), 300.

57. An act is not wrong simply because one hasn't gotten consent. As Arthur Ripstein observes, "I don't need your permission to admire your flowers as I walk past your garden." See "Beyond the harm principle," *Philosophy & Public Affairs* 34 (2006): 215–245, 221.

58. A. Buchanan and D. Brock, *Deciding for others,* (Cambridge: Cambridge University Press, 1989) 37.

59. *Ibid.*

60. J. Waldron, *Liberal rights,* (Cambridge: Cambridge University Press, 1993), 47.

61. Kleinig, "Consent," 300.

62. A. J. Simmons. *Moral principles and political obligations* (Princeton: Princeton University Press, 1979), 83.

63. See Wertheimer, *Consent to sexual relations,* 144.

64. H. Hurd, "The moral magic of consent," *Legal Theory* 2 (1996), 137.

65. P. Westen, *The logic of consent* (Burlington, VT: Ashgate Publishing Co) 2004.

66. This is based on a Texas case in which, at first, the grand jury refused to indict the defendant on the grounds that the victim consented when she proposed that the perpetrator use a condom. See the discussion in my *Consent to sexual relations,* 165.

67. Faden and Beauchamp, *History and theory,* 241.

68. *Ibid.* 280.

69. *Ibid.*

70. See A. Wertheimer, *Coercion* (Princeton: Princeton University Press, 1987).

71. The "gambler's fallacy" is the belief that the odds for something with a fixed probability increase or decrease depending upon recent occurrences—"It's been red four times in a row, so black is more likely to come up now."

72. "Dementia risk seen in players in N.F.L. study," *New York Times*, September, 29, 2009. http://www.nytimes.com/2009/09/30/sports/football/30dementia.html.

73. S. G. Stolberg, "The biotech death of Jesse Gelsinger," *New York Times*, November 28, 1999.

74. In other words, there are reasons to resist what Schneider has called "mandated autonomy" in research, as well as in medical care. C. Schneider, "Rethinking health law: After autonomy," *Wake Forest Law Review* 411 (2006): 413.

75. See Chapter 11 of my *Consent to sexual relations*.

76. G. Dworkin, *The theory and practice of autonomy* (Cambridge: Cambridge University Press, 1988), 20. The locus classicus is H. Frankfurt, "Freedom of the will and the concept of a person," *Journal of Philosophy* 68 (1971): 5–20.

77. I thank John Arras for suggesting that I clarify this point.

78. See C. Korsgaard, "The reasons we can share," *Social Philosophy and Policy* 10 (1993): 24–51, 46.

79. *History and Theory,* 339.

80. J. Rawls, *A theory of justice* (Cambridge, MA: Harvard University Press, 1971).

81. T.M. Scanlon, *What we owe to each other* (Cambridge, MA: Harvard University Press, 1998,) 189.

82. Scanlon, "The significance of choice," 184.

83. I thank Connie Rosati for helping me to formulate this point.

84. M. Cowart, "Understanding acts of consent: Using speech act theory to help resolve moral dilemmas and legal disputes," *Law and Philosophy* 23 (2004): 495–525, 509.

85. S. Horng and C. Grady, "Misunderstanding in clinical research," *IRB* (Jan-Feb, 2003): 11–16, 11.

86. Nuremberg. See http://ohsr.od.nih.gov/guidelines/nuremberg.html paragraph 1.

87. The Declaration of Helsinki, http://www.wma.net/e/policy/b3.htm, paragraph 21.

88. The Belmont Report, http://ohsr.od.nih.gov/guidelines/belmont.html, C.1.

89. Faden and Beauchamp, *History and theory*, 237.

90. Truog, et al. "Is informed consent always necessary . . . ?"

91. A. Applbaum, *Ethics for Adversaries* (Princeton: Princeton University Press, 1999), 117.

92. Department of Health and Human Services. Protection of Human Subjects. Code of Federal Regulations. 45*CFR*46, 1991. Sec 46. 116.

93. See F. Miller, et al. "Deception in research on the placebo effect," *PLoS Med.* 2 (9) (2005): e262.

94. 45 *CFR* 46.116.

95. See Emanuel, et al. "What makes clinical research ethical."

96. A. Wertheimer, *Exploitation* (Princeton: Princeton University Press, 1996).

Chapter 4

1. See S. Lederer, "Walter Reed and the Yellow Fever Experiments," in E. Emanuel, et al. (eds.) *The Oxford textbook of clinical research ethics* (New York: Oxford University Press, 2008) 9–17.

2. See http://en.wikipedia.org/wiki/TGN1412.

3. http://www.parexel.com/.

4. E. Emanuel and F. Miller, "Money and distorted ethical judgments about research: Ethical assessment of the TeGenero TGN1412 Trial," *American Journal of Bioethics* 7(2) (2007): 76–81.

5. http://rxgetpaid.com/.

6. http://guineapigzero.com/.

7. C. Elliott. "Guinea pigging," *The New Yorker,* January 7, 2008.

8. N. Dickert, E. Emanuel, and C. Grady, "Paying research subjects: An analysis of current policies," *Annals of Internal Medicine* 136 (2002): 368–73.

9. "Guinea pigging."

10. J. Harris, "Scientific research is a moral duty," *Journal of Medical Ethics* 31 (2005): 242–247, 246.

11. M. Wilkinson and A. Moore, "Inducements in research," *Bioethics* 11 (1997) 373–89, 373.

12. C. Grady, et al. "An analysis of U.S. practices of paying research participants," *Contemporary Clinical Trials* 26 (2006) 365–75.

13. R. Nozick, *Anarchy, State, and Utopia* (New York: Basic Books, 1974), 163.

14. See, for example, Elliott, "Guinea pigging."

15. Department of Health and Human Services. Protection of Human Subjects. Code of Federal Regulations. 45CFR46, 1991. §46.111.

16. Declaration of Helsinki, http://www.wma.net/e/policy/b3.htm, paragraph 18.

17. See Chapter 2. I owe the formulation of this point to Frank Miller.

18. N. King, "Defining and describing benefit appropriately in clinical trials," *Journal of Law, Medicine and Ethics* 28 (2000): 332–43.

19. I thank John Arras for pressing me on this point.

20. Lynn A. Jansen, "The ethics of altruism in clinical research," *Hastings Center Report* 39, (4) (2009): 26–36.

21. S. O. Hansson, "Weighing risks and benefits," *Topoi,* 12 (2004): 145–52.

22. I used the phrase "bad choice" trial in Chapter 1. Lynn Jansen uses the phrase "bad deal" trial in "A closer look at the bad deal trial: Beyond clinical equipoise," *Hastings Center Report* 8 (2005) 29–36.

23. D. Wendler and F. Miller, "Risk-Benefit Analysis and the Net Risks Test," in Emanuel, et al. *Oxford Textbook,* 503–14, 504.

24. Private communication.

25. E. Emanuel, "Undue inducements: Nonsense on stilts?" *American Journal of Bioethics* 5 (2005) 9–13, 11.

26. http://www.research.uci.edu/ora/hrpp/subjectselection.htm.

27. Syracuse University IRB Handbook, http://orip.syr.edu/sop/sop008.php.

28. Guidelines for Remuneration of Research Subjects in the Intramural Research Program and Registration in the Clinical Research Volunteer Program Office of Human Subjects Research, National Institutes of Health, http://ohsr.od.nih.gov/info/sheet20.html

29. http://www.fda.gov/oc/ohrt/irbs/toc4.html.

30. *Curb Your Enthusiasm*, Episode 50, first aired December 4, 2005.

31. R. Grant and J. Sugarman, "Ethics in human subjects research: Do incentives matter?" *Journal of Medicine and Philosophy* 29 (2004): 717–38, 726.

32. "The paradoxical case of payment as benefit to research subjects," *IRB* 11 (6) (1989): 1–3, 3.

33. See Wilkinson and Moore, "Inducements in research."

34. International Ethical Guidelines for Biomedical Research Involving Human Subjects, The Council for International Organizations of Medical Sciences, Guideline 7. http://www.cioms.ch/frame_guidelines_nov_2002.htm.

35. "You can get paid to catch malaria," *Seattle Times*, March 5, 2008.

36. See R. Steinbrook, "The Gelsinger Case," in *Oxford Textbook,* 110–20.

37. Grant and Sugarman, "Ethics in human subjects research," 720.

38. J. Lavery, et al. (eds) *Ethical issues in international biomedical research: A casebook* (New York: Oxford University Press, 2007), 281–84.

39. S. Edwards, "Restricted treatments, inducements, and research participation," *Bioethics* 20 (2006): 77–91, 84.

40. http://www.komonews.com/news/16316401.html.

41. R Titmuss, *The gift relationship* (New York: Pantheon, 1971).

42. N. Laceter, et al. "Will there be blood? Incentives and substitution effects in prosocial behavior," http://ftp.iza.org/dp4567.pdf.

43. http://money.cnn.com/2003/10/13/pf/dangerousjobs/.

44. *New York Times,* December 20, 2008.

45. Ibid.

46. R. Macklin, *Double standards in medical research in developing countries* (Cambridge: Cambridge University Press, 2004), 228.

47. "Guinea pigging"

48. P. McNeill, "Paying people to participate in research: Why not?" *Bioethics* 11 (1997): 390–96, 391.

49. *Ibid.*

50. H. Jonas, "Philosophical reflections on experimenting with human subjects," *Daedalus*, 98 (1969): 219–47, 230.

51. *Ibid.* 230.

52. *Ibid.* 228.

53. *Ibid.* 228.

54. L. Jansen, "The problem with optimism in clinical trials," *IRB* 28 (4) (2006): 13–19.

55. *Ibid.* 17.

56. http://www.hhs.gov/ohrp/informconsfaq.html.

57. C.L. Tishler and S. Bartholomae, "The recruitment of normal healthy volunteers: A review of the literature," *Journal of Clinical Pharmacology* 42 (2002): 363–73.

58. See A. Wertheimer, *Coercion* (Princeton: Princeton University Press, 1987), Chapter 10. Also see M. Berman, "The normative function of coercion claims," *Legal Theory* (2002), 8 (1):45–89.

59. Not quite. As I noted in Chapter 3, it may be argued that, in principle, it is legitimate for the society to coerce people into participating in research. But if so, we wouldn't have to rely on incentives.

60. See Wertheimer, *Coercion,* 127.

61. Macklin, "The paradoxical case,"1.

62. J. Feinberg, *Harm to self* (New York: Oxford University Press, 1986), 228–29.

63. *Ibid.* 242.

64. *Ibid.* 242.

65. Michael Sandel, "What Money Can't Buy," Tanner Lectures on Human Values (1998) http://www.tannerlectures.utah.edu/lectures/documents/sandel00.pdf, 111.

66. R. Goodin, "Volenti goes to market," *Journal of Ethics* 10 (2006): 53–74, 63.

67. For a contrary view, see A. J. London, "Justice and the human development approach to international research," *Hastings Center Report* 35 (1) (2005): 24–37. See Chapters 5 and 6 for a more extensive discussion of this point.

68. D. Rothman, "The shame of medical research," *The New York Review of Books,* November 30, 2000.

69. M. Nussbaum, "Taking money for bodily services," *Journal of Legal Studies* 27 (1998) 693–724.

70. The quotation is well known, but it appears that there is no agreement as to its source.

71. See *Coercion,* 222–225.

72. Department of Health and Human Services. Protection of Human Subjects. Code of Federal Regulations. 45CFR46, 1991. §46.

73. http://www.hhs.gov/ohrp/informconsfaq.html.

74. Syracuse University IRB Handbook, http://orip.syr.edu/sop/sop008.php.

75. See G. Ainslie, *Breakdown of will* (Cambridge: Cambridge University Press, 2001).

76. T. Lemmens and R. Nwabueze, "Culturally sensitive compensation in clinical research," in Lavery, et al. (eds) *Ethical issues,* 292.
77. I thank an anonymous reviewer for pressing me on this point.
78. CIOMS, http://www.cioms.ch/frame_guidelines_nov_2002.htm.
79. Grant and Sugarman, "Ethics in human subjects research," 727. Emphasis added.
80. B. Hale, "Risk, judgment, and fairness in research incentives," *American Journal of Bioethics* 7 (2007) 82–83, 83. Emphasis added.
81. E. Emanuel, et al., "Undue influence in clinical research in developing countries: Is it a worry?" *Lancet* 366 (2005):336–40.
82. W. Mischel, Y. Shoda, and M. L. Rodriguez, "Delay of gratification in children," *Science* 244 (1989): 933–938.
83. "The paradoxical case," 1.
84. Grant and Sugarman, "Ethics in human subjects research," 728.
85. *Ibid.*
86. B. Hale, "Risk, judgment, and fairness," 83.
87. 45 *CFR* 46, 1991. §46.
88. J. S. Mill, *On liberty* (Indianapolis: Hackett Publishing Co., 1978) Ch V.
89. J. S. Mill, [1848] 1965, *Principles of political economy*, in J. M. Robson (ed.), *Collected works of John Stuart Mill*, (Toronto: University of Toronto Press), 7th edition, vols. 2 and 3 book 5, chap. 11, sect. 12.
90. Syracuse University IRB Handbook, http://orip.syr.edu/sop/sop008.php.
91. http://www.research.uci.edu/ora/hrpp/subjectselection.htm.
92. http://www.uvm.edu/irb/researchmanual.htm.
93. http://www.circare.org/foia5/tgn1412_consentform.pdf.
94. Bloomberg News. "Parexel misled subjects sickened in London study, ethicists say," April 10, 2006 http://www.iconocast.com/News_Files/BNews6_18B_06/Biz3.htm.
95. Grant and Sugarman, "Ethics in human subject research," 729.
96. Aristotle, *The Politics* Book I, Part X.
97. "What money can't buy," 94. For reasons I do not understand, Sandel does not even cite the section "What money can't buy" in Michael Walzer's *Spheres of justice* (New York: Basic Books, 1983). Also see M. J. Radin, *Contested commodities* (Cambridge: Harvard University Press, 1996).
98. See E. Anderson, "Is women's labor a commodity?" *Philosophy & Public Affairs* 19 (1990): 71–92.
99. L. Kass, *Life, liberty and the defense of dignity* (San Francisco: Encounter Books, 2002), 195.
100. Macklin, "Paradoxical case," 3.
101. Elliott, "Guinea pigging."
102. Grant and Sugarman, "Ethics in human subject research," 730.
103. "What money can't buy," 104.

104. "Undue inducements and reasonable risks: Will the dismal science lead to dismal research ethics?" *American Journal of Bioethics* 5 (5) (2005): 29–32.

105. "What money can't buy," 100.

106. R. J. Sample, *Exploitation, what it is and why it is wrong* (Lanham, MD: Rowman and Littlefield). 2003: 4.

107. Grant and Sugarman, "Ethics in human subject research," 730.

108. I thank an anonymous reviewer for pressing me on this point.

109. "What money can't buy," 104.

110. "Undue inducements and reasonable risks," 29–32.

111. I thank an anonymous reviewer for helping to clarify these points.

112. See, for example, D. Satz, "Markets in women's sexual labor," *Ethics* 106 (1995): 63–85.

113. R. George, *Making men moral* (Oxford: Clarendon Press, 1993), 168.

114. "Undue inducements and reasonable risks," 31.

115. *Ibid.*

116. A. Smith, *An inquiry into the nature and causes of the wealth of nations* (1776) Vol I, Book I, Chapter II.

117. J. Rawls, *A theory of justice* (Cambridge: Harvard University Press, 1971), 57.

118. G. A. Cohen, *Self-ownership, freedom, and equality* (Cambridge: Cambridge University Press, 1995), 134–35.

119. I borrow this phrase from Richard Epstein, *Mortal peril* (Reading, MA: Addison-Wesley, 1997), 228.

120. A. J. London, "Reasonable risks in clinical research: A critique and a proposal for the integrative approach," *Statistics in Medicine* 25 (2006) 2869–2885, 2878.

121. *Ibid.*

122. *Ibid.* 2881

123. T.M. Scanlon, "Preference and urgency," *The Journal of Philosophy* 72 (1975): 655–669.

124. Rawls, *A theory of justice*, 187.

125. London, "Reasonable risks," 2878.

126. *Ibid.*

127. *Ibid.* 2879.

128. T. Beauchamp, et al., "Pharmaceutical research involving the homeless," *Journal of Medicine and Philosophy* 27 (2002): 547–64, 555.

129. J. McGregor, "Does the use of human subjects in research in developing nations violate their human rights?" *Journal of Social Philosophy* 37 (2006): 441–63, 452.

130. Peter Westen has argued that the principle of equality is substantively "empty." See "The empty idea of equality," *Harvard Law Review* 95 (1982): 537–84.

131. A. Shammoo and D. Resnik, "Strategies to minimize risks and exploitation in phase one trials on healthy subjects," *American Journal of Bioethics*, 6 (2006) w-1–w-13. w -10.

132. A. Wertheimer, *Exploitation* (Princeton: Princeton University Press, 1996), Ch7.

133. N. Dickert and C. Grady, "What's the price of a research subject? Approaches to payment for research participation," *New England Journal of Medicine* 341 (1999): 198–203.

134. *Ibid.*

135. 45CFR46, 1991. §46.111 (a) (3).

136. "Undue inducements: Nonsense on stilts," *The American Journal of Bioethics* 5(5) (2005):9.

137. http://ohsr.od.nih.gov/guidelines/belmont.html Belmont Report Part C 3.

138. *International ethical guidelines for biomedical research involving human subjects,* The Council for International Organizations of Medical Sciences, Guideline 12.

139. *Ibid.*

140. *Ibid.*

141. M. Kuczewski, "Is informed consent enough? Monetary incentives for research participation and the integrity of biomedicine," *American Journal of Bioethics* 1 (2) 2001: 50.

142. "Paradoxical case," 3.

143. F. Miller, et al. "Cosmetic surgery and the inner morality of medicine," *Cambridge Quarterly of Health Care Ethics* 9 (2000): 353–64.

144. Epstein, *Mortal peril,* 307.

145. Macklin, "Paradoxical case," 3.

146. *Ibid.*

147. Mill, *On liberty,* Chapter II.

Chapter 5

1. This chapter is a much expanded and revised version of a chapter in Jennifer Hawkins and Ezekiel Emanuel (eds.) *Exploitation and developing countries: The ethics of clinical research* (Princeton: Princeton University Press, 2008).

2. L. Kass, *Life, liberty and the defense of dignity* (San Francisco: Encounter Books, 2002), 2.

3. See E. Emanuel, et al. "What makes clinical research ethical?" *JAMA* 2000; 283: 2701–2711.

4. E. Emanuel, et al., "An ethical framework for biomedical research," in Ezekiel Emanuel, et al., *The Oxford textbook of clinical research ethics* (New York: Oxford University Press, 2008), p. 125.

5. E. Emanuel, "The paradox of exploitation" in James Lavery, et al. (eds.) *Ethical issues in international biomedical research: A casebook* (New York: Oxford University Press, 2007) 189.

6. http://www.igatecr.com/company/indiaadvantage/index.php

7. P. Lurie and S. Wolfe, "Unethical trials of interventions to reduce perinatal transmission of the human immunodeficiency virus in developing countries" 33 *New England Journal of Medicine* (1997):853–856.

8. Lavery (ed.) *Ethical issues in international biomedical research,* 151

9. G. Annas and M. Grodin, "Human rights and maternal-fetal HIV transmission prevention trials in Africa," *American Journal of Public Health* 88(1998): 560–63, 561.

10. R. Bayer, "The debate over maternal-fetal HIV transmission prevention trials in Africa, Asia, and the Caribbean: Racist exploitation or exploitation of racism," 88 *American Journal of Public Health* 88 (1998): 567–70, 569.

11. Z. Ahmed Bhutta, "Ethics in international health research: A perspective from the developing world, CMH working papers, Commission on Macroeconomics and Health, at 13. Available at http://www.emro.who.int/cbi/pdf/Ethics%20in%20 International%20Health%20Research.pdf

12. Council for International Organizations of Medical Sciences, *International ethical guidelines for biomedical research involving human subjects,* Revised draft, January 2002.

13. R. Crouch and J. Arras, "AZT trials and tribulations," *Hastings Center Report* 28 (1998): 26–34, 29.

14. Peter Lurie and Sidney Wolfe, "Unethical trials of interventions . . ."

15. "The ethics of research related to healthcare in developing countries," Nuffield Council on Bioethics.

16. See *Exploitation* (Princeton: Princeton University Press, 1996).

17. World Medical Association, Declaration of Helsinki. http://www.wma.net/e/ policy/b3.htm. This passage was revised in the 2008 version. Paragraph 32 now says "The benefits, risks, burdens and effectiveness of a new intervention must be tested against those of the best current proven intervention." This provision contains several exceptions, but they are irrelevant in the present context.

18. Allen Wood has argued that exploitation need not involve unfairness, that A exploits B when A uses something about B for A's own ends. See "Exploitation," *Social Philosophy and Policy* 12 (1995): 135–58, 136. It is not clear whether Wood's account is as fairness-free as he thinks, for he goes on to say that A exploits B when A uses B for A's own ends "by playing on some weakness or vulnerability in that person." This implies that A does not (wrongfully) exploit B if A uses B for A's own ends when A does not play on a weakness or vulnerability; that is, when the transaction is fair.

19. R. Arneson, "Exploitation," in Lawrence C. Becker (ed.). *Encyclopedia of ethics* (New York: Garland, 1992), 350.

20. The president of Stanford University claimed that big-time college athletics "reeks of exploitation," because the universities gain a great deal of revenue from the services of the athletes while the athletes (whose graduation rate is much

lower than that of non-athletes) gain little from their college experience. D. Kennedy, "So what if college players turn pro early?" *New York Times*, January 19, 1990, B7.

21. *USA Today* featured an article advocating the legalization of organ sales, whereby a person could be paid cash for a kidney. One reply maintained that such a policy would "open wide the door to exploitation." September 14, 1991.

22. See E. Anderson, "Is women's labor a commodity?" *Philosophy & Public Affairs* 19 (1990) 71–92.

23. The code of the American Psychiatric Association states that "the psychiatrist's ethics and professional responsibilities preclude his/her gratifying his/her own needs by exploiting the patient." From American Psychiatric Association, "Principles of medical ethics with annotations especially applicable to psychiatry," 1985, cited in Peter Y. Windt, et al., eds. *Ethical issues in the professions* (Englewood Cliffs, NJ: Prentice-Hall, 1989), 567.

24. A. Buchanan, *Ethics, efficiency, and the market* (Totowa, NJ: Rowman and Allanheld, 1985), 87.

25. N. Holsmstrom, "Exploitation," *Canadian Journal of Philosophy*, 7 (1997): 353–69, 357.

26. J. Farr Tormey, "Exploitation, oppression and self-sacrifice," *Philosophical Forum* 5 (1974), 207–08.

27. S. Benn, *A theory of freedom* (Cambridge: Cambridge University Press, 1988), 138.

28. J. Feinberg, *Harmless wrongdoing* (Oxford: Oxford University Press, 1988), 176–79.

29. S. Munzer, *A theory of property* (Cambridge: Cambridge University Press, 1990), 171.

30. A. Levine, *Arguing for socialism* (London: Verso, 1988), 66–67.

31. J. L. Hill, "Exploitation," *Cornell Law Review* 79 (1994): 631–699, 637.

32. A. Carse and M. Little, "Exploitation and the enterprise of medical research," in Hawkins and Emanuel (eds.) *Exploitation and developing countries,* 211.

33. See *Harm to others* (New York: Oxford University Press, 1987).

34. See John Moore v. Regents of the University of California, 51 Cal 3rd 120; 271 Cal. Rptr. 146; 793 P.2d 479 (1990).

35. A. Buchanan, *Marx and justice* (Totowa, NJ: Rowman and Allanheld, 1984), 44.

36. See C. Korsgaard, "The reasons we can share," *Social Philosophy and Policy* 10 (1993): 24–51, 40.

37. See Wertheimer, *Exploitation,* Chapter 7.

38. I borrow the phrase "pure procedural justice" from John Rawls, *A Theory of Justice* (Cambridge: Harvard University Press, 1971), 85. Rawls does *not* argue that the fairness of a transaction is a matter of pure procedural justice. Christopher Boorse does take this view in "The myth of pure exploitation," unpublished mss on file with author.

39. Joan McGregor, "Does the use of human subjects in research in developing nations violate their human rights?" *Journal of Social Philosophy* 37 (2006) 441–63, 452.

40. Allen Wood, "Exploitation," *Social Philosophy and Policy*, 12 (1995), 147.

41. D. Orentlicher, "Universality and its limits: When research can reflect local circumstances," *Journal of Law, Medicine and Ethics* 30 (2002): 403–10, 407.

42. See *Exploitation,* Chapter 7.

43. I say *might*. See Matt Zwolinski, "The ethics of price gouging," *Business Ethics Quarterly,* 18 (2008) 347–378.

44. Robert Mayer, "What's wrong with exploitation," *Journal of Applied Philosophy,"* 24 (2007): 137–150.

45. Jacobellis v. Ohio, 378 U.S. 184, 197 (1964).

46. See Anderson, "Is women's labor a commodity?"

47. I set aside the argument that surrogacy harms the children that result from the surrogacy arrangement. Since these children would otherwise not exist, it is difficult to see how they are made worse off as a result of being conceived.

48. See E. Anderson, "Is women's labor a commodity?"

49. "Hockey helmets, concealed weapons, and daylight saving: A study of binary choices," *Journal of Conflict Resolution* 17 (1973): 381–428.

50. http://en.wikipedia.org/wiki/Baby_M

51. Joel Feinberg refers to some wrongs as "free-floating evils." See *Harmless wrong-doing* (New York: Oxford University Press, 1990).

52. S. Shiffrin, "Paternalism, unconscionability doctrine, and accommodation," *Philosophy & Public Affairs* 29 (Summer 2000): 205–250, 234.

53. *Ibid.* 224.

54. L. B. Murphy, *Moral demands in non-ideal theory* (New York: Oxford University Press, 2000), 5.

55. As John Rawls puts it, ideal theory "works out the principles that characterize a well-ordered society under favorable circumstances." *A theory of justice,* 8.

56. See J. Rawls, *The law of peoples* (Cambridge, MA: Harvard University Press, 1999).

57. This is the wording of Paragraph 32 in the 2008 version. http://www.wma.net/e/policy/b3.htm

58. SR. Levine, "The best proven therapeutic method" Standard in clinical trials in technologically developing countries," *IRB* 20 (1998): 5–9, 6.

59. Needless to say, similar issues arise with respect to the affluent and the poor in developed societies.

60. S. Shah, *The body hunters: Testing new drugs on the world's poorest patients* (New York: New Press, 2006), 19.

61. P. Lurie and S. Wolfe, "The developing world as the 'answer' to the dreams of pharmaceutical companies: The Surfaxin story," in Lavery, et al, (eds.) *Ethical issues in international biomedical research,* 164.

62. See P. Litton and F. Miller, "A normative justification for distinguishing the ethics of clinical research from the ethics of medical care," *The Journal of Law, Medicine and Ethics* 33 (2007): 566–574.

63. See H. Morreim, "The clinical investigator as fiduciary: Discarding a misguided idea," *Journal of Law Medicine and Ethics* (2005) 33: 586–598. Also see P. Litton and Franklin G. Miller (2005). "A normative justification for distinguishing the ethics of clinical research from the ethics of medical care."

64. A. Ballantyne, "HIV intervention and clinical research: Exploitation and risk," *Bioethics* 19 (2005): 476–491, 487.

65. *Ibid.* 479.

66. An old chestnut used by game theorists asks how a rich man and a poor man should agree to share $200. "The rich man could argue for a $150–$50 split in his favor because it would grieve the poor man more to lose $50 than the rich man to lose $150." H. Raiffa, *The art and science of negotiation* (Cambridge: Harvard University Press, 1982), 52. Raiffa also observes that an arbitrator might suggest the reverse split because the poor person needs the money more and adds that the rich man might also argue for an even split on the grounds that it is wrong to mix business with charity.

67. Bayer, "The debate over maternal-fetal HIV transmission prevention trials in Africa, Asia, and the Caribbean: Racist exploitation or exploitation of racism."

68. A famous mathematician once challenged Nobel Prize winning economist Paul Samuelson to name one theory in all the social sciences that is both true and nontrivial. Samuelson responded with the theory of comparative advantage, "That it is logically true need not be argued before a mathematician; that it is not trivial is attested by the thousands of important and intelligent men who have never been able to grasp the doctrine for themselves or to believe it after it was explained to them." P.A. Samuelson (1969), "The way of an economist," in P.A. Samuelson, ed., *International economic relations: Proceedings of the Third Congress of the International Economic Association* (London: Macmillan), 1–11.

69. James Surowiecki notes that low income Americans consume more low cost goods produced in China than do high income Americans. As consumers, although perhaps not as workers, low income Americans are primary beneficiaries of free trade. http://www.newyorker.com/talk/financial/2008/05/26/080526ta_talk_surowiecki

70. A. Smith, *The wealth of nations* (1776) IV.ii.12.

71. "In praise of cheap labor," *Slate*, March 21, 1997.

72. *Ibid.*

73. M. Wolf, *Why globalization works* (New Haven: Yale University Press, 2004), 185.

74. F. Teson and J. Klick, "Global justice and trade: A puzzling omission" http://papers.ssrn.com/sol3/papers.cfm?abstract_id=1022996, 54

75. *Ibid.* 76.

76. A. Shamoo and D. Resnik, "Strategies to minimize risks and exploitation in Phase One trials on healthy subjects," *The American Journal of Bioethics* 6(3): W1–W13, 2006, w8.

77. P. Lurie and S. Wolfe, "Letter to Tommy Thompson," February 22, 2001. *The Public Citizen.*

78. Annas and Grodin, Human rights and maternal-fetal HIV transmission prevention trials in Africa," 562.

79. International Ethical Guidelines for Biomedical Research Involving Human Subjects, The Council for International Organizations of Medical Sciences, Guideline 7.

80. Shamoo and Resnik, "Strategies to minimize risks and exploitation in Phase One trials on healthy subjects," W8.

81. D. Rothman, "The shame of medical research," *The New York Review of Books,* November 30, 2000.

82. C. Weijer, "Protecting communities in research: Philosophical and pragmatic challenges," *Cambridge Quarterly of Healthcare Ethics* 8 (1999): 501–13, 503.

83. Annas and Grodin, "Human rights and maternal-fetal HIV transmission prevention trials in Africa."

84. Guideline 10.

85. "Fair benefits for research in developing countries" *Science* 13 (2002): Vol. 298. no. 5601: 2133–2134.

86. *Ibid.*

87. W. Chiong, "The real problem with equipoise," *American Journal of Bioethics* 6 (2006) 37–47, 46.

88. E. Emanuel, "Addressing exploitation: Reasonable availability versus fair benefits," in Jennifer Hawkins and Ezekiel Emanuel (eds.) *Exploitation and developing countries: The ethics of clinical research,* p. 307.

89. I thank John Arras for pressing me on this point.

90. Crouch and Arras, "AZT trials and tribulations," 28.

91. T. Pogge, *World poverty and human rights* (Oxford: Polity Press, 2002).

92. R. Gilpin, *U.S. power and the multinational corporation* (New York: Basic Books, 1975), 289.

93. R. Temple, "Benefit to trial participants or benefit to the community?" in Lavery, et al. eds, *Ethical issues in international biomedical research,* 157.

94. A. London, "Justice and the human development approach to international research," *Hastings Center Report* 35 (205) 24–37, 27.

95. *Ibid.*

96. *Ibid.* 28.

97. *Ibid.* 32.

98. Temple, "Benefit to trial participants or benefit to the community?" 91.

99. National Bioethics Advisory Commission, *Ethical and policy issues in international research: Clinical trials in developing countries,* Chapter 4, (2001) 65. http://bioethics.georgetown.edu/nbac/clinical/Chapter4.pdf.

100. "Testing our drugs on the poor abroad" in Emanuel and Hawkins, *Exploitation and developing countries,* 105–141.

101. *Ibid.* 111.

102. *Ibid.* 116.

103. "The *locus classicus* is Peter Singer, "Famine, affluence, and morality,"*Philosophy & Public Affairs* 1, (1972), 229–243.

104. Murphy, *Moral demands in nonideal theory,* 127.

105. Pogge 122.

106. Pogge Ibid.

107. M. Lockwood, "Sins of omission? The non-treatment of controls in clinical trials," *Proceedings of The Aristotelian Society,* Supp Vol LVII 1983, 207–22.

108. "The toxin puzzle" *Analysis* 43, (1983): 33–36.

109. D. Gauthier, "Assure and threaten" *Ethics* 104, (1994): 690–721.

110. Pogge, "Testing our drugs on the poor abroad" in Emanuel and Hawkins, *Exploitation and developing countries,* 122–23.

111. T. B. Newman, et al. "Effects and costs of requiring child-restraint systems for young children traveling on commercial airplanes," *Arch Pediatr Adolesc Med* 2003;157: 969–974.

112. Lurie and Wolfe, "The developing world as the 'answer' to the dreams of pharmaceutical companies: The Surfaxin story," 166.

113. "Researchers' obligations to uninfected partners in discordant couples in an HIV-1 Transmission Trial I the Rakai District, Uganda," in Lavery, et al. (eds.) *Ethical issues in international biomedical research* 345.

114. P. Lurie and S. Wolfe, "Unethical trials of interventions to reduce perinatal transmission of the human immunodeficiency virus in developing countries."

115. *Ibid.*

116. Marcia Angell, "The ethics of clinical research in the Third world," *New England Journal of Medicine* 337 (1997): 847–49, 848.

117. "Research that is unacceptable in one society because its risks outweigh the risks posed by the disease may have a favorable risk-benefit ratio in another society where the risks posed by the disease are significantly greater. Adapting these requirements to the identities, attachments, and cultural traditions embedded in distinct circumstances neither constitutes moral relativism nor undermines their universality, doing so recognizes that while ethical requirements embody universal values, the manner of specifying these values inherently depends on the particular context." E. Emanuel, D. Wendler, C. Grady, "What makes clinical research ethical?" *JAMA* 283 (2000): 2701–11, 2708.

118. I thank an anonymous reviewer for pressing me to be clear as to what I am and am not addressing here.

Chapter 6

1. S. Scheffler, *Boundaries and allegiances* (Oxford: Oxford University Press, 2001), 49. On "natural duties," see John Rawls, *A theory of justice* (Cambridge, MA, 1971), 114–117.

2. I say "the state" here because the coal mining company might have contractual or moral obligations towards their employees.

3. It appears, for example, that a high proportion of Malaysian workers are immigrants that "have been fooled hook, line and sinker" by labor brokers who tricked them into paying high placement fees for jobs that yield a net income of close to zero and from which they cannot extricate themselves. They are trapped in virtual servitude. *Newsweek*, March 24, 2008. Some may raise questions as to whether those in poverty can actually give valid consent to such work. I have considered those issues elsewhere in Chapters 3, 4, and 5, and so for present purposes, I shall simply assume that it is possible to do so.

4. The contrast between the obligations of Nike and Hike is mirrored by arguments about the obligations of consumers who indirectly benefit from workers. Those who think they should boycott Nike products are typically more concerned about the plight of the Nike laborer who works for $1.00 per hour than with the peasant who works for $.50 per hour because the consumer would otherwise benefit from the Nike laborer whereas she does not benefit from the peasant's labor. P. Krugman, "In praise of cheap labor," *Slate*, March 21, 1997.

5. It might be argued that Nike has indirectly "used" the prospective employees that it did not hire, for the "reserve army of labor" drives down the wages that Nike must pay those that it does hire.

6. As quoted in M. Specter, "The vaccine: Has the race to save Africa from AIDS put western science at odds with western ethics?" *New Yorker*, February 3, 2003, 54.

7. http://en.wikipedia.org/wiki/Tobacco_Master_Settlement_Agreement.

8. P. Singer, "Famine, affluence, and morality," *Philosophy & Public Affairs*, 1, (1972), 229–243; Thomas Pogge, *World poverty and human rights: Cosmopolitan responsibilities and reforms* (Cambridge, UK: Polity Press 2002); John Rawls, *The law of peoples* (Cambridge, MA: Harvard University Press, 1999).

9. International Ethical Guidelines for Biomedical Research Involving Human Subjects, The Council for International Organizations of Medical Sciences, Guideline http://www.cioms.ch/frame_guidelines_nov_2002.htm.

10. "Fair benefits for research in developing countries" *Science* 13 December 2002: Vol. 298. no. 5601, pp. 2133–2134.

11. http://govinfo.library.unt.edu/nbac/clinical/execsum.html

12. Paragraph 17, Declaration of Helsinki, The World Medical Association, 59th WMA General Assembly, Seoul, October 2008.

13. E. Emanuel, "The paradox of exploitation" in James Lavery, et al. (eds.) *International issues in international biomedical research, A casebook* (New York: Oxford University Press, 2007), 189.

14. M. Wolf, *Why globalization works* (New Haven: Yale University Press, 2004), 237.

15. P. Lurie and S. Wolfe, "Letter to Tommy Thompson," February 22, 2001, *The Public Citizen.* http://www.pharm.chula.ac.th/vsuntree/news/apr/Surfactan_6apr.htm

16. L. Gostin, "Ethical principles for the conduct of human subject research: Population-based research and ethics," *Law, Medicine and Ethics* 19 (1991): 191–201, 198.

17. http://www.wma.net/e/policy/b3.htm - note2.

18. R. Macklin, *Double standards in medical research in developing countries* (Cambridge: Cambridge University Press, 2004), 80.

19. Z. Zong, "Should post-trial provision of beneficial experimental interventions be mandatory in developing countries?" *Journal of Medical Ethics* 2008; 34: 188–192, 190.

20. D. Rothman, "The shame of medical research," *The New York Review of Books,* November 30, 2000.

21. "The obligation to ensure access to beneficial treatment for research participants at the conclusion of clinical trials," in E. Emanuel, et al. (eds) *The Oxford textbook of clinical research ethics* (New York: Oxford University Press, 2008), 701.

22. The National Institutes of Health, "Regarding guidance for addressing the provision of antiretroviral treatment for trial participants following their completion of NIH-funded HIV antiretroviral treatment trials in developing countries" (emphasis added). http://grants.nih.gov/grants/policy/antiretroviral/QandA.htm

23. *Double standards in medical research in developing countries,* 228.

24. Lavery, "The obligation to ensure access to beneficial treatment for research participants at the conclusion of clinical trials," 701.

25. M. Merritt and C. Grady, "Reciprocity and post-trial access for tarticipants in antiretroviral therapy trials," *Aids (*2006) 20: 1792–94, 1791.

26. P. E. Cleaton-Jones, "An ethical dilemma: Availability of antiretroviral therapy after clinical trials with HIV-infected patients are ended," *BMJ* 314 (1997):887

27. *Ibid.*

28. P. Busse, "Strident but essential: The voices of people with AIDS," *BMJ* 1997; 314:888 (22 March).

29. P. E. Cleaton-Jones, "An ethical dilemma: Availability of antiretroviral therapy after clinical trials with HIV-infected patients are ended".

30. Zong, "Should post-trial provision of beneficial experimental interventions be mandatory in developing countries?", 190.

31. H. Richardson, "Incidental findings and ancillary-care obligations," *The Journal of Law, Medicine & Ethics* 36, (2008): 256–270, 259.

32. H. Richardson and L. Belsky, "The ancillary-care responsibilities of medical researchers," *Hastings Center Report* 34 (2004): 25–33, 29.

33. *Ibid.* 26.

34. *Ibid.* 27.

35. Richardson, "Incidental findings and ancillary-care obligations," 264.

36. On the distinction between "pure procedural" justice and "imperfect procedural" justice, see John Rawls, *A theory of justice,* pp. 83ff.

37. Henry Sidgwick, The Methods of Ethics, London: Macmillan, 1874, p. 234.

38. H. Richardson, "The special obligations of beneficence: The case of medical researchers' ancillary-care obligations," unpublished mss on file with author, 26.

39. J. Thomson, *The realm of rights* (Cambridge: Harvard University Press, 1990), 283.

40. See my *Exploitation* (Princeton: Princeton University Press, 1996) and *Consent to sexual relations* (Cambridge: Cambridge University Press, 2003).

41. See Chapter 5.

42. Richardson, "The special obligations of beneficence: The case of medical researchers' ancillary-care obligations", 18.

43. *Ibid.*

44. See Chapter 2.

45. Richardson, "The special obligations of beneficence: The case of medical researchers' ancillary-care obligations", 20.

46. "Fair benefits for research in developing countries".

47. G. Annas and M. Grodin, "Human rights and maternal-fetal HIV transmission prevention trials in Africa," *American Journal of Public Health* 88(1998): 560–63, 561.

48. Rawls was embarrassed about the possibility that the difference principle might be used to justify supporting the "malibu surfer." See *Political liberalism* (New York: Columbia University Press, 1993). 181–2.

49. R. Sample, *Exploitation: What it is and why it's wrong* (Lanham, MD: Rowman and Littlefield, 2003), 69.

50. "The myth of pure exploitation" Unpublished mss on file with author.

51. D. Parfit, "Acts and outcomes: A reply to Boonin-Vail," *Philosophy & Public Affairs* 25 (1996): 308–17.

52. See "Independence of irrelevant alternatives," http://en.wikipedia.org/wiki/Independence_of_irrelevant_alternatives. An anecdote which illustrates a violation of this property has been attributed to Sidney Morgenbesser: After finishing dinner, Sidney Morgenbesser decides to order dessert. The waitress tells him he has two choices: apple pie and blueberry pie. Morgenbesser orders the apple pie. After a few minutes the waitress returns and says that they also have cherry pie at which point Morgenbesser says, "In that case I'll have the blueberry pie." There are cases in which the addition of an option changes the meaning of a previous option. Suppose A is considering (1) not marrying B and (2) marrying B

with the possibility of divorcing B and prefers (2), but that the state now adds the option of "covenant marriage" (3) in which divorce is very difficult. (2) has now become a less committed form of marriage and A might now prefer (1) to (2) because the meaning of (2) has changed.

53. G.A. Cohen, "Incentives, inequality, and community," in Grethe B. Peterson (ed.), *The Tanner lectures on human values*, Vol 13 (Salt Lake City: University of Utah Press, 1992), 305

54. D. Kahneman, et al., "Fairness and the assumptions of economics," *Journal of Business* 59 (1986) S-285–300.

55. *Exploitation: What it is and why it's wrong* p. 57.

56. *Ibid.* p. 60.

57. See A. Sen, "Rights and agency," in *Consequentialism and its critics*, ed. Samuel Scheffler (Oxford: Oxford University Press, 1988), 187–223.

58. B. Herman, "The scope of moral requirement," *Philosophy & Public Affairs*, 30 (2001) 227–56.

59. *Exploitation: What it is and why it's wrong,* 68.

60. *Ibid.* 71.

61. A. Applebaum, *Ethics for adversaries* (Princeton: Princeton University Press, 2000).

62. T.M. Scanlon, *What we owe to each other* (Cambridge, MA: Harvard University Press, 1998), 105.

63. Frances Kamm, *Morality, mortality*, V. II, (Oxford University Press, 1996), p. 296. I thank Govind Persad for bringing this case to my attention.

64. J. Brand-Ballard, "Contractualism and deontic restrictions," *Ethics* 114 (2005): 269–300, 274.

65. F. Kamm, *Intricate ethics* (New York: Oxford University Press, 2007), 26.

66. T. M. Scanlon, *What we owe to each other*, 153.

67. See the entry on contractualism in the *Stanford encyclopedia of philosophy.* http://plato.stanford.edu/entries/contractualism/

68. R. Arneson, "The end of welfare as we know it," *Social Theory and Practice* 28 (2002) 315–336, 327.

69. J. Brand-Ballard, "Contractualism and deontic restrictions," p. 275.

70. Ibid.

71. L. Temkin, "Equality, priority, and the leveling down objection" in Matthew Clayton and Andrew Williams (eds.) *The ideal of equality* (New York: MacMillan, 2000), 126–61.

72. *Ibid.* 136.

73. *Ibid.* 139.

74. J. Bentham, *The principles of morals and legislation* (Amherst: Prometheus Books, 1988).

75. Derek Parfit, *Climbing the Mountain*, Unpublished mss. 59.

76. See Chapter 5.

77. Something like this occurred in Episode 30 of the television show Curb Your Enthusiasm. Episode 30. First aired November 17, 2002.

78. *Boundaries and allegiances*, 36–37.

79. Bernard Williams famously objected to the two-level approach, suggesting that to think that one can save one's wife rather than two strangers because the preference for one's wife can be justified from an impartial point of view is to provide the agent "with one thought too many." *Moral Luck* (Cambridge: Cambridge University Press, 1981). Brian Barry has remarked, in response, that he is "inclined to doubt that anything very informative is to be gained by asking what is the optimal number of thoughts for a person to have in any given situation." *Justice as impartiality* (Oxford: Clarendon Press, 1995), 231.

80. See L. Fuller, *The morality of law* (New Haven: Yale University Press, 1964).

81. See World Medical Association, Declaration of Helsinki (2008), Paragraph 33: "At the conclusion of the study, patients entered into the study are entitled to be informed about the outcome of the study and to share any benefits that result from it, for example, access to interventions identified as beneficial in the study or to other appropriate care or benefits."

82. *Boundaries and allegiances*, 56.

83. *Ibid.* 87.

84. M. Kurjanska and M. Risse, "Fairness in trade II: Export subsidies and the fair trade movement," http://papers.ssrn.com/sol3/papers.cfm?abstract_id=939648, 26.

85. D. Kahneman, J. Knetsch, and R. Thaler. "Experimental test of the endowment effect and the Coase Theorem," *Journal of Political Economy* 98 (1990); 6: 1325–1348.

86. L. Forer, *Criminals and victims* (New York: W.W. Norton, 1981), 5.

Index